Disability in Ancient Egypt and Egyptology

This book explores disability across time and space – from 'ancient Egypt' as a culture to Egyptology as a contemporary field – to go beyond simply identifying disability, encouraging readers to thoughtfully consider the history of disabled people in ancient Egypt and Egyptology.

Through a critical investigation, this volume reshapes often-overlooked narratives of disability within the discipline of Egyptology and Egyptian Archaeology. Chapters explore evidence of disability, the historiographical ways in which disability has been approached, and how disability histories are (mis)represented in various contemporary spaces. Coverage stretches across Egypt and Nubia from the Predynastic to the Roman periods, as well as receptions of these cultures and disability in museums. Its editors and many of its authors are disability community members who are experts in their respective professions, comprising an international authorship and including voices from typically underrepresented groups. Contributors range from early career researchers to senior scholars, as well as those working outside and adjacent to academia. While focusing on ancient Egypt and Egyptology, this volume offers new ways to consider disability in the broadest possible sense. It uses terminology informed by the disability community and offers guidance for disability inclusivity in curatorial and pedagogical museum and university contexts. It prioritises disability as an essential area of research in ancient world studies, and platforms both ancient and modern disabled voices. The deep, detailed exploration into disability in the past and in our discipline offered by this book inspires readers to further explore and appreciate the infinite diversity of the human experience in all its infinite combinations.

The first book-length treatment of the subject, *Disability in Ancient Egypt and Egyptology* provides a much-needed resource for students and scholars of ancient Egypt, Egyptology, and disability in the ancient world. It is also suitable for researchers in disability studies, practitioners in broader ancient world studies, and museum and heritage professionals.

Alexandra F. Morris is a disabled Egyptologist, lecturer, and disability activist tying the past to the present. Her research is on disability in ancient Egypt, the Classical world, and creating inclusive museums. She holds many roles in academic, disability, heritage, and government sectors. She has cerebral palsy and dyspraxia.

Hannah Vogel is an archaeologist researching ableism and disability in the ancient world and the disciplines of History and Archaeology. Her research interests include Disability Studies, Bioarchaeology, and Egyptology. She is an advocate for accessibility and has worked in museums, public outreach, and inclusive pedagogies.

Routledge Studies in Ancient Disabilities

Routledge Studies in Ancient Disabilities is a series dedicated to the investigation of new perspectives, the application of new approaches, and the promotion of period-based and cross-cultural investigations of disability throughout antiquity. Extending beyond the core disciplines of ancient history, archaeology and classical studies, the series aims to provide a forum for scholars with diverse backgrounds, including bioarchaeology, biblical studies and contemporary disability studies, to explore the evidence for disabilities within communities extending from the Bronze Age to late Antiquity. Encouraging cross-disciplinary studies, the series aims to bring questions of disability and impairment into dialogue with those concerning status, gender, sexuality, ethnicity, and other lived experiences, as well as to consider how successive generations have received, appropriated, or reworked these forms of identity. Ultimately, the series seeks to expand the geographical, cultural, and chronological scope of work on ancient disabilities and broaden our understandings of physical impairment and mental and intellectual disabilities (and related conditions).

For further information about contributing to the series, please contact Dr Emma-Jayne Graham at emma-jayne.graham@open.ac.uk

Disability Studies and the Classical Body
The Forgotten Other
Edited by Ellen Adams

Disability in Ancient Egypt and Egyptology
All Our Yesterdays
Edited by Alexandra F. Morris and Hannah Vogel

For more information on this series, visit: https://www.routledge.com/Routledge-Studies-in-Ancient-Disabilities/book-series/ANCDIS

Disability in Ancient Egypt and Egyptology

All Our Yesterdays

Edited by Alexandra F. Morris and Hannah Vogel

Routledge
Taylor & Francis Group
LONDON AND NEW YORK

First published 2025
by Routledge
4 Park Square, Milton Park, Abingdon, Oxon OX14 4RN

and by Routledge
605 Third Avenue, New York, NY 10158

Routledge is an imprint of the Taylor & Francis Group, an informa business

British Library Cataloguing-in-Publication Data
Names: Morris, Alexandra F., editor. | Vogel, Hannah, editor.
Title: Disability in Ancient Egypt and Egyptology : all our yesterdays / edited by Alexandra F. Morris and Hannah Vogel.
Description: Abingdon, Oxon ; New York, NY : Routledge, 2025. | Series: Routledge studies in Ancient disabilities | Includes bibliographical references and index.
Identifiers: LCCN 2024028688 (print) | LCCN 2024028689 (ebook) | ISBN 9781032576480 (hardback) | ISBN 9781032576503 (paperback) | ISBN 9781003440369 (ebook)
Subjects: LCSH: People with disabilities—Egypt—History—To 1500. | Disabilities—Egypt—History—To 1500.
Classification: LCC HV1559.E5 D57 2025 (print) | LCC HV1559.E5 (ebook) | DDC 362.40932—dc23/eng/20241023
LC record available at https://lccn.loc.gov/2024028688
LC ebook record available at https://lccn.loc.gov/2024028689

ISBN: 978-1-032-57648-0 (hbk)
ISBN: 978-1-032-57650-3 (pbk)
ISBN: 978-1-003-44036-9 (ebk)

DOI: 10.4324/9781003440369

Typeset in Times New Roman
by Apex CoVantage, LLC

Contents

Figures

Contributors

Livia Bergerot is a doctoral student in Egyptology at Paul-Valéry University Montpellier 3 under the supervision of Professor Marc Gabolde. Her PhD work is titled *Bes, from Prototype to Archetype: Forms and Functions of a God.*

Michele R. Buzon is a professor of Anthropology at Purdue University, USA. Her publications focus on identity transformation and lifeways using a bioarchaeological approach in the ancient Nile Valley, particularly at the Third Cataract site of Tombos, Sudan.

Ilaria Cariddi, PhD at Ca' Foscari University (Italy), specialized in Egyptian literary texts, autobiographies, and silence studies, is a contract lecturer of Egyptology and research fellow at University of Florence (Italy), curating the Istituto Papirologico Vitelli's collection of Egyptian Roman-age papyri from the Tebtynis temple library.

Aidan Dodson is honorary professor of Egyptology at the University of Bristol, UK, where he has taught since 1996, a fellow of the Society of Antiquaries of London, and a former chairman of the Egypt Exploration Society. He is the author of thirty books.

Stephanie Evelyn-Wright is a researcher who focuses on the osteoarchaeological study of disability. She received her PhD in Archaeology from the University of Southampton (UK) in 2022. Her most recent publication was a disability-based critique of the Archaeology of the Senses for the *Theoretical Roman Archaeology Journal.*

Scott D. Haddow is a Canadian bioarchaeologist based at the University of Copenhagen (Denmark) who works on human skeletal remains from the prehistoric to the Roman period in southwest Asia and northeast Africa.

Rosalind Janssen is honorary lecturer in Education at UCL's Faculty of Education and Society, UK. She currently teaches Egyptology classes and summer schools at Oxford University's Department of Continuing Education and London's City Lit. She co-authored *Growing Up and Getting Old in Ancient Egypt* (2007).

Kyle Lewis Jordan is a freelance disabled curator and archaeologist based in the United Kingdom, having studied Egyptology and the archaeology and heritage of Egypt and the Middle East at UCL. He most recently curated for the Ashmolean Museum and Pitt Rivers Museum in Oxford.

Lucas Justinian is an independent scholar based in the UK, with an academic background in philosophy and antiquity.

Samar Kamal is professor of Egyptology, Faculty of Tourism and Hotels, Minia University, Egypt. Samar is also Vice Dean of Post Graduate Studies and Research Affairs.

Ella Karev is a senior lecturer in Egyptology in the Department of Archaeology and Ancient Near Eastern Cultures at Tel Aviv University, Israel. Her forthcoming monograph (*Physical Descriptions, Biometrics, and Eikonographia in Graeco-Roman Papyri from Egypt*) discusses the use of physical descriptions in documentary identification.

Karen L. Kobylarz is a seventh-grade teacher at Unity Junior High in Cicero, Illinois, USA, near Chicago. She holds degrees in elementary Education, curriculum and instruction, and writing, and is also a board member for her local chapter of the American Research Center in Egypt.

Bénédicte Lhoyer is an assistant curator at the Musée de Picardie (Amiens, France) and lecturer at the Ecole du Louvre (Paris). Her research, which favours a historical anthropological approach, draws on texts, iconography, and material culture, and focuses on disability studies and art history.

Roisin Mackie is currently a digitiser at the Natural History Museum, England, and previously gained a MSc in Archaeology, specialising in Bioarchaeology, from the University of Southampton.

Uroš Matić is a lecturer at the Institute for Ancient History and Ancient Near Eastern Studies of the University of Innsbruck (Austria) and Institute for Classics of the University of Graz (Austria). He specializes in war, violence, and gender in ancient Egypt.

Alexandra F. Morris is a disabled Egyptologist, lecturer, and disability activist tying the past to the present. Her research is on disability in ancient Egypt, the Classical world, and creating inclusive museums. She holds many roles in academic, disability, heritage, and government sectors. She has cerebral palsy and dyspraxia.

Hana Navratilova is research fellow in Egyptology, Harris Manchester College, University of Oxford, United Kingdom; Egyptologist, historian, epigrapher; editor of *Who Was Who in Egyptology*, and member of the Egyptian expedition to Dahshur, the Metropolitan Museum of Art; recently published *A Citizen of Nowhere,* biography of J. Černý.

Nicola Reggiani teaches Papyrology at the University of Parma (Italy). Her research mainly focuses on the edition of Greek papyri from Ptolemaic and Roman Egypt, the Greek papyri with medical content, digital Papyrology (textual encoding and AI), and the modern reception of ancient Egyptian themes.

Emily Smith-Sangster is a PhD candidate at Princeton University, USA, and associate director of the Abydos South Project in Egypt. Her dissertation examines the expression of post-mortem identity at the Ahmose North Cemetery and more broadly across Upper Egypt, in the early New Kingdom.

Steven M. Stannish is an associate professor of History at SUNY Potsdam in the United States. His research focuses on the myths, religions, and philosophical systems of the ancient Mediterranean.

Hannah Vogel is an archaeologist researching ableism and disability in the ancient world and the disciplines of History and Archaeology. Her research interests include Disability Studies, Bioarchaeology, and Egyptology. She is an advocate for accessibility and has worked in museums, public outreach, and inclusive pedagogies.

Katie M. Whitmore earned her PhD from Purdue University examining health in the ancient Nile Valley. She is a forensic anthropologist with SNA International supporting the Defense POW/MIA Accounting Agency, and a lecturer at the University of Nebraska, Lincoln in the United States.

Sonia R. Zakrzewski is a bioarchaeologist based at University of Southampton (UK), focusing primarily on aspects of identity seen in the human body, including ethnicity, migration, religion, and disability. This has mostly involved Egyptians, medieval Islamic individuals from Spain, and early Saxons in England.

Michael R. Zimmerman, MD, PhD, is a retired anthropologist and pathologist researching mummy Paleopathology. He was adjunct professor of Biology at Villanova University. He is a consulting scholar at the University of Manchester's KNH Centre for Biomedical Egyptology and the Penn Museum. For 45 years he was a faculty member at the University of Pennsylvania.

Introduction

Alexandra F. Morris and Hannah Vogel

Welcome to our volume, *Disability in Ancient Egypt and Egyptology: All Our Yesterdays*. In it we explore disability across time and space, focusing on ancient Egypt and the associated disciplines that explore this culture. The aim of this book is to critically investigate the often-overlooked histories of disability in ancient Egypt and within the fields Egyptology and Egyptian Archaeology. We identify many instances of disability, but more than that, we encourage readers – you – to thoughtfully consider the history of disabled people in ancient Egypt and how their histories are represented in various contemporary spaces. This volume reshapes narratives of disability experiences, and disability within the discipline of Egyptology and Egyptian Archaeology itself. It challenges approaches towards terminology and tone in the field of ancient Disability Studies and offers guidance for disability inclusively in research, and in curatorial and pedagogical museum and university contexts. Beyond ancient Disability Studies, our engagement with the disability paradigm, disabled scholars, and community members as well as international perspectives on what can be considered 'disability history' are important contributions towards the study of our human past(s). This volume, while focusing on ancient Egypt and Egyptology, offers new ways to consider 'disability' in the broadest possible sense. We hope this collection of works will encourage future critical investigations in ways that are culturally contextualised.

For this book, we have explicitly used language guided and deemed appropriate by the disability community at the time of writing. This includes the use of identity-first language ('disabled person') over people-first language ('person with disability'), although we have also respected individual author choice for our disabled authors. It is our aim to set the standards for accepted language within this emerging field. See both Vogel's and Justinian's chapters for a further discussion on disability terminology, language use, and the harm that inappropriate language can cause.

Further building on the point of terminology, the subtitle, "All Our Yesterdays," was a deliberate reaction to the subtitle "The Forgotten Other" of the first volume in this series (*Routledge Studies in Ancient Disabilities*) and is reflexive of the shifting viewpoint this book provides. *We are neither forgotten, nor an other*. Disabled people have always existed and have always been part of the very fabric of society and the human experience. The title is also a *Star Trek* reference stemming from

DOI: 10.4324/9781003440369-1

the original series, namely an episode "All Our Yesterdays" that involved Captain Kirk and the crew of the Starship *Enterprise* travelling backwards in time to the ancient past through a library archive. The show, in its first iteration, was about creating and striving for a more inclusive future, literally, "infinite diversity in infinite combinations," and actively showed disabled people as part of that future. In striving for that more inclusive future, perhaps we should look to our ancient past for guidance of what that future could look like.

Furthermore, this volume was created with a deliberate incorporation of 'Crip Time,' and community care, that we feel ultimately led to a better book. Crip Time – time travel – is a nebulous concept developed by the disabled community that includes a way of viewing time more flexibly.[1] Our contributors include early career researchers, senior scholars, and people outside academia. Many of our contributors are disabled people writing on subjects that combine their professional expertise and lived experience. Additionally, our contributors are from a wide variety of international backgrounds and perspectives. This book is the product of an inclusive approach to editing, and it is important to outline what this looks like. Significant advancements in the ancient Disability Studies movement are led by PhD students and early career scholars, and so we have incorporated voices from various countries, communities, and career stages, with some early career scholars directly solicited, others welcomed by an open call. From the outset, we as editors carefully addressed accessibility. We created built-in extensions in terms of deadlines and multi-format media, and offered individualised support to contributors as needed. It was important to us to be flexible as to what that support looked like. In some cases, the editors provided virtual writing consultation, peer writing sessions, resources, reading recommendations and sourcing, English language assistance, and making in-person house calls. For some contributors we had to be even more flexible than our pre-established extended deadlines and adapted accordingly. Therefore, this book is not only about a minority group, but it was also created by an inclusive practice.

Because this is the first comprehensive book on ancient Egypt and disability, the temporal scope of this work spans from the Predynastic to the Roman period.[2] Time in ancient Egypt is traditionally split into the following periods and dynasties: Predynastic, *c.* 4000–2686 BCE (Naqada I, II, III, and the early dynastic also known as the Thinite period, namely Dynasties 0–3); Old Kingdom, *c.* 2686–2160 BCE (Dynasties 3–6); First Intermediate period, *c.* 2160–2055 BCE (Dynasties 6–early 11); Middle Kingdom, *c.* 2055–1650 BCE (Dynasties 11–13); Second Intermediate period, *c.* 1650–1550 BCE (Dynasties 14–17); New Kingdom, *c.* 1550–1069 BCE (Dynasties 18–20, which includes the Amarna period); Third Intermediate period, *c.* 1069–664 BCE (Dynasties 21–24, and the Nubian period); Late period, *c.* 664–332 BCE (Dynasties 26–31); Argead period, *c.* 332–323 BCE (Dynasty 32); Ptolemaic Egypt 323–30 BCE (Dynasty 33); and finally Roman Egypt 30 BCE–300 CE (Dynasty 34).

We have encouraged authors to consider disability and neurodiversity in the broadest possible sense. You will find considerations of disabled embodiment in visual and material culture, human remains, and textual sources from ancient and modern times. The use of 'disability' here includes physical, mental, and intellectual embodiments, bodily differences (visually apparent or not), mobility and sensory disabilities, bodily modifications (or in two chapters bodily mutilation), congenital and acquired disease, and various states of human diversity.

While we editors and many of the disabled scholars who have contributed to this volume have a personal preference for identity-first language, there are a range of preferences within the disability community and scholarship. As such, some chapters will use different disability terminology according to the author's preferences. In each instance, this is noted in the chapter text, endnotes, or an author's note. For the same reasons we have not prescribed a model to address disability (see Chapter 1 by Vogel which covers a brief outline of some of the models of disability). While it could be suggested that the different approaches to disability within this volume may seem disjointed, we argue that this instead reflects the diversity of experiences and realities of human variation within the field, and in societies past and present.

This volume addresses two broad themes delineated by sections. Theme 1 considers disability and disabled experiences in the discipline of Egyptology, museums, and pedagogy. This section includes chapters about disabled scholars and reception studies, including the perception and display of disability, and accessibility in museums and archives as well as in pedagogical contexts. Theme 2 considers disability and bodily difference within the historical and social contexts of ancient Egypt and Nubia. Although these themes are artificially constructed boundaries, we encourage the reader to question if disability in ancient Egypt is fundamentally separate from disability history in the modern discipline of Egyptology. The way ancient Egyptian disability is presented in museums, classrooms, and scholarly literature is inherently influenced by the researchers who disseminate that research. Of course, this is not to suggest that conceptualisations or experiences of disability in ancient Egypt were the same as today – in any time or place. Fundamentally, as the various models, definitions, and approaches throughout this book explore, disability is incredibly complex and contextual. We welcome this complexity and hope that this volume will promote further research in this space.

Section 1, which focuses on disability in Egyptology, starts with an introduction to the history of Disability Studies, provides brief overview of how Egyptological works have engaged with the disability paradigm, and outlines some key disability history works in broader ancient world studies. In this chapter Hannah Vogel outlines the activist origins of Disability Studies, and in doing so, highlights its importance in the disciplines of history and archaeology and within the present volume. In the second chapter, Lucas Justinian explores the close connections between the origins of Egyptology and the pseudoscientific eugenic paradigm. This chapter challenges readers and Egyptologists to address the problematic impact of eugenics, and the ableism generated by its legacy in Egyptology. Chapter 3 is by Alexandra F. Morris and Kyle Lewis Jordan. This team of scholars and disability activists explore historiographical approaches to the famous New Kingdom pharaohs Akhenaten and Tutankhamun. They call for reconsideration in the way scholars view, and thus communicate, ableist biases that are especially prevalent in discussions surrounding these two pharaohs. In Chapter 4 Steven M. Stannish furthers this discussion by focusing on the various retrospective diagnoses and ableist gaze that scholars have used to 'diagnose' Akhenaten. This chapter calls for reconsideration of earlier diagnosis attempts, especially considering modern religious lenses and an Enlightenment aesthetic, which centred on 'health'-based values. Hana Navratilova continues the historiographical approach in Chapter 5, and explores the experiences of a prominent disabled archaeologist, Jaroslav Černý. This chapter focuses on disability within the Egyptological field during the twentieth century, rather than evidence of disability in the ancient past.

Chapter 6 by Roisin Mackie shifts focus away from the discipline of Egyptology to the ways disability is presented to the public in museums. Mackie uses a case study of ancient Egyptian human remains in the British Museum to explore the ways in which disability is often overlooked in the reception of ancient Egypt by the public. The chapter challenges the ways that human remains are curated and displayed in museums, especially the language used, and accessibility given to disabled visitors, to call for more disability inclusion in this space. The final chapter in Section 1 is by Karen L. Kobylarz, which uses a pedagogical lens to explore to the extent to which museums are accessible and if/how disability is represented. This analysis in Chapter 7 is conducted from the perspective of a teacher and considers how one could plan a successful learning experience (via a fieldtrip or virtual visit) to a museum. In doing so, Kobylarz calls for greater disability representation in museum spaces and educational resources.

Section 2 explores different embodiments of disability in both ancient Egyptian and ancient Nubian contexts. Chapter 8 starts the section with a survey by Samar Kamal, which examines artistic representations of physical disability as related to occupation in private tombs. In Chapter 9, Bénédicte Lhoyer details in depth a variety of artistic, skeletal, and sculptural evidence related to individuals with spinal disabilities from the Naqada period to the Middle Kingdom. Emily Smith-Sangster in Chapter 10, examines prior analyses of dwarfism in the Old Kingdom and argues for a more realistic and humanistic interpretation of the evidence that does not see them as separate from society or as an "other." Livia Bergerot examines depictions and past interpretations of the dwarf god Bes, and similarly argues for a new interpretive paradigm, mapping the ways in which older analyses were influenced by colonialism, eugenics, and racism. Katie M. Whitmore and Michele R. Buzon continue the discussion on dwarfism through an analysis of a case study of an individual with dwarfism from the New Kingdom site of Tombos in Sudan (Nubia) utilising a Bioarchaeology of Care and Index of Care approach. What is unique about their chapter is that they apply this approach to a less 'severely limiting' example of disability, meaning this individual was an active participant both in society and perhaps in provisioning their own care. In Chapter 13, Michael R. Zimmerman similarly examines a case study of a man with a clubbed foot from the Dakleh Oasis and speculates on what we can learn about the treatment for individuals with the same disability today.

These contributions are followed by chapters in which authors use the expertise of their embodiments of their own disabilities to explore analyses of that embodiment in the past. Aidan Dodson uses the embodiment of his own disability to re-examine and reinterpret artistic and skeletal evidence relating to cerebral palsy in ancient Egypt. Alexandra F. Morris also uses the embodiment and understanding of her own disability to argue for a re-examination and reinterpretation of evidence concerning the god Harpocrates and cerebral palsy. This is followed by discussions of textual evidence, which offer an important balance to the emphasis in previous chapters on visual and material sources in preceding chapters. In Chapter 16, Ilaria Cariddi surveys textual evidence related to deafness and those who were hard of hearing in ancient Egypt. Ella Karev examines evidence for disability as biometric modalities in papyri from the Greco-Roman period. Nicola Reggiani explores evidence for physical impairment in Greek papyri from Roman Egypt.

The volume is concluded by more creative interpretations of disability and masculinity. Rosalind Janssen in Chapter 19 combines Egyptological, Ancient Near Eastern, feminist, gerontological, and textile studies with Disability Studies for an interdisciplinary take on baldness as a disability. Uroš Matić in Chapter 20 examines cases of Libyan genital mutilation in contexts of warfare in New Kingdom Egypt to argue for the idea of a disabled masculinity. Lastly, in Chapter 21, Sonia R. Zakrzewski, Stephanie Evelyn-Wright, and Scott D. Haddow explore the use of fictive narrative as a means of illuminating the lives of eunuchs from the Greco-Roman period, and additionally consider eunuchs as falling under the umbrella of disability.

This book reflects the diversity of the disabled experience and, in many ways, can be read as a celebration of the disabled experience both ancient and modern. While a variety of very serious and complex topics are covered, there is also a sense of joy and humour that is especially highlighted in Janssen's chapter. Disability, as discussed in more modern disability history, is not a tragedy, nor should it be viewed as such just because the context is ancient. Furthermore, as Dodson, Kobylarz, Jordan, Justinian, Mackie, and Morris demonstrate, using the embodiment of one's impairment and the expertise of lived experience creates more thorough and complex histories that better reflect the lived experience of ancient people and helps to further humanise them.

Disability history in the ancient world is a rapidly emerging space and we warmly welcome you, the reader, to expand on our arguments, views, and studies. This is the first step in what will become a more nuanced and rich discussion. It is hoped that this book will cause you to reflect on and think about disability in new ways and in places that you may not have considered it before, for example as you wander a gallery, stroll/roll through a museum, or peruse an archive. Perhaps you will take a moment to consider disability as you excavate or explore an archaeological site, to think about its context and use or how a disabled peer might experience the same site. Disability is also present in your classrooms and offices – the students you teach and colleagues you work with. Disability is and has always been everywhere: we just need to open our minds enough to acknowledge it. If you are a disabled person, we hope that you feel our community is represented fairly and respectfully – with academic rigor but also with meaningful efforts to avoid hurtful stereotypes and generalisations. This book demonstrates disability solidarity and shows that accessibility is not just possible; it genuinely betters our scholarship. We hope that this deep, detailed exploration into disability in the past and in our discipline will inspire you to further explore the infinite diversity of the human experience in all its infinite combinations.

Notes

1 Sheppard (2020, 39–47).
2 Dates after Shaw (2000).

Bibliography

Sheppard, E. "Performing Normal but Becoming Crip: Living with Chronic Pain." *Scandinavian Journal of Disability Research* 22, no. 1 (2020): 39–47.
Shaw, Ian. *The Oxford History of Ancient Egypt.* Oxford: Oxford University Press, 2000.

Part One

Disability in Egyptology

Reception Studies, Museums, and Pedagogy

1 Disability Studies

An Introduction for Egyptology

Hannah Vogel

Author's Note

This research was carried out under the auspices of the Commonwealth Funded Australian Government Research Training Program and a scholarship awarded by Department of History and Archaeology funded by anonymous donor to the Rundle Foundation of Egyptian Archaeology under the auspices of the Australian Centre for Egyptology, Macquarie University.

Disability Studies – What Is It?

Disability Studies (DS) is an umbrella term for a field of study aimed at examining the nature, implications, and consequences of disability in contemporary society.[1] Much of the recent scholarly work in DS is actively intersectional. Scholars draw from feminist theory, critical race theory, queer theory, and other frameworks to consider how aspects of identity (including disability) are co-constitutive, always interacting with each other.[2] Disability Studies, despite the range of models and approaches, centres the experiences of disabled people (note that terminology is variable) and emphasises the role of the disability community.[3]

Disability Studies was the academic result of social and political activism during the disability rights movement(s) of the late twentieth century. The academic discipline had substantial theoretical development from its political foundation in the 1960s to early 1970s and is now a multidisciplinary field.[4]

The activist origins of this field are important motivations for its use in and expansion to other disciplines. These activist origins are often called upon by DS scholars to reinforce models and develop new frameworks for addressing disability.[5] It is important to note the origins of the field were built by disability activists from many Western European countries, including the United Kingdom, Scandinavia, and the United States of America who campaigned for change in the way disability was understood in society. Activists demanded the re-definition of disability from a medical and individual problem to a political issue.[6] Sociology and anthropology are typically where Disability Studies is now situated. Disability Studies aims to bring disability into an arts/humanities framework, rather than a medical 'problem'. Fundamentally, Disability Studies rejects overmedicalisation.

DOI: 10.4324/9781003440369-3

The field was founded via rejection of the medical model. The 'medical model' is based in modern Western medicine and pathologizes physical and mental impairments, as well as other 'deviations' from an idealised bodily 'norm' of Western society, as functional limitations.[7] Disability activists called for reconsiderations of ableist assumptions about the existence and treatment of disability. They did so by challenging the presumed historical oppression and exclusion of disabled people, as the 'normal' experience and reaction to disability throughout time and place. Integral to the redefinition of disability was to contest overmedicalised accounts of disability.[8] To really engage with the development of the Disability Studies field, it is important to recognise the three key elements of early DS agendas. Firstly, activists challenged that disabled people are a "marginalised and disadvantaged constituency".[9] This contributed to the second claim that disabled people were a minority group. During early DS (1970s to early 2000), disability was framed as a minority worth theoretical consideration, in the same way women and 'race' were being redefined in academic and social contexts. Thirdly, activists argued that disability should be 'reconstructed' not as a medical problem, but rather as a social issue. Critical Disability Studies, especially from 2015 to present, rejects the second notion of 'minority'. Recent scholarship instead argues disabled people are not a minority, given that most (if not all) people experience disability at some point in their lifetime. The existence of disability is not in question in either framework, only the lens in which it is theoretically viewed.

The conceptualisation of disabled people as a disadvantaged group within the social model was the focus of much early DS scholarship. The social model is a dominant theoretical approach in the United States of America and the United Kingdom. The social model is the most famous re-definition of disability, and was based on the political ideology of the Union of the Physically Impaired Against Segregation (UPIAS). This model provided the structural analysis of disabled people's social exclusion.[10] It distinguishes *impairment* from *disability*: impairment is a biological or physiological feature of an individual's physical body and/or their intellectual capabilities, whereas disability is a socially and culturally constructed phenomenon implied or imposed on an individual with an impairment. The social model is often perceived as a dichotomy, placing the medical model *vs* the social model. These 'first wave' DS perspectives were centralised on economic considerations, materialist analysis, and supporting the politicisation of disability.[11]

While the social model was once the most commonly employed approach, it is not the only alternative to the medical model in the disability paradigm.[12] Some other conceptualisations of disability include, but are not limited to:[13]

1. The *charity model* is widely rejected in most scholarship, but sometimes features in interpretations of the pre-industrial world. This model views disabled people as 'victims' deserving of pity.
2. The *moral model* of disability is rejected in Disability Studies but sometimes features in historical scholarship, especially in works of the eighteenth and nineteenth centuries in which assumptions were made that in the past, disability was viewed by the person or their parents as the product of witchcraft or the consequences of divine intervention (namely punishment).

3. The *social constructivist model* is predominantly from the United States of America and refers to the view that differentness causes 'normal' people to stigmatise people with disabilities and construct their identity from this 'otherness'. The most frequently cited statement of this model is by Goffman,[14] although it is first found in earlier works and is a highly prominent model of disability in the 1970s to early 1980s.[15]
4. The *impairment model* was highly cited in the 1990s in critiques of the social model. This model argued that impairment and personal experiences are missing from the social model and instead suggested that the impairment (i.e., physiological bodily or mental difference) is what distinguishes the person.[16]
5. The *oppressed minority (political) model*, also known as the *social political model of disability*, is a model that argues that disabled people face discrimination and are an oppressed minority group.[17] This model includes the social model definition of disability and impairment but seeks to normalise the minority experience of disability as no more deviant than other minority groups. This model views discrimination as caused by the society majority.
6. The *independent living model* of the disability paradigm views disabled persons as responsible decision makers and sees problems with the professional structures and services engaging with disability. This conceptualisation of disability was highly used in activist movements – "nothing about me, without me."[18]
7. The *post-modern, post-structuralism, humanist, experience, existentialism inspired models*. While there are a range of conceptualisations of disability in these frameworks, the common thread is the notion that culture is a social and political construct and that the experience of disability itself can be deconstructed. Namely this approach deconstructs enlightenment ideas of progress, knowledge, and human rational actors. This approach has been critiqued as highly theoretical and for having limited practical application.
8. The *human variation disability model* argues that while disabled people experience discrimination similar to racial or ethnic minorities (for example) the disability community's experience of discrimination is exacerbated by the way society reacts to disability.[19] This model focuses on the multidimensional nature of disability and argues that discrimination is compounded by limitations in standardised social institutions. Some critiques of this model are that it requires the concept of 'normal' which is culturally contextual.[20]
9. Also commonly cited within disability related literature is the *International Classification of Functioning, Disability, and Health* (ICF), developed by the World Health Organisation.[21] In this model disability is conceptualised via assessments of functioning, although it does consider environmental factors and social, cultural, and political systems.[22] The ICF has widespread use as an epidemiological tool in medicine and policy, but has been criticised in Disability Studies.[23] Bickenback has extensively covered the responses to this model with the basis of most critiques being that the ICF reflects a 'medical model' of disability and that, as a tool for classification, it does not adequately cover the multidimensional aspects of disability.[24]

Despite the range of models, the close ties of disabled people's political movements and organisations stretched across disciplinary boundaries. This has made DS international and multidisciplinary. The history of this field, and the work by activists, academics, and allies, has resulted in the establishment of new paradigms of disability that are an intellectual challenge to the way disability is theorised and understood.

Critical Disability Studies

The central tenet of many DS approaches is that disability is not universal; rather it refers to historically and culturally specific phenomena.[25] As DS has grown and gained academic interest, many concepts have attracted increased critical scrutiny with demands for greater academic validity.[26] Since the 1990s many DS scholars have questioned first wave studies by highlighting the need to move beyond largely economic and materialist arguments, and to critically unpack notions of normalcy, ableism, and the categorical construction of disabled people as the 'other'.[27] The term 'Critical Disability Studies' (CDS) has since been applied to scholarly work of the twenty-first century that challenges aspects of DS.[28] Critical Disability Studies has been motivated by the need to overcome challenges to the social model, include post-modernist ideas and Foucauldian concepts of biopower, incorporate intersectionality, and explicitly contest the universalising tendency of Western scholarship. Critical Disability Studies problematises dichotomies critiquing both disablism *and* ableism.[29] In CDS, disability is a lived reality and a lens (or identity) through which disabled people interpret their place in the world. Critical Disability Studies also views disability as a social and political definition based on experience and societal power relations.[30]

(C)DS: Why Is It Important to Egyptology?

The focus of academic research, including the themes, topics, and identities we as scholars chose to research can be considered a reflection of the priorities of academia at large. Researching disability legitimises disability identity as an incredibly important aspect of humanity, thus deeming it worthy of greater scholarly research.

Challenging ableism or ableist preconceptions in our disciplines is fundamentally important because it contests the acceptance of ableism in all aspects of academic praxes, ontologies, and epistemologies, including our universities, libraries, archives, museums, and pedagogy. This is activism that brings public attention to disability as a fundamental reality. Disability Studies, and in this volume, Disability Studies in Egyptology, shapes disabled people's heritage, history, and identity. While experiences of disability have been overlooked in the past, disability is *not* invisible. Disability *is* important and worthwhile. Disability research has been understudied because of research agendas, not an absence of evidence. The range of evidence that can be viewed through the DS lens presented in this volume makes clear why this field is so important to integrate into Egyptology.

Disability (and by extension Disability Studies) intersects with all aspects of identity. Exploring ancient disability rejects retrospective application of modern ableism to the past. Disability Studies adds to a more complex past, and this complexity is more reflective of the reality of human experience.

How Has Disability Studies Been Used in Ancient World Studies?

Studies on disability, particularly ones that engage with the disability paradigm, are becoming increasingly prevalent throughout studies of the ancient world. A full literature review of disability throughout the ancient past is beyond the scope of this chapter. However, some more recent works that are commonly cited and/or are particularly innovative in their DS or CDS engagement are addressed here to encourage readers to explore this emerging field in different geographical and cultural contexts of the past.

Firstly, we will consider the 2021 volume *Disability Studies and the Classical Body: The Forgotten Other,* edited by Ellen Adams from the same series as the present volume, *Routledge Studies in Ancient Disabilities*. This volume is an edited collection in four parts that addresses disability in relation to the modern reception of the 'classical body'. Adams uses the term 'classical body' for three purposes, referring to lived bodily experiences, the notion of ideal classical form, and the corpus of scholarship that shaped modern and Western culture and intellectual traditions.[31] This collection of chapters includes, in Part 1, two chapters that use a medical humanities and classical reception approach to study illness, impairment, and chronic pain. Both chapters in this part consider the role of the 'patient' in clinical or medical consultations. Part 2 includes four chapters focused on "using, creating and showcasing disability support and services".[32] Several of the chapters consider the types and use of prostheses[33] and the display of prosthetics in museum contexts.[34] Within the same part, Adams's own chapter explores opportunities for learning from engaging with blind people in the appreciation of visual art, focusing especially on audio descriptions.[35] Part 3, "Real bodies and retrieving senses: Disability in the ritual record", focuses on archaeological evidence from funerary contexts and bodily experiences. The chapter by Emma-Jayne Graham especially challenges the use of 'abled body' norms in sensory experiences and seeks greater acknowledgment of human diversity, including disability.[36] The final part of the book includes two juxtaposing chapters on "Classical reception as the gateway between Classics and disability studies".[37] The volume as a whole challenges readers to consider Disability Studies as an important, productive, and exciting avenue of future research. It also demonstrates that there are many different avenues from which to engage with disability in the context of Classics and cognate disciplines that study the ancient Greek and Roman worlds. The work itself makes a bold claim (self-admitted by Adams) that disability is the "forgotten other". As discussed in this book's introduction, we challenge the notion of 'other' in relation to disability.

Debby Sneed is a key scholar in ancient Greek Disability Studies, who has published on access ramps in healing temples and infanticide. Sneed's research directly challenges medicalised approaches by removing disability from the biomedical lens as the sole framework of study and dissociates her interpretations from approaches that estimated ability via modern medical models.[38] Sneed, in both articles, advocates for a theoretical approach that incorporates Disability Studies. She argues that some disabled ancient Greeks were accommodated through inclusive design by accessibility ramps, which were a feature in temple architecture, particularly in healing sanctuaries.[39] The article successfully advocates for an approach informed by DS to re-assess archaeological sites and promote new understandings of ancient lives.[40] In her second article "Disability and Infanticide in Ancient Greece", Sneed challenges the widespread assumption that disability constituted valid grounds for infanticide in ancient Greece.[41] This is achieved via a re-examination of commonly cited literary sources, placing them back in their literary (and temporal) contexts, as well as material culture and bioarchaeological evidence to address ableist assumptions of disability in ancient Greece. This article rejects a scholarly 'apparent willingness' to accept that all disabled children were 'unwanted'.[42] The article, while focused on the ancient evidence, does much to challenge modern scholarship's ableism. Sneed also comments on the contemporary impact of ancient world studies when addressing the value of a human life.[43] Disability Studies and CDS are fundamental theoretical foundations to these publications. In these works, disability is addressed as a reality, but without typical assumptions of medicalisation and marginalisation. Disability is explored without a lens of 'compassion' or stigmatisation, which is prevalent in some academic work.[44]

As demonstrated by Sneed, disability can be considered via evidence for the development and use of assistive technology. Draycott has published extensively across various cultural and temporal contexts about the use of prosthetics. *Prosthetics and Assistive Technology in Ancient Greece and Rome* is one of the most comprehensive studies of this topic for the classical world in antiquity.[45] Draycott explores prosthetics and their users via a range of documentary, literary, archaeological and bioarchaeological evidence. Given the focus on impairment that is addressed separately to notions of disability (deemed as disadvantage), Draycott follows a social model approach, although this is not explicitly stated. The author does well at balancing the focus on the material of the prosthesis – its manufacture, purpose, and functionality – but also its use and user. Critical consideration is given to the way these assistive tools were embodied, and in relevant cases, how prosthetics can be used in conjunction with other assistive technology such as walking sticks, crutches, canes, *et cetera*.[46] Importantly, the scope of the volume is beyond that of limb and facial prosthetics (i.e., extremities, limbs, teeth, nose, and eyes) by considering the use of wigs and hair pieces. The study of materials used for 'beautification' are well attested, but it is somewhat unique to explore them in the context of prosthetics.

In Draycott's edited volume, Finch explores prosthesis use in an ancient Egyptian context. Finch discusses the manufacture and use of two prosthetic toes from ancient Egyptian mummified remains which were previously proven to have been used during the individual's lives. The study used experimental archaeology to re-create as accurately as possible the toes and some sandals, utilising two volunteers to test their use in a clinical setting.[47]

In the conclusion of this volume Draycott demonstrably engages with DS approaches. Draycott states, "Ancient assistive technologies were not only an extension of the body but also an extension of the self."[48] This is highly reflective of the way many disabled community members talk about their bodies and aides: for example, the way disability activist, the late Engracia Figueroa considers her wheelchair an extension of her body.[49] The performative use of assistive technologies and the agency enacted in their commission is incredibly important to humanise the study of disability in the past.

The way Draycott considered the materiality of impairment and prosthetics together offers bodily agency and a sense of humanisation. Many previous studies of impairment (using Draycott's terminology) are heavily medicalised.[50] Medicalised approaches to prosthetics consider "how useful" they were and make judgments on the quality of life of the disabled person without appropriately considering the individual's agency in the prosthesis acquisition and use (or decision to use at all).[51] This is especially important in instances in which prosthetics do not add to 'quality of life', which have been useful and/or only cosmetic. For instance, a replacement eye does not 'work' in the ancient world, in that it does not restore vision to the orbital cavity, but the decision to acquire one is an important expression of bodily agency. Also noteworthy is Draycott's chapter on "living prothesis" which considers animals and other people who supplemented and/or rendered manufactured prosthetic use unnecessary.[52] A similar theme of care provision and support sought by disabled people from animals is explored in Section 3 of *Care in the Past: Archaeological and Interdisciplinary Perspectives.*[53] Although dealing with a range of temporal and geographical contexts, no ancient Egyptian evidence is addressed.[54]

Volume one of the multi-volume series *A Cultural History of Disability*, dealing with 'antiquity', is edited by Laes. The book is a multiauthor approach to disability, or rather impairment, given that the volume has variable acceptance (and mostly rejection) of the word 'disability'. The chapters seem to broadly take a social model approach, although this is not explicitly identified. Most chapters address ancient classical antiquity from the Greek and Roman worlds.[55] There is no chapter within the *Cultural History of Disability in Antiquity* to consider ancient Egyptian contexts.

Laes's edited volume is one of the most cited historical studies of disability in the ancient world.[56] This multidisciplinary work is separated into five parts and each contributor examined 'disability' from a range of historical, theoretical, and sociological perspectives. Part one is a six-chapter section that covers seven ancient cultures: the Hittites,[57] Mesopotamia and Israel,[58] Persia,[59] Egypt,[60] India,[61] and China.[62] Parts two and three are the most substantial segments of the volume with six Greek and seven Roman chapters. Parts four and five have a geographical range of studies in the later ancient world.

The use of inverted commas for 'disability' here is deliberate, since Laes argues in the introduction that "disability is a recent term, one which profoundly characterises attitudes and approaches of modern Western civilisation."[63] Laes argued that 'infirmity', drawing the term from the Latin word *infirmitas*, is a more appropriate term for physical impairment in pre-modern societies. 'Infirmity', to Laes, is variable, mostly defined by social role and was related to a body's physical or mental deviance.[64] While the use of categorisations of bodily and mental impairments is a fair way to consider ancient evidence within the scope of the volume, this author rejects that "disability is simply unsuitable to describe concepts and conditions of people in the ancient world".[65] Disability itself is inherently variable. The construction of the concept of disability is complex and difficult to define. However, Laes rejects its use based on an assumption that disability is and always was a negative experience. This creates an exclusionary binary. Namely that the experience of disability is restricted to the modern world's use of eugenics, public health, and an able/disabled dichotomy. One could argue that all concepts, disability included, are troubled by anachronisms. Yet in scholarship, both the researchers producing the work and the readers who engage with it do not exist in isolation. There is no 'objective truth' to the past, and to simplify the experience of disability as 'infirmity' is to reduce the agency of disabled people (past and present). While this is a landmark volume in engaging with ancient evidence of disability, the terminology of the volume does not appropriately engage with modern Disability Studies, evidenced Laes's repeated use of the offensive 'r-word' slur on the very first page.[66] Laes does critique the modern and prominently Western use of 'healthy', which is indeed relevant criticism continued in the present volume. However, his approach to disability as only negative and modern concepts is rejected in our work. Our volume, by contrast, critiques notions of 'health' and disability by actively engaging with the lived experiences of disabled scholars and community members. Our volume focuses on embodiment, as well as on terminology that is inclusive of the modern disability community. 'Disabled' is a complex term, yet it does not mean 'unable'. Disabled is not the opposite of 'abled'. To repeat the phrase used by contemporary disabled people, "[D]isability is not a dirty word".[67] Disability in our volume is a complex set of embodiments that interact with other forms of identity. Disabled experiences can be bodily or intellectual differences that are reflective of human variation, and sometimes include congenital or pathological disease, impairments, and bodily functions.

The only chapter in *Disability in Antiquity* that covers an ancient Egyptian context is by David. David's chapter is comprehensive in terms of evidence variety. The chapter explores many instances of disease and/or bodily difference (disability is not defined) in human remains, artistic representations, and textual sources. This also includes an extensive survey of artefacts and texts, including mostly medical-magical papyri that conceivably include a form of disability. However, this catalogue is highly clinical. There is a distinct lack of engagement with the disability paradigm. Revisitation of this data with greater theoretical engagement with DS/CDS would be incredibly beneficial to challenge underlying ableist presumptions. For example, there is an overuse of generalisations for disabled experiences which fails to consider agency and how disability interacts with other identities. David states:

> Egyptian attitudes to death and the afterlife undoubtedly influenced their perception of physical anomalies. They were probably more willing to accept and tolerate deformity and disability because of the belief that no one could achieve perfection in this world.[68]

However, this immediately assumes that disability was an exceptional case, rather than (as statistically relevant) a highly likely bodily reality. Later in the chapter, when making a case for disability 'integration', David suggests that social acceptance would be equated to instances in which the Egyptians did not prescribe medical/magical treatments. Also, there is an implicit assumption that infanticide of disabled children was the norm across antiquity, and therefore that the evidence for disability makes ancient Egypt the 'exception' (noting this generalisation of Egypt as a monolithic culture across time and space). This fails to appropriately consider realities of human variation. It is also an ableist notion, namely that disability is avoided in all cases and that "acceptance" is unusual. Where treatment and care are addressed in the chapter there are some useful forms of evidence that are underrepresented in previous literature. However, the focus is entirely on the care of the disabled person and the 'burden' towards the community rather than any consideration of whether individual were enacting their own agency in care provision.

Egyptology has long associations with the analysis of human remains from a biomedical framework. The cognate disciplines of bioarchaeology, paleopathology, and physical anthropology have had many applications on ancient Egyptian human remains, many of which include the study of disabled individuals, although disability is rarely explicitly mentioned. There are, however, some more recent theoretical engagements within bioarchaeology with the disability paradigm.

Bioarchaeology, outside an ancient Egyptian context, has increasingly engaged with the study of disability and impairment. For instance, the landmark publication by Byrnes and Muller collates CDS, bioarchaeology, and social theory, although not in an ancient Egyptian context.[69] *Bioarchaeology of Impairment and Disability* is a collection of studies that offer innovative engagements between theory, method, and data; notably CDS and bioarchaeology.[70] Some of the chapters engage with a modified social model, by addressing 'disability' as a part of social identity that is only partially based on biological differences.[71] There has also since been further research into disability and impairment at a population scale analysis by Bohling, Croucher, and Buckberry via a medically influenced social model.[72]

Tilley and Oxenham proposed the 'Bioarchaeology of Care', which included consideration of psycho-social, emotionally supportive care.[73] Tilley and Cameron published the 'Index of Care', which is an online four-stage method for reproducible interpretation of caregiving, values, and social norms within a particular time and culture.[74] The application of this index was demonstrated by an individual from Neolithic Vietnam.[75] The Bioarchaeology of Care continues to develop and offer new research avenues, although greater engagement with Disability Studies would encourage a more agency-centred approach. The focus on caregivers, via the care receiver, that is made possible by this index risks the recipient of care (and potentially disabled person) being reduced to a passive role, rather than being an active party in caregiving. Tilley and Schrenk published additional case studies and expanded the theory with *New Developments in the Bioarchaeology of Care*[76] as well as incorporating the Bioarchaeology of Care framework with 'mummy studies' to extend the interpretive significance of palaeopathological data.[77]

There is a variety of catalogue style studies that address bodily difference, including disability in visual culture, such as Mahran and Kamal who surveyed Old Kingdom tomb wall scenes.[78] There is also a range of studies which address certain bodily experiences and/or disabilities. For instance, Dasen compared dwarfism in ancient Egypt and Greece using artistic, textual, and bioarchaeological data, and Kozma surveyed bioarchaeological evidence for dwarfism in human remains.[79] I also acknowledge an extensive number of studies which conceivably cover disability in ancient Egypt, including but not limited to publications relating to human remains, excavation reports, studies of medicine and magic, and studies of textual or visual evidence. The existence of disability is well proven and ever present; as such, a comprehensive review of the academic literature that considers disability is beyond the scope of this chapter. While many of these studies explore human variation – including bodily, intellectual, or mental difference that can be considered disability or potentially disabled embodiments – few directly use the word disability or engage with DS/CDS.

The following three works are select examples of published research that *does* directly engage with CDS/DS in relation to ancient Egyptian contexts. Draycott and Finch[80] have engaged with earlier DS in two case studies. Draycott explores disability via a social model approach, namely defining disability as disadvantage and discrimination imposed on an individual.[81] Draycott's chapter utilises the WHO's definition of disability in the case study, which criticises overly medicalised approaches to explore petitions written by a man with a vision impairment – *Gaius Gemellus Horigenes* from Karanis (Roman period).[82] Finch also used a case study approach to explore an artificial upper limb included in the mummified remains of an individual most likely from Akhmim in the early Ptolemaic period.[83] While it was innovative for the time to theoretically consider disability as a bodily identity, Finch's use of disability definitions is now an outdated approach. Finch considered disability (and prosthesis in the case study) as solely a bodily difference and questioned the embalmers' addition of the limb shape to the mummified remains to be a commentary about bodily completeness reflective of social inclusion. Finch cited the definition of deformity and disability by Garland from 1995, which refers mostly to bodily differences as resulting in social marginalisation.[84] This approach focuses on deformity as deviation from "normal appearances" which will "marginalize the individual".[85] This notion that "society's perception of this deviation from the norm that dictates how far the individual is excluded or becomes disabled in his or her daily life"[86] is based on a limited range of possible experiences of disability. The statement is followed by a highly social model view that "this impact is imposed by others which is so often extremely difficult to determine".[87] However, disability does not equate to a dichotomy of inclusion or exclusion, and thus fails to negotiate the complex interplay of factors throughout different stages of lifespan, social and identity factors, geographical and temporal space, and many more.

The 2020 article by Morris is one of the first to comprehensively analyse the material and visual culture within Tutankhamun's tomb, alongside a study of his human remains to explicitly argue about disability.[88] The paper considers material culture and its placement in the pharaoh's tomb to convincingly argue that Tutankhamun was disabled, and that several accommodations were made for him in his tomb. Morris suggests that artistic representations of the king being supported by others and the placement of many chairs and stools, walking sticks, and medicinal plants and herbs were deliberately positioned to make the afterlife readily accessible to the pharaoh, especially when considering medical studies of Tutankhamun's physical remains. The article makes a strong case for such deliberate accommodations, but also challenges why so many people, public and scholars alike, avoid disability associations. Morris questions why most museum exhibitions and public literature ignore the presence, or even possibility, of disability. As posited by Morris, "Does making him able-bodied say more about our society today, than it does about the man himself?"[89] This argument is further explored by Morris and Jordan in Chapter 3 of this volume.

The 2023 article by Vogel and Power is a comprehensive historiographical review of approaches to the study of disability in Egyptology and Egyptian archaeology.[90] The paper uses a CDS approach with embodiment theory and consideration of appropriate terminology to argue for better awareness of ableist assumptions relating to disability. It challenges readers to implement greater inclusivity in terminologies and research in ancient world studies.[91] Vogel and Power aimed to determine "whether ableist assumptions permeate" approaches to bodily differences and disability in Egyptology and Egyptian archaeology by focusing on ableism rather than disability.[92] The paper covers a range of published research on disability and has a broad scope including "bodily differences, namely physical bodily differences that are visually apparent in either human remains or visual representations, and present at birth or throughout the individual's life" and "disabilities of varied aetiologies and durations".[93] Works reviewed in the paper are categorised into four approaches, namely, "1. Cataloguing and studying disease, 2. Cataloguing disabilities and bodily differences, 3. 'Othering' disability and bodily differences, and 4. Engaging with the disability paradigm".[94] The authors stress that the article does not focus on particular scholars but instead considers the ways Egyptological scholarship has addressed studies of disability and calls for reconsideration of many ableist assumptions that it demonstrates are present in much academic work. The article encourages the problematisation of ableist methodologies and argues that disability has experienced limited theoretical development in Egyptology, with the dominant approach having been focused on medicalised examinations and retrospective diagnosis.[95] Ableism, the focus of the study, is demonstrated through the overuse of medicalisation, the use of dehumanising dualisms (such as mind;body, subject;object, normal;abnormal) and presumptions of disability automatically equalling social exclusion or marginalisation. It is also worth noting that much of the research for this paper provided inspiration for the present volume. The prevalence of ableism and disablism explored by Morris and by Vogel and Power underscores our call for more theoretically engaged research. The study of disability requires a deep understanding of both disabled experience and disability history.

Conclusions and Future Studies

The ways our disciplines address these topics is inherently affected by our context and time. The disabled community of today deserve a history which considers the inevitable existence of human variation in a light that is not marred by ableism or founded in medicalised and eugenics ideals. The typical argument against 'disability' in the ancient world is based on the contextual nature of disability; namely, that people in the past do not view disability the same way 'we' do today. However, disability is not viewed the same for any person. Disability is complex. It is variable in duration and type, and interacts with other aspects of identity, materiality, access, and community. We can acknowledge that disability is variable for different people, places, and times in the past. This acceptance of variation is not a hindrance to research. Instead, it creates a multifaceted range of research avenues. While this complexity challenges the assumptions we can make, and at some point, will result in variable interpretations, we do have a responsibility to conduct ethical, informed, and considered engagement with the ancient world. This complexity is more authentic to our modern communities. Overmedicalisation or attempts at an objective 'truth' are not appropriate means to study disability because they neglect the agency and experience of the past person, while simultaneously actively excluding contemporary disabled people.

Engagement with CDS and DS offers Egyptology more complex but more authentic interpretations of the past. It seeks to view humanity. This is not to reject the possibility of marginalisation, stigmatisation, objectification, or discrimination a disabled person might experience, either now or in the ancient past. The theoretical engagement with DS and/or CDS that I am calling for asks scholarship to consider as many possible experiences of disability as the evidence may reveal. As demonstrated in other fields and disciplines engaging with feminist theory, critical race theory, queer theory, embodiment theory, and relevant communities, theoretical approaches offer a deeper understanding and a different (or additional) lens to view past evidence, as well as see other and new evidence beyond what was previously considered. Our experiences will always influence the way we see the world around us, and construct the world of the past. Embracing such an embodied view of the world will open possibilities for the past, and therefore increase inclusivity for the present. It is hoped this volume will contribute to a more inclusive future for our disciplines.

Notes

1 Southwell-Wright (2013, 67).
2 McRuer (2020) *s.v.* "Disability Studies".
3 "What is Disability Studies?" *Disability Studies, University of Washington*, last modified 2023, accessed May 27, 2023, https://disabilitystudies.washington.edu/what-is-disability-studies.
4 Battles (2011, 107).
5 Roulstone, Thomas, and Watson (2012, 3).
6 Roulstone, Thomas, and Watson (2012, 3).
7 Byrnes and Muller (2017, 2).
8 Shakespeare (2010, 214).
9 Roulstone, Thomas, and Watson (2012, 3).
10 The re-definition of disability was inspired by what Mark Oliver termed the "social model" in 1983; *cf.* Shakespeare (2010, 215).

11 Feminist disability activists named this disadvantage as social oppression; entering the concept of 'disablism' alongside 'sexism' and 'racism'; Roulstone, Thomas, and Watson (2012, 4).
12 For further discussions of these models see Pfeiffer (2001, 29–52).
13 Pfeiffer (2001, 29–52).
14 Goffman (1963).
15 Pfeiffer (2001, 32).
16 See French (1993, 17–25) for examples.
17 Pfeiffer (2001, 35–37).
18 Pfeiffer (2001, 37–38).
19 Scotch and Schriner (1997, 148–59).
20 Pfeiffer (2001, 40).
21 Bickenbach (2012, 55).
22 Altman (2001) has extensively covered the development of the WHO's models and classifications of disability, including their application.
23 Bickenbach (2012, 57).
24 See further: Ibid., 51–66.
25 Shakespeare (2010, 215).
26 Roulstone, Thomas, and Watson (2012, 4).
27 Roulstone, Thomas, and Watson (2012, 4).
28 Shakespeare and Watson (2001), Shuttleworth and Meekosha (2017, 50).
29 Shuttleworth and Meekosha (2017, 25).
30 Reaume (2014, 1248).
31 Adams (2021a, 2).
32 Adams (2021a, 89).
33 Draycott (2021, 93).
34 Goggins (2021, 117–29).
35 Adams (2021b, 130–59).
36 Graham (2021, 165–91).
37 Hall (2021, 215), King (2021, 237–63).
38 Sneed (2018, ii).
39 Sneed (2020).
40 Sneed (2020, 1016).
41 Sneed (2021, 748).
42 Sneed (2021, 748).
43 Sneed (2021, 767).
44 For example, compare the way Garland (2010) has approached disability in ancient Greece.
45 Draycott (2022).
46 Draycott (2022, 38).
47 Finch (2018).
48 Draycott (2022, 173).
49 Spoccia, "Disabled Activist Dies after United Airlines Destroyed Her Custom Wheelchair," *The Independent*, November 5, 2021, accessed May 2, 2023, https://www.independent.co.uk/news/world/americas/crime/disabled-activist-death-united-airlines-b1952152.html?r=84962.
50 For example, see Brier et al. (2015).
51 See Vogel and Power (2023) for an overview of medicalisation in Egyptology removing agency, although not in relation to prosthetics.
52 Draycott (2022, 38).
53 Powell, Southwell-Wrigh, and Gowland (2017).
54 Garland (2010).
55 Laes (2020).
56 Laes (2017).
57 Beal (2017).

58 Kellenberger (2017, 47–60).
59 Coloru (2017).
60 David (2017).
61 Miles (2017).
62 Milburn (2017).
63 Laes (2017, 4).
64 Laes (2017, 4).
65 Laes (2017, 6).
66 Laes (2017, 1).
67 Andrews et al. (2019).
68 David (2017, 86).
69 Byrnes and Muller (2017).
70 Byrnes and Muller (2017, v).
71 For example: Cormier and Buikstra (2017).
72 Bohling, Croucher, and Buckberry (2022).
73 Tilley and Oxenham (2011). See also Tilley (2015).
74 Tilley and Cameron (2014).
75 Tilley and Oxenham (2011, 35–42).
76 Tilley and Schrenk (2017).
77 For example: see Nystrom and Piombino-Mascaii (2017), Nystrom and Tilley (2019).
78 Mahran and Kamal (2016, 169–92).
79 Dasen (1993), Kozma (2008, 3104–12), Kozma (2006, 303–11).
80 Finch (2013, 111–32).
81 Draycott (2015, 190).
82 Draycott (2015, 190).
83 Finch (2013, 115–16).
84 Garland (2010), Finch (2013, 129).
85 Finch (2013, 126–27), *cf.* Kelley (2007, 33).
86 Finch (2013, 126–27).
87 Finch (2013, 126–27).
88 Morris (2020, 53–72).
89 Morris (2020, 62).
90 Vogel and Power (2023).
91 Vogel and Power (2023, 11).
92 Vogel and Power (2023, 1).
93 Vogel and Power (2023, 4).
94 Vogel and Power (2023).
95 Vogel and Power (2023, 9).

Bibliography

Adams, Ellen, ed. *Disability Studies and the Classical Body: The Forgotten Other*. Milton Park: Routledge, 2021a.

Adams, Ellen. "New Light on 'the Viewer' Sensing the Parthenon Galleries in the British Museum." In *Disability Studies and the Classical Body: The Forgotten Other,* edited by E. Adams, 130–59. London: Routledge, 2021b.

Altman, Barbara M. "Disability Definitions, Models, Classification Schemes, and Applications." In *Handbook of Disability Studies*, edited by Gary L. Albrecht, Katherine Seelman, and Michael Bury, 97–122. Thousand Oaks: Sage Publications, 2001.

Andrews, E., Anjali J. Forber-Pratt, Linda R. Mona, Emily M. Lund, Carrie R. Pilarski, and Rochelle Balter. "#SaytheWord: A Disability Culture Commentary on the Erasure of Disability." *Rehabilitation Psychology* 64, no. 2 (2019): 111–18.

Battles, Heather. "Towards Engagement: Exploring the Prospects for an Integrated Anthropology of Disability." *vis-à-vis: Exploring Anthropology* 11, no. 2 (2011): 107–24.

Beal, Richard H. "Disabilities from Head to Foot in Hittite Civilisation." In *Disability in Antiquity*, edited by Christian Laes, 27–46. Abingdon: Routledge, 2017.

Bickenbach, Jerome E. "The International Classification of Functioning, Disability and Health and its Relationship to Disability Studies." In *Routledge Handbook of Disability Studies*. 1st ed., edited by Nick Watson, Alan Roulstone, and Carol Thomas, 51–66. Abingdon: Routledge, 2012.

Bohling, Solange, Karina Croucher, and Jo Buckberry. "The Bioarchaeology of Disability: A Population-Scale Approach to Investigating Disability, Physical Impairment, and Care in Archaeological Communities." *International Journal of Paleopathology* 38 (2022): 76–94.

Brier, Bob, Phuong Vinh, Michael Schuster, Howard Mayforth, and Emily J. Chapin. "A Radiologic Study of an Ancient Egyptian Mummy with a Prosthetic Toe." *The Anatomical Record* 298 (2015): 1047–58.

Byrnes, Jennifer F., and Jennifer L. Muller, eds. *Bioarchaeology of Impairment and Disability: Theoretical, Ethnohistorical, and Methodological Perspectives*. Ann Arbor: Springer, 2017.

Coloru, Omar. "Ancient Persia and Silent Disability." In *Disability in Antiquity*, edited by Christian Laes, 60–74. Abingdon: Routledge, 2017.

Cormier, Aviva, and Jane Buikstra. "Impairment, Disability, and Identity in the Middle Woodland Period: Life at the Juncture of Achondroplasia, Pregnancy, and Infection." In Bioarchaeology of Impairmen*t and* Disability: Theoretical, Ethnohistorical, *and* Methodological Perspectives, edited by Jennifer F. Byrnes and Jennifer F. Muller, 225–48. Cham: Springer, 2017.

Dasen, Véronique. *Dwarfs in Ancient Egypt and Greece*. Oxford: Clarendon Press, 1993.

David, Rosalie. "Egyptian Medicine and Disabilities: From Pharaonic to Greco-Roman Egypt." In *Disability in Antiquity*, edited by Christian Laes, 75–89. Abingdon: Routledge, 2017.

Draycott, Jane. "Reconstructing the Lived Experience of Disability in Antiquity: A Case Study from Roman Egypt." *Greece and Rome* 62, no. 2 (2015): 189–205.

Draycott, Jane. "Prostheses in Classical Antiquity: A Taxonomy." In *Disability Studies and the Classical Body: The Forgotten Other*, edited by Ellen Adams, 93–116. Milton Park: Routledge, 2021.

Draycott, Jane. *Prosthetics and Assistive Technology in Ancient Greece and Rome*. Cambridge, UK: Cambridge University Press, 2022.

Finch, Jacky. "The Complex Aspects of Experimental Archaeology: The Design of Working Models of Two Ancient Egyptian Great Toe Prostheses." In *Prostheses in Antiquity*. 1st ed., Vol. 1, edited by Jane Draycott, 29–48. London, UK: Routledge, 2018.

Finch, Jacqueline L. "The Durham Mummy: Deformity and the Concept of Perfection in the Ancient World." *Bulletin of the John Rylands Library Manchester* 89 (2013): 111–32.

French, Sally. "Disability, Impairment or Something in Between." In *Disabling Barriers-Enabling Environments,* edited by John Swain, Vic Finkelstein, Sally French, and Mark Oliver, 17–25. London: Sage, 1993.

Garland, Robert. *The Eye of the Beholder: Deformity and Disability in the Graeco-Roman World*. 2nd ed. New York: Bloomsbury Publishing, 2010.

Goffman, Erving. *Stigma: Notes on the Management of Spoiled Identity*. Englewood Cliffs, NJ: Prentice-Hall, 1963.

Goggins, Sophie. "Displaying the Forgotten Other in Museums: Prostheses at National Museums Scotland." In *Disability Studies and the Classical Body: The Forgotten Other*, edited by Ellen Adams, 117–29. Milton Park: Routledge, 2021.

Graham, Emma-Jayne. "Interactional Sensibilities: Bringing Ancient Disability Studies to Its Archaeological Senses." In *Disability Studies and the Classical Body: The Forgotten Other*, edited by Ellen Adams, 165–91. Milton Park: Routledge, 2021.

Hall, Edith. "The Immortal Forgotten Other Gang: Dwarf Cedalion, Lame Hephaestus, and Blind Orion." In *Disability Studies and the Classical Body: The Forgotten Other*, edited by Ellen Adams, 215–36. Milton Park: Routledge, 2021.

Kellenberger, Edgar. "Mesopotamia and Israel." In *Disability in Antiquity*, edited by Christian Laes, 47–60. Abingdon: Routledge, 2017.

Kelley, Nicole. "Deformity and Disability in Greece and Rome." In *This Abled Body. Rethinking Disabilities in Biblical Studies*, edited by Hector Avalos, Sara J. Melcher, and Jeremy Schipper, 31–45. Atlanta: Society of Biblical Literature, 2007.

King, Helen. "A History of Our Own? Using Classics in Disability Histories." In *Disability Studies and the Classical Body: The Forgotten Other*, edited by Ellen Adams, 237–63. Milton Park: Routledge, 2021.

Kozma, Chahira. "Dwarfs in Ancient Egypt." *American Journal of Medical Genetics* 140 (2006): 303–11.

Kozma, Chahira. "Skeletal Dysplasia in Ancient Egypt." *American Journal of Medical Genetics* 146 (2008): 3104–12.

Laes, Christian, ed. *Disability in Antiquity*. Abingdon: Routledge, 2017.

Laes, Christian, ed. *A Cultural History of Disability*. Vol. 1. London: Bloomsbury Academic, 2020.

Mahran, Heba, and Samar Mostafa Kamal. "Physical Disability in Old Kingdom Tomb Scenes." *Athens Journal of History* 2, no. 3 (2016): 169–92.

McRuer, Robert. *Oxford Research Encyclopedia of Literature: s.v. "Disability Studies"*. Edited by Robert McRuer. Oxford: Oxford University Press, 2020.

Milburn, Olivia. "Disability in Ancient China." In *Disability in Antiquity*, edited by Christian Laes, 106–18. Abingdon: Routledge, 2017.

Miles, M. "India: Demystifying Disability in Antiquity." In *Disability in Antiquity*, edited by Christian Laes, 90–105. Abingdon: Routledge, 2017.

Morris, Alexandra F. "Let That Be Your Last Battlefield: Tutankhamun and Disability." *Athens Journal of History* 6, no. 1 (2020): 53–72.

Nystrom, Kenneth C., and Dario Piombino-Mascaii. "Mummy Studies and the Soft Tissue Evidence of Care." In *New Developments in the Bioarchaeology of Care: Further Case Studies and Expanded Theory*, edited by Lorna Tilley and Alecia A. Schrenk, 199–218. Cham: Springer, 2017.

Nystrom, Kenneth C., and Lorna Tilley. "Mummy Studies and the Bioarchaeology of Care." *International Journal of Paleopathology* 25 (2019): 64–71.

Pfeiffer, David. "The Conceptualization of Disability." In *Exploring Theories and Expanding Methodologies: Where* We Are *and* Where We Need *to* Go. Vol. 2, edited by Sharon N. Barnartt and Barbara M. Altman, 29–52. Bingley: Emerald Group Publishing, 2001.

Powell, Lindsey, William Southwell-Wright, and Gowland Rebecca, eds. *Care in the Past: Archaeological and Interdisciplinary Perspectives*. Oxford: Oxbrow Books, 2017.

Reaume, Geoffrey. "Understanding Critical Disability Studies." *CMAJ: Canadian Medical Association Journal* 186, no. 16 (2014): 1248–49.

Roulstone, Alan, Carol Thomas, and Nick Watson. "The Changing Terrain of Disability Studies." In *Routledge Handbook of Disability Studies*, edited by Alan Roulstone, Carol Thomas, and Nick Watson, 3–11. Abingdon: Routledge, 2012.

Scotch, Richard K., and Kay Schriner. "Disability as Human Variation: Implications for Policy." *The ANNALS of the American Academy of Political and Social Science* 549, no. 1 (1997): 148–59.

Shakespeare, Tom. "The Social Model of Disability." In *The Disability Studies Reader*. 3rd ed., edited by Lennard J. Davis, 214–21. New York: Routledge, 2010.

Shakespeare, Tom, and Nick Watson. "The Social Model of Disability: An Outdated Ideology?" In *Exploring Theories and Expanding Methodologies: Where We Are and Where We Need to Go*. Research in Social Science and Disability, Vol. 2, edited by Sharon N. Barnartt, 9–28. Bingley: Emerald Group Publishing Limited, 2001.

Shuttleworth, Russell, and Helen Meekosha. "Accommodating Critical Disability Studies in Bioarchaeology." In *Bioarchaeology of Impairment and Disability: Theoretical, Ethnohistorical, and Methodological Perspectives*, edited by Jennifer F. Byrnes and Jennifer F. Muller, 19–38. Cham: Springer, 2017.

Sneed, Debby. "The Life Cycle of Disability in Ancient Greece." PhD diss., University of California, 2018.

Sneed, Debby. "The Architecture of Access: Ramps at Ancient Greek Healing Sanctuaries." *Antiquity* 94, no. 376 (2020): 1015–29.

Sneed, Debby. "Disability and Infanticide in Ancient Greece." *Hesperia: The Journal of the American School of Classical Studies at Athens* 90, no. 4 (2021): 747–72.

Southwell-Wright, William. "Past Perspectives: What Archaeology Can Offer Disability Studies?" In *Emerging Perspectives on Disability Studies*, edited by Matthew Wappett and Katrina Arndt, 67–95. New York: Palgrave Macmillan, 2013.

Spoccia, Gino. "Disabled Activist Dies after United Airlines Destroyed Her Custom Wheelchair." *The Independent,* November 5, 2021. Accessed May 2, 2023. https://www.independent.co.uk/news/world/americas/crime/disabled-activist-death-united-airlines-b1952152.html?r=84962.

Tilley, Lorna. *Theory and Practice in the Bioarchaeology of Care*, 35–42. Cham: Springer, 2015.

Tilley, Lorna, and Tony Cameron. "Introducing the Index of Care: A Web-Based Application Supporting Archaeological Research into Health-Related Care." *International Journal of Paleopathology* 6 (2014): 5–9.

Tilley, Lorna, and Mark F. Oxenham. "Survival against the Odds: Modeling the Social Implications of Care Provision to Seriously Disabled Individuals." *International Journal of Paleopathology* 1, no. 1 (2011): 35–42.

Tilley, Lorna, and Alecia A. Schrenk, eds. *New Developments in the Bioarchaeology of Care: Further Case Studies and Expanded Theory*. Cham: Springer, 2017.

University of Washington. "What is Disability Studies?" Last modified 2023. Accessed May 27, 2023. https://disabilitystudies.washington.edu/what-is-disability-studies.

Vogel, Hannah, and Ronika K. Power. "Recognising Inequality: Ableism in Egyptological Approaches to Disability and Bodily Differences." *World Archaeology* 54 (2023). https://doi.org/10.1080/00438243.2023.2170911.

2 Challenging the Eugenic Paradigm in Egyptology

Lucas Justinian

Author's Note

Throughout this chapter I will use the term *impairment* to refer to physical, psychological and sensory conditions which can be functionally limiting, and *disabled* to refer to someone experiencing marginalisation through the sociostructural limitations imposed upon them as a result of their impairments. I will be working with a definition of *ableism* as any discrimination against people perceived to be, or known to be, disabled. Though this unnuanced definition is not always suitable to wider discourse, it serves for the discussion in this chapter. I use the word *ableism* because it is the common term, but acknowledge that *disablism* can be preferred. Please also be aware that while I am myself disabled, I have made the stylistic choice to refer to disabled people collectively in the third person.

What is the Eugenic Paradigm?

Eugenics is a pseudoscience dating to the nineteenth century, based upon elementary genetic principles applied simplistically to complex human traits. While selective breeding is as possible for humans as for any other sexually reproducing organism, traits considered desirable in humans are highly subjective and, often, genetically more complex than the colour of a flower's petals or the sugar content of fruit. Selectively breeding for eye colour is one thing: selectively breeding for imprecisely and tendentiously defined traits such as intellectual ability, beauty or a kindly disposition is another.

While it is historically true that eugenics emerged as a scientific manifestation of ableism and white supremacy,[1] and that these were existing concepts in the late nineteenth century, modern ableism now exists in the light of the *paradigm* of eugenics. Placing ableism not as a form of bigotry but as a form of concern motivated by medically objective facts grants it legitimacy and empowers injustices which, viewed through other lenses, such as race, would be openly regarded as bigotry. Referring to the over-diagnosis of underperforming Black students as intellectually disabled and placing them in separate classrooms or schools from others as segregation,[2] for instance, would not be in line with the view that such actions are intended for compassionate reasons. Yet, segregation is a precise descriptor of

DOI: 10.4324/9781003440369-4

this practice, given the explicit racial component of such cases. Likewise, the word *eugenics* itself is unpopular because it is falsely assumed to only refer to practices such as clinical murder and forced sterilisation, and not to subtler assumptions about the heritability and worthiness of certain traits. It is these latter principles, and the dressing up of racism, classism and ableism in scientific language while focusing almost entirely on the biomedical aspects of disability and race, that constitute what I term the *eugenic paradigm* throughout this chapter. The distinction between eugenics as a philosophical position and the eugenic paradigm is fine, but important: even those who know little of eugenics historically, politically or technically will tend to use eugenic reasoning or language when justifying ableist instincts.

This paradigm saturates not only scholarship but also popular discourse, two arenas that necessarily inform and reflect one another, so I will examine both scholarly and wider cultural sources in this chapter. It is important to note, particularly while exploring the most unpleasant real-world consequences of the paradigm, that my intention is not to point the accusatory finger at any particular field of study. Rather, it is to demonstrate that a wider cultural prevalence of certain ideas necessarily impacts scholarship, and that the very nature of these ideas is to hide in plain sight as reasonable positions when unexamined. Likewise, since scholarship feeds into the wider consciousness, certain ideas can be heightened or given weight that perhaps ought not to be, because of unexamined biases shared by most people within any given culture.

One arena in which the eugenic paradigm is employed is when discussing consanguinity and inbreeding. This is relevant to Egyptologists, since consanguineous marriage was a common pharaonic practice.[3] Prominently, Tutankhamun has been argued to be born from sibling incest, and to have produced two children with his own sibling.[4] As a pharaoh from whom we have derived a good deal of biomedical data but whose personal narrative is incomplete, Tutankhamun is an ideal example of how the eugenic paradigm prevents Egyptology from addressing the full history of a person or period. His health concerns are increasingly known, both those supposed to be hereditary and those acquired later in life,[5] and this focus on his biomedical history creates a specific image of him whereby he is viewed not as a fully embodied man, but as a sickly boy.

The direct consequence of the medicalisation of disability via the eugenic paradigm is that disabled people are seen primarily, or even entirely, in the context of their visible or socially impactful impairments,[6] which with the ability to screen for certain traits during pregnancy can begin antenatally. These value judgements on the worthiness of life, when made devoid of the context of full embodiment (that is, a full conceptualisation of someone including their subjectivity, agency and personhood),[7] have historically come at a grave cost to disabled people.

Eugenics and Egyptology

The eugenic paradigm must be challenged if justice for disabled people is to be achieved. Of course, Egyptology is not commonly seen as the front line in the struggle for disability liberation, but it is an anthropological discipline with the power to connect living people with those who lived millennia ago. Even so, before we can discuss Egyptology's relationship to the eugenic paradigm as a field within anthropology, we must address its specific relationship to the pseudoscience of eugenics *per se.*

Flinders Petrie scarcely needs an introduction to any archaeologist. His exacting methodology for cataloguing his discoveries is often considered the foundation of archaeology as a true scientific discipline. This tendency for precision and diligence was one which Petrie credited to his childhood education, and he reported being horrified by the "rough shovelling" he once witnessed at a site on the Isle of Wight, only eight years old.[8] Precision of observation and diligence in the handling of evidence were key to the scientific method, and key to Petrie's archaeological method in turn. Not all of Petrie's applications of these principles were laudable.

One of his defining working partnerships was with Francis Galton, a polymath with a particular interest in the application of statistical principles to the human mind. Petrie's relationship with Galton began in earnest in the 1880s, when his reputation for diligence caused Galton to ask him to retrieve human remains from Egypt as part of an ongoing anthropometric study.[9] The purpose of this project was ultimately the 1887 publication of *Racial Photographs from the Egyptian Monuments*, a documentation of the various ethnic groups ancient Egypt encountered or conquered.[10] Petrie developed, from this time onward, an express interest in biometrics and selective human breeding that has been dismissed in later scholarship as Galton's influence on Petrie, rather than an ideology Petrie himself possessed.[11] In fact, Petrie affirmatively believed that, for example, "it is obviously possible by selective action to increase or diminish not only the bodily activity but also the mental ability seen in the whole community".[12] Intriguingly, while in places Petrie demonstrates an understanding that most want of ability emerges from want of opportunity, he also proposes an education system which strictly medicalises academic ability, and derives profit from the diversion of the labour of the underserved:

> The finest 5 per cent, both mentally . . . and physically as well, should be premiated by assisted higher education of suitable type. The worst 10 per cent should be remanded to a training school where physical and mental development would be scientifically carried out, and as much profit as possible be made from their labour toward self-support.[13]

This proposed policy becomes immediately and explicitly eugenic:

> The best half of the most able should receive . . . free support for all children they may have after they have reached the age of twenty-five. The worst half of the most incapable . . . should be . . . informed that if they had any children they must pay a heavy fine, or else go into servitude.[14]

Petrie suggests augmenting this policy by allowing women who are among the "most incapable" to undergo voluntary sterilisation, in order to avoid lifelong government monitoring.[15] In these arguments, it is clear that Petrie was directly contributing to translating eugenics out of the purely biological or medical realms and into the socio-political. Although no policy was enacted in Britain precisely as Petrie would design it, the parallel American eugenic movement led by Charles Davenport would influence United States policymakers to the extent that decades of eugenic injustices would come to pass, including court-mandated sterilisations of criminal defendants.[16]

Petrie remains a pillar of modern Egyptology, somewhat unavoidably. The discipline benefits from methodologies and discoveries with a direct lineage to his. In short, eugenics and Egyptology are themselves consanguineous. Therefore, in benefitting directly from the same founding principles as would later inform Petrie's eugenic arguments and racist constructions of history, Egyptology would seem to have a special obligation to address the eugenic paradigm within anthropology.

This obligation is increasingly being upheld. In 2011, the Petrie Museum of Egyptian Archaeology in London hosted an exhibition and events programme called *Typecast: Flinders Petrie and Francis Galton*, exploring Petrie and Galton's scholarship of race, heredity and archaeology.[17] In a paper reflecting on the exhibition, curator Debbie Challis discussed numerous past efforts to bring to light Petrie's ideas regarding eugenics and race, and iterated that the particular goal of the *Typecast* exhibition was to direct that light upon the Petrie Museum itself and how its collection, cataloguing and display standards have historically reflected the racial and eugenic beliefs of its namesake.[18] As part of the events programme, debates among audience members often became heated about issues of race, and there was considerable resistance to the idea that Egyptology had an inherent kinship with the scientific racism of Petrie and Galton.[19] This strongly indicates that more reflection on the conjoined history of Egyptology and the eugenic paradigm needs to take place within academic and curatorship circles.

The Limits of Palaeopathology

The embodiment of a person is a full conception of them including their physical, psychological, social and experiential states. Though a term increasingly used within anthropological contexts, embodiment is part of the everyday activity of comprehending the inhabitants of the world as we interact with them. In archaeology there are barriers to embodiment that have often proven convenient to ignore, such as a relative paucity of societal context and everyday documented lives, resulting in embodiments based upon incomplete or unreliable material evidence.

Egyptology is particularly associated with one class of material evidence through the idiosyncratic Egyptian practice of mummification. That practice has left behind astoundingly intact remains given their age, and this wealth of biomedical data can tempt us to frame ancient people in a biomedical way. This, however, is a very limited means of embodying an ancient person. While a corpse, whatever the state of preservation, can provide hints about some aspects of the living person, our remains record neither our joy, nor our anguish, nor the granular richness of our experiences.

Though there are social mores and even laws concerning the dignified treatment of the recently deceased, those mores seem to no longer apply once human remains are sufficiently ancient. It is unlawful in many jurisdictions for a laboratory to make use of an undonated corpse for research, yet ancient remains are less strictly monitored, notwithstanding efforts to devise non-destructive means of examination, which apply as much to human remains as they do to papyrus or fabric. All corpses are both objects and former people, assuming a materialist stance, yet the history of these objects *as* former people is part of what defines them. It is dehumanising, even if strictly accurate, to regard human remains as artefacts or specimens,[20] and contributes to the eugenic paradigm through the over-medicalisation of deceased and disabled people.

The social model of disability, arguably the model most compatible with the human rights of disabled people,[21] asks researchers and legislators to bear in mind that disability results from opportunity loss *arising from* biomedical impairment and not solely from impairment.[22] It is here that the largest obstacle is faced in the quest to embody ancient people alleged to have been disabled, because disability defined this way cannot be established solely on the basis of biomedical data. The assumption that ability and disability exist on a strict binary, and that any impairment is inherently disabling, is itself ableist.[23] We lack a full awareness of the social context of an ancient person, and the ability to state definitively which opportunities, if any, they were denied on account of their impairments. This tenet should be applied cautiously, of course, and never used to infer that disability was absent from the past, even when the historical record is silent about it.

Tutankhamun is a useful case study in the embodiment of an ancient person who may have been disabled. Whether we find ourselves able to grant him the label *disabled* or not, as a prominently impaired ancient person Tutankhamun is necessarily part of any discussion which includes Egyptology and critical Disability Studies. It is known that Tutankhamun possessed notable structural irregularities in his feet, in particular necrosis in his left,[24] and that he had been infected with malaria on at least two separate occasions.[25] We do not have the evidence to suggest that Tutankhamun's life (or even death) was defined by his experience of these impairments, but nonetheless they form a large component of modern embodiments of the king, even outside academic circles. Since the harmful impact of the eugenic paradigm is in large part measured by the popularity of its tenets in wider society, we should consider the perception of an ancient person in non-academic circles, which by definition concern themselves far less with academic rigour.

A prominent *National Geographic* article from 2010, for example, directly calls Tutankhamun "Disabled, Malarial, and Inbred" in its title, and uses phrases such as "frail", "weak", "plagued by malaria" and "forced . . . to walk with a cane".[26] These descriptors are highly emotionally charged, and seem deliberately chosen to evoke whatever combination of pity, disgust and even sardonicism (given that Tutankhamun was royalty) to which the reader's inclinations dispose them. In addition, the article refers to Tutankhamun as a boy three times and never once as a man, despite his death at the adult age of 19. This is a common term employed to refer to Tutankhamun, despite his survival of childhood. Infantilising Tutankhamun, particularly when pairing the word *boy* with words such as *frail*, can dehumanise him by deliberately evoking pity. This tendency to infantilise someone as part of an ableist perception of them persists, and is not a question of harmless semantics. A recent and abhorrent example is found in the Ashley X case of 2004, in which a six-year-old was forced to undergo several procedures including a hysterectomy and hormone therapy. The aim of these procedures was to forestall her adulthood because it was deemed by her parents and physicians that she would be easier to care for if she remained biologically a child.[27] Infantilising the disabled is part of an overall narrative of victimhood which justifies paternalistic endeavours to medicalise them, almost all of which take the form of profound and intimate violence.

It is common to characterise Tutankhamun as "sickly" and infer that he "suffered" from his physical conditions.[28] In fact, while it is defensible to suggest that a certain medical condition that tends to cause suffering in people living today may have done so in historical people, it is problematic to reserve the use of the word *suffering* for people with chronic illnesses and other impairing conditions. Such usage supports the ableist assumption that disabled people's default state is one of suffering, and that their suffering is by definition more than the suffering non-disabled people experience.

The power of such assumptions is particularly pertinent when discussing ancient cultures, whose medical paradigm was different from the modern (Eurocentric) one. Normality is, broadly, a relationship with averages such that abnormality represents statistical distance from a given average. Put simply, ancient Egyptian expectations of normality, assuming such expectations existed at all, would have been different from those of modern Western cultures.[29] A lack of definitively modern medical innovations such as vaccinations and antibiotics, as well as the chemical knowledge required to produce the hundreds of medications deemed by the World Health Organisation to be essential,[30] would have given an ancient Egyptian very different expectations of their own health than a modern Egyptian might have. Because impairment is as likely to result from injury and illness as it is through genetics (indeed, much more likely the longer someone lives), an ancient Egyptian can be reasonably supposed to accept that variation in the form and function of the human body was entirely ordinary. Seen this way, Tutankhamun's age at his death might be reframed not as remarkably young but, given his medical circumstances, remarkably old.

It is not incidental to a eugenic embodiment of Tutankhamun that his consanguinity is commonly referred to in a pejorative sense. While it is counterintuitive to castigate someone on the circumstances of their parentage (one element of a person's history for which the person has no responsibility), *inbred* continues to be used as an insult. In one biography of Tutankhamun, the word is used as a comparable adjective:

> [G]iven how inbred King Tut[ankhamun] was . . . it led to other problems. Such problems include that he couldn't raise any heirs, due to miscarriages, thus ending his bloodline. His genealogy was also responsible for his other genetic defects.[31]

It is not inevitable that close inbreeding results in impairments for the offspring. Inbreeding can result in the replication of recessive and co-dominant genes, some of which may correlate with detrimental phenotypes, but not always. One kinship community known for its close inbreeding but not for producing offspring with notable impairments is the Ptolemaic dynasty. According to the conventional genealogy of the dynasty, Cleopatra VII and at least ten of her ancestors were the product of close consanguineous union, the majority of which were brother-sister.[32] As Sheila Ager asks, with flair, "Should the [Ptolemaic] family not simply have imploded in a welter of birth defects, mental deficiency and cultural-emotional malaise and wretchedness?"[33] Cleopatra VII is famous for her political manoeuvring, and her desperation to survive repeated encounters with the Roman Republic in the person of several of its foremost citizens, but she is not known for any biomedical anomalies. She produced four children of her own, none known to have possessed any distinctive or life-defining medical conditions. The key difference between Tutankhamun's embodiment and Cleopatra's is that for the latter we have no physical remains, and so her embodiment has been constructed through her personal and political history. For Tutankhamun, almost the opposite is true: he reigned on the cusp of an era of Egyptian civilisation almost fully erased from later histories, leaving only his tomb and remains as an account of his character and deeds.

A pharaonic tomb, seen as an extension of the person of the king, must be part of the embodiment of the pharaoh in question, though only to a certain degree because funerary customs imperfectly reflect a person's reception by those tasked with burying them. It remains important to take direct material evidence into consideration, however, and Tutankhamun's tomb housed a considerable collection of mobility aids, chiefly in the form of walking sticks though there is evidence of adaptations made to chairs as well.[34] While the presence of mobility aids ought not be a surprise to anyone with knowledge of Tutankhamun's physiology, their prominence in the tomb (the walking sticks numbering well over 100, and placed in numerous locations) suggests the importance of mobility and independence in the pharaoh's life, and gives an indication that these needs were thoroughly met.

Caution must be exercised in imparting intentionality to the collection of walking sticks found in KV62. Someone with impaired mobility is not, in the *National Geographic* phrase, "forced" to use mobility aids,[35] but through their use is granted increased mobility. It is not customary to use similar terminology in relation to spectacles or contact lenses to aid vision, for example, and it is noteworthy that myopia, trivially adjusted for up to a certain severity, is not generally considered a disability in popular discourse. It would be absurd to append the biography of a deceased person with the sentence, "They were, sadly, afflicted with myopia and confined to the use of glasses." In other words, the tools used to correct impaired vision are sufficiently pervasive in society and trivial to equip each day that they would not usually be considered as part of a person's embodiment. Likewise, we have no firm evidence that Tutankhamun's walking sticks were of any more significance to his day-to-day life than implied by their designed function, taken up each morning and scarcely considered again until the time came to choose another one, perhaps on functional or aesthetic grounds. The sheer number of them could reflect a tiresome tendency for obsequious courtiers to make gifts of them, or an enthusiasm for collecting them, or any other explanation: their number alone tells us little of Tutankhamun's subjective relationship with them.

Palaeopathology is not purely a biomedical discipline and can provide contextual evidence that points towards disabled people being cared for. It is possible, for instance, to observe evidence of healing that would ordinarily require the intervention of others.[36] Yet disablement is far more complex a matter than whether a person received the minimum support required to survive. Survival alone tells us little of how an injured or chronically ill person might have been treated. Anthropologist Katherine Dettwyler gives an account of two disabled people she observed in Mali, who survived into adulthood but were still subject to daily derision and abuse.[37] With cases such as this in mind, the subject of the so-called palaeopathology of care must be approached with caution: even when we encounter distinct evidence of healing and survival, intentionality and wider context can be elusive. Just as it is not enough to call Tutankhamun disabled on the sole basis of his demonstrable impairments, it is not enough to conclusively say that he was not disabled on the sole basis that he seemed to receive a given level of support.

Palaeopathology is, even with these limitations in mind, a valuable tool in the embodiment of ancient people. With access to mummified remains, Egyptologists have the potential to generate data not available to palaeopathologists restricted to osteological sources. Yet the relative richness of this evidence must not tempt researchers to either derive spurious connotations about the quality of life of people studied, or to undervalue insights from other parts of the discipline about personal history and wider societal factors which may have impacted their lived experience.

Impact of the Eugenic Paradigm

In the eugenic paradigm, all impairments are called disabilities, and both words are synonymous with flaws of such scale and nature as to be a differentiator between strictly disabled people and strictly normal people, framed not as a social phenomenon but as a personal tragedy.[38] In turn, this narrative of personal tragedy to be avoided at any cost leads to the perception that disability and disabled people are a problem which need to be solved.[39] Cases such as Ashley X and others demonstrate that drastic measures including imposed medical procedures and even homicide are not unheard of as interventions against disabled people. Medical homicide has been lawful in the Netherlands since the early twenty-first century, and in a 2018 review of cases involving intellectual impairment and neurodivergence, researchers discovered that euthanasia candidacy criteria were not easily applied in such cases.[40] The researchers recommended that reasonable adjustments must be in place to ensure that the criteria which, if met, result in the physician-imposed termination of a patient's life, are not applied to a patient who may have difficulty understanding or communicating their medical situation.[41]

There has also been a growth in a certain kind of impairment prevention, in the form of antenatal screening.[42] In an outline of the rising trend of such screening, Caplan noted that even in cases in which a pregnant person would never choose to terminate, screening still took place, potentially indicating that the forthcoming child would be viewed primarily as an impaired person.[43] Even if one does not equate the termination of a pregnancy on grounds of impairment with the killing of a born child on the same grounds,[44] it does show that value judgements can be made on the worthiness of a life before that life has definitively begun. Caplan does not clearly account for the idea that some parents may choose to screen so that they can make preparations in case of impairment, for accessibility adjustments and meeting health needs, but it is important to keep in mind that this is a benign motivation for screening, since lack of environmental accommodation can be disabling.

There are impairments that result in suffering of various kinds in and of themselves, but as discussed previously it is inappropriate to associate impairment *per se* with suffering. Viewing disability as a continual trial of suffering and therefore as a kind of life less (or not) worth living is what leads to cases such as that of Ashley X, and some of the cases examined in the review of Dutch euthanasia. In the latter, the researchers identified that many of the challenges of neurodivergence and intellectual disability arise from "difficulties with integration in society", rather than just the intrinsic quality of the patients' impairments.[45] In the Netherlands, the euthanasia of young children is generally unlawful; however, using a set of criteria called the Groningen Protocol, newborns may be killed in a clinical context without a resulting prosecution.[46] These decisions are made on the grounds of assumed unbearable suffering on the part of patients who cannot express the extent or quality of their suffering, and with parental permission, which cannot be grounded in objectivity. Such protocols, argues bioethicist Eric Kodish, fortify two assumptions that compromise medical ethics: firstly that children are the property of their parents to dispose of as they wish; and secondly that euthanasia is universally motivated by the goal of ending the *patients'* suffering, rather than that of their caregivers.[47] What these arguments highlight is the need to consider not only suffering, but wider personhood and the embodiment of patients.

Disability theorist Fiona Campbell wrote of an interviewer's surprise to discover that the conjoined twins he was speaking with were happy and well-adjusted, since the default assumption is that nobody living under such circumstances ought to be.[48] So negative is the light in which the concept of disability is cast that the label *disabled* is not applied in cases in which one might, for consistency's sake, expect to see it. Earlier I gave the example of myopia not being seen as a disability because of its prevalence; another example is old age. Old age correlates with limitations to mobility, autoimmune function, cognitive performance and so on, but only in the cases of extreme examples are such conditions considered beyond the norm for old age.[49] In other words, while someone in their eighties experiencing limited mobility is generally considered part of the acceptable continuum of human ability, someone in their teens experiencing the same might be viewed as a tragic case.

The connotation of *disabled* as a negative descriptor is important, because language use is not simply a reflection, but an action with the power to guide the construction of our social reality. As such, the language of disability directly shapes perceptions of disabled people.[50] A 2017 overview of Turkish proverbs examined 45 common idioms featuring words to do with impairment or disability.[51] In many of the examined proverbs, disabled people are inferred to be untrustworthy, unfortunate or inauspicious, and one equated poor mental health with death, with the authors explaining a common attitude that while the death of a loved one is tragic, the mental incapacity of a loved one is worse because they must live with great suffering.[52]

Since a change in chosen language may be a way to prevent interpersonal awkwardness, it is tempting to address the marginalisation of disabled people through idiom as a problem in itself. Yet changing the specific words used to describe an impairment, or a group of disabled people, or disabled people in general, does not change the underlying oppressive function of those words.[53] The eugenic paradigm drapes itself in the language of compassion and decency, so as standards of decency and compassionate language evolve, the paradigm is empowered to continue notwithstanding such changes. Once it was decent to refer to someone as an idiot, but the word gained enough negative connotations to become exclusively an insult.[54] At present the word *psychotic* is employed colloquially to describe someone who is emotionally unpredictable or malicious, yet it is a medical term for a specific set of symptoms, with no intended moral connotations. One can imagine how difficult the word must be to use, however technically accurate, should the time come for one's mental health needs to be disclosed. The approach of challenging language alone is what Rose Galvin describes as an "elementary semiotic approach",[55] which does not address the root oppressive paradigm that such polite language masks, and in masking protects. It is the eugenic paradigm which must be challenged, not only individual instances of marginalising language and behaviour.[56]

The association of disability with unfavourable quality of life is not only upheld in the popular consciousness, but by cultural institutions including galleries and museums. In a 2004 review of the display and interpretation of museum collections relating to the lives of disabled people, it was found that disabled people and disability generally were associated with concepts such as poverty, failure and victimhood.[57] Museums also have the power to normalise the conception of visibly impaired people as spectacle,[58] which is an existing concern for many. Lesley Ellis, a researcher into the lives of women with dwarfism, reviewed findings suggesting that the life of people with visibly atypical body types can be, in the age of the ubiquitous smartphone camera, a panopticon.[59] Such behaviours are not always subtle, since the abled gaze is normalised by the assumption that someone with an atypical body type is inherently worthy of scrutiny, and on occasion encounters of this kind are hostile and include physical and sexual threats.[60] The difficulty in finding a balance between appropriate inclusion of disabled people in history and the inadvertent normalisation of the abled gaze has resulted in several curators preferring to stay away from disability representation altogether, which speaks to a clear need for representation in museum and gallery curation, and other academic spaces.

The Vital Role of Academic Subjectivity

Academia is not wholly separate from wider culture, but as a major generator and refiner of shared knowledge it can serve to consolidate and reinforce mores and schemas which are less examined in everyday contexts, for better and worse. Academia overall is a challenging environment for disabled researchers, faculty and students. In a 2022 review of studies examining ableism in academic institutions, as many as 35% of faculty in Canada reported receiving ableist treatment as recently as 2021.[61] The impact of this is clear, since the proportion of academics self-identifying as disabled in countries such as the UK, Canada and Australia was found to be much lower than the proportion of disabled people within the general population. The explanation given for this was that although inclusiveness was a principle espoused by institutions for the purposes of faculty recruitment, lack of institutional support thereafter led to low retention of researchers.[62]

The link between lack of institutional support for disabled researchers and low retention is not only a matter of speculation. In some instances, of the faculty members who identified themselves as disabled to researchers, as few as 4% disclosed their accessibility needs to their employing institutions, and many opted to try to pass as non-disabled, so that their competency would not be questioned. Rates of disclosure were higher in institutions where the culture of both interpersonal and official support was more inclusive.[63]

Academia is therefore part of a cycle in which stigma against disability, derived from the eugenic paradigm which causes non-disabled people to assume diminished competence in their disabled peers, has a muting effect on disabled voices. This in turn leads to disability scholarship lacking what Dodd et al. called "an authoritative voice on the representation of disability",[64] which normalises the otherness that leads to the silencing of disabled voices, *ad infinitum*. To break this cycle, academia must all the more embrace a maxim which has become common in the wider disability rights movement: "Nothing about us without us."

The embodiment (including the subjective experiences) of those studied *by* researchers has already been discussed, and now it is important to consider the subjectivity of the researchers themselves. This is usually anathema within scholarly circles, particularly in disciplines which are considered by their contributors to be scientific. Yet for any scientific endeavour to properly address its subject matter, it must use the appropriate tools and metrics. I have established that a total embodiment of a person cannot be achieved only through their biomedical facts, and I have argued that, manifestly, the embodiment of disabled people by non-disabled people has overall not been successful in producing fair outcomes. This has been the case even when disabled people have been directly asked to relay their experiences, as in the case of the surprised journalist and his conjoined interviewees.[65] It is tempting to pretend that what is subjective is not as likely to be true as what is objective, but this is predicated on a simplistic view of subjectivity. A pertinent example in this instance is pain. The firing of a certain chain of neurons is not pain, unless those neurons are part of a conscious person able to interpret that firing in a subjective way. This makes it subjective, but nonetheless a state with a truth value. It is *ontologically subjective*, to borrow a phrase from philosopher John Searle, who elaborates:

> The pain in my toe is ontologically subjective, but the statement '[John] now has a pain in his toe' is not epistemically subjective. It is a simple matter of (epistemically) objective fact, not a matter of (epistemically) subjective opinion.[66]

Crucially, what this entails is that not every perspective is equal in all matters, even ones which involve questions of (epistemically) objectively true or false statements. There exists no expert, for example, who can override a person's experience of their own pain. Each person is the sole necessary and sufficient authority on whether they feel the pain (making the determination subjective), but the pain either exists or does not, and is not a matter of opinion on the part of the person feeling it (making the determination ontological).

We might here remember Tutankhamun, who had skeletal irregularities and needed assistance with his mobility. We might infer that he suffered, because we think we would in a similar position, but our inference can never produce certainty. Both impairment and disablement have predominantly subjective elements but are absolutely ontologically real.[67] The tendency to prefer detachment in academia does not always serve justice, and this is something which Debbie Challis discusses in her reflections on the *Typecast* exhibition. Challis gives the example of the BBC's portrayal of Apartheid in South Africa as neutral to the point of excess, and explores the idea that too much detachment in the study of history can create distance between the past and present which serves to underplay ongoing injustice.[68] It is important for researchers and particularly curators to take note of Challis's regret that she did not employ more of her own subjectivity when implementing *Typecast.*[69]

Egyptology, when it seeks to construct biographies or make sociological models of ancient Egypt, is an anthropological discipline. Its subjects are subjects in all senses. One does not measure the mass of an electron by use of an interview process, or rate someone else's pain by waving a Geiger counter over a wound. Likewise, one cannot cleave to ontologically objective facts alone to fully embody and thereby do justice to an ancient (or still living) person. Yet, while the subjectivity of Tutankhamun and his contemporaries is unavailable to us, the subjectivity of researchers in similar biomedical and social states is not.

In their recommendations for exploring appropriate language to use when speaking with autistic adults, Kristen Bottema-Beutel and her colleagues recommended considering first the question: "Would I use this language if I were in a conversation with an autistic person?"[70] Let us likewise consider whether if we were in a conversation with Tutankhamun we would refer to his daughters, buried with the same customs used for many royal children, using the *National Geographic*'s phrase, "stillborn fetuses". Let us consider whether we would stand before someone with the responsibility to secure a nation's military, economic and religious future and call him "frail" and "inbred", or before a 19-year-old who survived malaria twice and call him a "boy". Until the eugenic paradigm is banished, and the answer to these questions is unanimously negative, Egyptologists are failing their subjects, their disabled colleagues and disabled people generally.

Conclusion

The eugenic paradigm of medicalising disabled people pervades anthropology and sustains the perception that atypical physical, psychological and sensory states universally constitute life-ruining flaws. Egyptology has a particular relationship with this paradigm, both through sharing a parent in Flinders Petrie and in its incomparable access to ancient soft tissue data.

The necessity of ridding Egyptology of its eugenic tendencies is not a question of avoiding speaking ill of the dead, nor of more general politeness and good taste. Egyptology is one of the most publicly accessible and popular anthropological disciplines, attracting hobbyists, armchair enthusiasts, students and career researchers. Not to address the eugenic paradigm is to place unwarranted barriers to entry for future scholars, and to thereby hamper the ability of future Egyptologists to construct personal and social histories of the ancient culture and its inhabitants. Additionally, and more gravely, it is to participate in a wider culture which marginalises, degrades and endangers people with impairments and biomedical differences.

Upon any occasion in which an underlying current of some form of prejudice or bigotry is discussed, there is a temptation among those participating to feel a sense of accusation, but it is not my intention to cast the field of anthropology in a grim light. It is very important when discussing the eugenic paradigm to remember that although there are historic figures (such as Petrie) who prominently held abhorrent views, the nature of a *paradigm* is that so many of its tenets are unconsciously held, even by people with sound principles operating with the very best of intentions. So, while guilt or innocence are not applicable concepts in important discussions of this kind, the liberation of any marginalised group requires a truthful appraisal of all wrongs done, intentionally and otherwise. Momentary personal discomfiture is a small price to pay to make cases such as that of Ashley X harder to repeat.

It is my hope that recent efforts to examine and address these offences will continue not by considering instances of ableism one by one, but by recognising the paradigm which generates and nurtures them and taking active steps towards its eradication. Flinders Petrie was cautious of the idea of radical and decisive reform, preferring change which took place gradually over many generations.[71] Given the grave nature of the problem and the demonstrated failure of attempts to evolve away from society-wide ableism, I am forced to conclude that this is another area in which Petrie was mistaken.

Notes

1 Powell (2021, 623).
2 Smith (2004).
3 Albeit consanguineous breeding is considerably less well evidenced, and it is important to remember the ceremonial and political aspects of royal marriage.
4 Hawass et al. (2010, 639–41).
5 Ibid., 642–44.
6 Scott-Hill (2004, 90).
7 Dornan-Fish (2012, 280–81).
8 Petrie (1969, 8).
9 Sheppard (2010, 18).
10 Petrie (1887).

11 Sheppard (2010, 22–23).
12 Petrie (1907, 4).
13 Ibid., 87.
14 Ibid., 88.
15 Ibid., 88–89.
16 Lombardo (2008, 62).
17 Challis (2013, 15).
18 Ibid., 18.
19 Ibid., 24.
20 Vogel and Power (2023, 10).
21 Lawson and Beckett (2021, 369–71).
22 Oliver (2013, 1024).
23 Vogel and Power (2023, 5–7).
24 Hawass et al. (2010, 642–43).
25 Ibid., 643–44.
26 Than (2010).
27 Powell (2021, 617).
28 Antanovskii (2020).
29 Vogel and Power (2023, 7).
30 World Health Organisation (2021).
31 Mardon et al. (2021, 33).
32 Ager (2006, 168).
33 Ibid., 171.
34 Morris (2020, 54–56).
35 Than (2010).
36 Battles (2011, 110).
37 Dettwyler (1991, 382).
38 Hevey (1993, 118).
39 Barton (1993, 242).
40 Tuffrey-Wijne et al. (2018, 19).
41 Ibid., 19–20.
42 Caplan (2004, 291).
43 Ibid., 292.
44 For the avoidance of misunderstanding: I do not.
45 Tuffrey-Wijne et al. (2018, 19).
46 Verhagen and Sauer (2005, 961–62).
47 Kodish (2008, 893).
48 Campbell (2000, 60).
49 Abberley (1987, 17).
50 Bottema-Beutel et al. (2021, 20).
51 Kesgin and Karakoç (2017, 140).
52 Ibid., 141.
53 Galvin (2003, 160–61).
54 Ibid.
55 Ibid.
56 The term 'neurodivergent' and its relatives may be examples of neologisms which *do* challenge the eugenic paradigm, since their correct use seems to constitute an admission by the speaker that traits found in, e.g., ADHD and autism exist on a natural continuum of human ability. More work is needed but is outside the scope of this chapter.
57 Dodd et al. (2004, 13).
58 Ibid., 15.
59 Ellis (2018, 232).
60 Ibid., 231.
61 Lindsay and Fuentes (2022, 179).

62 Ibid.
63 Ibid., 183.
64 Dodd et al. (2004, 14).
65 Campbell (2000, 60).
66 Searle (1998, 44–45).
67 Battles (2011, 112).
68 Challis (2013, 17–18).
69 Ibid. (29).
70 Bottema-Beutel (2021, 25).
71 Petrie (1907, 40–44).

Bibliography

Abberley, Paul. "The Concept of Oppression and the Development of a Social Theory of Disability." *Disability, Handicap & Society* 2, no. 1 (1987): 5–19.

Ager, Sheila L. "The Power of Excess: Royal Incest and the Ptolemaic Dynasty." *Anthropologica* 48, no. 2 (2006): 165–86.

Antanovskii, Robyn. "Unmasking Tutankhamun: The Figure Behind the Fame." *Heritage Daily,* Last modified March 5, 2020. Accessed February 9, 2023. https://www.heritagedaily.com/2020/03/unmasking-tutankhamun-the-figure-behind-the-fame-2/99143.

Barton, Len. "The Struggle for Citizenship: The Case of Disabled People." *Disability, Handicap & Society* 8, no. 3 (1993): 35–48.

Battles, Heather. "Towards Engagement: Exploring the Prospects for an Integrated Anthropology of Disability." *Vis-á-vis: Explorations in Anthropology* 11, no. 1 (2011): 107–24.

Bottema-Beutel, Kristen, Steven K. Kapp, Jessica Nina Lester, Noah J. Sasson, and Brittany N. Hand. "Avoiding Ableist Language: Suggestions for Autism Researchers." *Autism in Adulthood* 3, no. 1 (2021): 18–29.

Campbell, Fiona A. K. "Eugenics in Disguise? Law, Technologies, and Negotiating the 'Problem' of 'Disability'." *Australian Feminist Law Journal* 14, no. 1 (2000): 55–70.

Caplan, Helen. "Genetics, Disability and Bioethics." In *Disabling Barriers – Enabling Environments.* 2nd ed., edited by John Swain, Sally French, Colin Barnes, and Carol Thomas, 291–96. London: SAGE Publications, 2004.

Challis, Debbie. "Creating Typecasts: Exhibiting Eugenic Ideas from the Past Today." *Museum Management and Curatorship* 28, no. 1 (2013): 15–33.

Dettwyler, Katherine A. "Can Paleopathology Provide Evidence for 'Compassion'?." *American Journal of Biological Anthropology* 84, no. 4 (1991): 375–84.

Dodd, Jocelyn, Richard Sandell, Annie Delin, and Jackie Gay. *Buried in the Footnotes: The Representation of Disabled People in Museum and Gallery Collections*. Leicester: Research Centre for Museums and Galleries, 2004.

Dornan-Fish, Jennifer. "Motive Matters: Intentionality, Embodiment, and the Individual in Archaeology." *Time and Mind* 5, no. 3 (2012): 279–98.

Ellis, Lesley. "Through a Filtered Lens: Unauthorised Picture-Taking of People with Dwarfism in Public Spaces." *Disability & Society* 33, no. 2 (2018): 218–37.

Galvin, Rose. "The Making of the Disabled Identity: A Linguistic Analysis of Marginalisation." *Disability Studies Quarterly* 23, no. 2 (2003): 149–78.

Hawass, Zahi, Yahia Z. Gad, Somaia Ismail, Rabab Khairat, Dina Fathalla, Naglaa Hasan, Amal Ahmed, et al. "Ancestry and Pathology in King Tutankhamun's Family." JAMA 303, no. 7 (2010): 638–47.

Hevey, David. "The Tragedy Principle: Strategies for Change in the Representation of Disabled People." In *Disabling Barriers – Enabling Environments.* 1st ed., edited by John Swain, Vic Finkelstein, Sally French, and Mike Oliver, 116–21. London: SAGE Publications, 1993.

Kesgin, Yıldıray, and Elif Karakoç. "Turkish Proverbs as a Reproduction of Ableist Language in Social Memory." In *Research on Communication*, edited by Christian Ruggiero,

Hasan Arslan, and Mehmet Ali Icbay, 135–43. Bialystok: International Association of Social Science Research, 2017.

Kodish, Eric. "Paediatric Ethics: A Repudiation of the Groningen Protocol." *The Lancet* 372, no. 9616 (2008): 892–93.

Lawson, Anna, and Angharad E. Beckett. "The Social and Human Rights Models of Disability: Towards a Complementarity Thesis." *The International Journal of Human Rights* 25, no. 2 (2021): 348–79.

Lindsay, Sally, and Kristina Fuentes. "It is Time to Address Ableism in Academia: A Systematic Review of the Experiences and Impact of Ableism among Faculty and Staff." *Disabilities* 2, no. 2 (2022): 178–203.

Lombardo, Paul A. "Disability, Eugenics, and the Culture Wars." *Saint Louis University Journal of Health Law & Policy* 2, no. 1 (2008): 57–79.

Mardon, Austin, Suad Alad, Gurman Barara, Ishpreet Chana, Irene Falade, Rokya Harun, Jamie Johnson, Amy Li, Jennifer Pham, and Noah Varghese. *King Tut*. Edmonton: Golden Meteorite Press, 2021.

Morris, Alexandra F. "Let That Be Your Last Battlefield: Tutankhamun and Disability." *Athens Journal of History* 6, no. 1 (2020): 53–72.

Oliver, Mike. "The Social Model of Disability: Thirty Years On." *Disability & Society* 28, no. 7 (2013): 1024–26.

Petrie, W. M. Flinders. *Racial Photographs from the Egyptian Monuments*. London: R.C. Murray, 1887.

Petrie, W. M. Flinders. *Janus in Modern Life*. London: Archibald Constable, 1907.

Petrie, W. M. Flinders. Seventy Years in Archaeology. New York: Greenwood and Henry Holt, (1932) 1969.

Powell, Robyn M. "Confronting Eugenics Means Finally Confronting Its Ableist Roots." *William & Mary Journal of Race, Gender and Social Justice* 27, no. 3 (2021): 607–33.

Scott-Hill, Mairian. "Impairment, Difference and 'Identity'." In *Disabling Barriers – Enabling Environments*. 2nd ed., edited by John Swain, Sally French, Colin Barnes, and Carol Thomas, 87–93. London: SAGE Publications, 2004.

Searle, John R. *Mind, Language and Society*. New York: Basic Books, 1998.

Sheppard, Kathleen L. "Flinders Petrie and Eugenics at UCL." *Bulletin of the History of Archaeology* 20, no. 1 (2010): 16–29.

Smith, Phil. "Whiteness, Normal Theory, and Disability Studies." *Disability Studies Quarterly* 24, no. 2 (2004).

Than, Ker. "King Tut Mysteries Solved: Was Disabled, Malarial, and Inbred." *National Geographic,* Last modified February 17, 2010. Accessed February 7, 2023. https://www.nationalgeographic.com/culture/article/100216-king-tut-malaria-bones-inbred-tutankhamun.

Tuffrey-Wijne, Irene, Leopold Curfs, Ilora Finlay, and Sheila Hollins. "Euthanasia and Assisted Suicide for People with an Intellectual Disability and/or Autism Spectrum Disorder: An Examination of Nine Relevant Euthanasia Cases in the Netherlands (2012–2016)." *BMC Medical Ethics,* no. 19 (2018): 1–21.

Verhagen, Eduard, and Pieter J. J. Sauer. "The Groningen Protocol – Euthanasia in Severely Ill Newborns." *The New England Journal of Medicine* 352, no. 10 (2005): 959–62.

Vogel, Hannah, and Ronika K. Power. "Recognising Inequality: Ableism in Egyptological Approaches to Disability and Bodily Differences." *World Archaeology* (2023): 1–14.

World Health Organisation Model List of Essential Medicines – 22nd List. Geneva: World Health Organisation, 2021. Accessed February 8, 2023. https://www.who.int/publications/i/item/WHO-MHP-HPS-EML-2021.02.

3 The Measure of a Man

Akhenaten, Tutankhamun, and the (Pseudo)science of Disability in Egyptology

Alexandra F. Morris and Kyle Lewis Jordan

Ask yourself these questions: *What does "disability" mean to me? How does it make me feel? How does it affect my understanding of history?* It is important to confront your assumptions about disability. If your internalised rationality towards disability is that it is an inherently 'lesser' standard of life, then you have limited yourself to seeing it in those terms. This leads to the binary assumption that capacity and capability are intrinsically linked to ability/disability, as are notions of pain and suffering. Egyptology is full of these types of binaries. However, disability is not a binary, but a spectrum of lived experiences. As stated by Vogel and Power: "The generalised assessment of inclusion and acceptance continues a notion of a dichotomous experience, namely included;excluded and able;disabled."[1]

As authors we both identify as disabled people. We both came into Egyptology from a young age out of love for the ancient Egyptians. However, as we experienced first-hand the disablism that is prevalent in society, it was not lost on us how ableism was embedded within the discipline's scholarship from its foundation. This correlates to the beginnings of an industrialised age that saw people's bodies and minds reduced to their capacity, giving rise to the medical model of disability (later critiqued by the social model). Disability models are covered by Vogel's chapter in this volume; by acknowledging them, we highlight why this dichotomy is so prevalent within historical scholarship.

However, the impairments that are often classified under the label of disability today existed before either model. Disability, in this chapter, follows Dubourg's definition, a social-cultural model of disability "constituted by social and cultural processes, mechanisms which . . . shape representations of the impaired body."[2] In this model, "the body becomes a social and historical object," wherein individuals experience "disability as a social, religious, and cultural phenomenon."[3]

Akhenaten and his son, Tutankhamun, have been the subject of countless popular histories and retellings that have continually sensationalised their lives and afterlives.

Author's Note: The authors of this chapter regard themselves as joint first-authors of this piece, and request that this be acknowledged. Co-authorship is an invaluable process that provides access to and ensures credit for the work of disabled scholars, and we firmly believe that academia is better served by disavowing the perception that the creation of ideas has been, or can only ever be, a sole endeavour.

DOI: 10.4324/9781003440369-5

This is unsurprising for Egyptology, which historically has been a reception of ancient Egypt in the eyes of a predominantly Western, non-disabled gaze. There is an inescapable emphasis on the condition of the ancient Egyptian physique and psyche, which is used repeatedly to justify certain actions of our ancient subjects.[4] These ableist biases, which link the physical body with morality in Egyptological scholarship, have a long and harmful history. These biases are part of the subject's foundations that continue to reassert themselves within scholarly publications and public discourse.

Critical approaches to the study of ancient Egypt are becoming more prevalent. Yet within the public consciousness outdated approaches and terminology still loom large. Theories that have largely been disproven are still stated as fact.[5] Outdated terminology, obsolete since the passage of the *Americans with Disabilities Act* (1990) and the *UK Disability Discrimination Act* (1996), is still being used. The continued use of offensive language lies both with the authors of these pieces and with the publishers who continue to publish them without engaging with the numerous style guides. These guides inform how to talk about disability, and have been published by various organisations, activists, and fellow scholars.[6] While such scholars have pointed out this language as problematic,[7] offensive language still occurs regularly within the field and in publicly accessible publications,[8] demonstrating a sustained ignorance of the disabled community.

While there are more robust approaches happening in Egyptology, scholarly arguments about Akhenaten and Tutankhamun have remained inconsistent, sensationalised by profiteering Egyptomania. This chapter examines the fallacies of this phenomenon through a disability paradigm, demonstrating that the attributions of impairments for Akhenaten are ever tenuous, and the clear evidence for Tutankhamun's impairments necessitates bringing his embodiment into dialogue with disability. It also argues the need for Egyptology to engage with Disability Studies and discuss how this impacts our view of disabled people in antiquity, as well as the public view of disabled people today. The use of modern labels on ancient peoples is fraught with unknowns. At present, this leads to circular arguments that have more to say about modern society's discomfort with the lives of disabled people than it does about the embodiment of disability in the ancient past.

Any conversation concerning the health and capacities of past peoples can only be effective when incorporating a 'disability paradigm.' We cannot hope to fully appreciate the circumstances of either Akhenaten, Tutankhamun, or any ancient persons' lives if we do not afford them the full range of human experience, which ultimately includes disability. Both the haphazard attribution of impairments, and the dogged resistance to the idea of any impairments at all, obscures any chance of seeing either pharaoh as men.

Akhenaten

It must be acknowledged that Egyptologists at the time of the discoveries of Akhenaten and Tutankhamun had their own agendas that directly influenced how they interpreted the material. Prominent theories that influenced major Egyptologists of the time were laden with eugenics, racism, ableism, and sexism.[9] W.M. Flinders Petrie infamously was wedded to the idea of a "Dynastic Race" who ruled over an entirely subservient African caste.[10] Forcing these pharaohs and ancient people into this worldview necessitated Akhenaten being a deviant, and for Tutankhamun to be non-disabled.

John Gardner Wilkinson was the first Egyptologist to comment on the art found at the site of Amarna in 1824 remarking that it was "of a very peculiar style" and argued that "from their features it is evident they were not Egyptians."[11] Richard Lepsius in a 1845 letter connected the site specifically to Akhenaten, stating it was the "fourth Amenophis, that royal Puritan who persecuted all the gods of Egypt and would only permit the worship of the Sun's disc."[12] Petrie was the first Egyptologist to publish remarks on various theories relating to Akhenaten in 1894, which were based solely on art. The main theories surrounding Akhenaten at the time were that he was a eunuch or a woman masquerading as a man. There was no consensus on whether Amenhotep IV and Akhenaten were even the same person.[13] Petrie proposed that Akhenaten was Amenhotep IV and dismissed both theories:

> Is it credible that the most uxorious king of Egypt who appears with his wife on every monument . . . that this king was either a woman in masquerade or an eunuch?. . . It is needless to further consider these fantastic hypotheses which are flatly contradicted by every distinctive fact.[14]

The supposed mummified remains of Akhenaten (there is still no consensus) were found in tomb KV55 in 1907 by the Anglo-American team of Edward R. Ayrton and Theodore M. Davis, along with antiquities service representative Joseph Lindon Smith, and Arthur Weigall. Most relevant to our discussion is that when the body and tomb were identified, they were initially believed to be that of a woman and were therefore published by Davis as *The Tomb of Queen Tiyi*.[15] The mistake was later realised, and Davis and fellow Egyptologist Gaston Maspero addressed this in the publication, but Davis opted to publish their findings using the incorrect title. Davis concluded that "Khuniantonu's mummy was buried in it by mistake":[16]

> [T]he wrappings of the mummy were entirely removed, exposing the bones. . . . I concluded to have them examined and reported upon by two surgeons who happened to be in the "Valley of the Kings." They . . . reported that the pelvis was evidently that of a woman. Therefore, everyone . . . accepted the sex, and supposed that the body was doubtless that of Queen Tiyi. Some time thereafter, the bones were sent to Dr. G. Elliot Smith, Professor of Anatomy in the Egyptian Government School of Medicine, Cairo, for his inspection and decision. Alas! Dr. Smith declared the sex to be male. It is only fair to state that the surgeons were deceived by the abnormal pelvis and the conditions of the examination.[17]

From the beginning Akhenaten's body seems to have been pathologised by those that examined him, with Dr. Smith writing:

> When these bones were sent to me for examination . . . I reported that they formed the greater part of the skeleton of a young man, who, judged by the ordinary European standards of ossification, must have attained an age of about twenty-five or twenty-six years at the time of his death . . . it is highly improbable that he could have attained thirty years if he had been normal. The cranium, however, exhibits in an unmistakable manner the distortion characteristic of a condition of hydrocephalus. The bones, therefore, cannot be regarded as those of a perfectly normal person.[18]

However, Akhenaten's body seems to be subject to the same ideological tug-of-war to which we will see Tutankhamun's body has been subject. The identity of his supposed remains changes, as does their age, and shifts between healthy and pathologised depending upon who examines them. Smith identified Akhenaten's body as showing signs of hydrocephalus and possible disability, but in later examinations, seems to shift between non-disabled and disabled. Anatomist Douglas Derry (who also examined Tutankhamun and concluded he was nondisabled) found no evidence of hydrocephalus in 1931.[19] Pathologist Andrew Sandison with Cyril Aldred in the late 1950s to early 1960s, working from photographs of the body, stated that it showed signs of an endocrine disorder known as Fröhlich's syndrome and did not rule out hydrocephalus.[20] Akhenaten's body was re-examined by anatomist Ronald Harrison in 1963–1966 who found no evidence of hydrocephalus or of any other disorder.[21] He was then examined again in 2000 by Egyptologists Joyce Filer and Nasry Iskander, who again found "no evidence of pathology."[22] The most recent examination of the body was by Zahi Hawass and a team of Egyptologists in 2010, who again stated that there were no signs of pathology, and reasserted the mummified remains were Akhenaten.[23] Their study has been critiqued by many Egyptologists, who point out that a selective reading of DNA evidence is erroneous. To date, there is no consensus.[24] As historian Ronald T. Ridley states:

> It is by now obvious that faced with this dilemma, scholars since Petrie have thrown the most basic cautions of historical method to the winds, and indulged in pure fantasy . . . And here another fundamental principle of historical method applies: when we do not have evidence, we must admit it.[25]

American James Henry Breasted was one of the first Egyptologists to publish on Akhenaten. His *A History of Egypt: From the Earliest Times to The Persian Conquests* was published in 1909. He describes Akhenaten as

> a young dreamer, who, in spite of unprecedented greatness in the world of ideas, was not fitted to cope with a situation demanding an aggressive man of affairs and a skilled military leader . . . the young and inexperienced son

> of Amenhotep III and the queen Tiy, was indeed strong and fearless in certain directions, but he failed utterly to understand the practical needs of his empire.[26]

These descriptions are such a contrast to later disability-linked descriptions of Akhenaten, that one must wonder how much of the negativity we see directed at Akhenaten is *precisely because* he is associated with disability. "Disability" quite wrongly puts a negative connotation because of modern societal biases that sees disability as a tragedy, linking it with evil and negativity. Additionally, Breasted does not seem to agree about Akhenaten being disabled: "[T]he strange treatment of the lower limbs by Ikhnaton's artists is a problem which remains unsolved and cannot be wholly accounted for by supposing a malformation of the king's own limbs."

Weigall was one of the first to link Akhenaten explicitly with disability. In his 1922 publication about the pharaoh, he states that "his skull was misshapen, and he must have been subject to occasional epileptic fits" and "the misshapen skull was pronounced to be that of a man who . . . was probably subject to hallucinations."[27] This analysis was based on skeletal evidence without consensus, meaning there is no confirmation that the skeleton identified prior and discussed earlier is Akhenaten.[28] It was also partially built on the racist and eugenicist idea that one could tell the personality of someone through the examination of the skull (phrenology).[29] Weigall's interpretations of Akhenaten were biased by his somewhat hostile relationship with Howard Carter and Lord Carnarvon. More importantly, this was the beginning of explaining Akhenaten's art and religious revolution through the idea of disability, since there had to be something 'abnormal' about the man who sparked such radical change. As Amelia Edwards wrote, "We are accustomed to a certain amount of courtly exaggeration on the part of those who record with pen or pencil the great deeds of the Pharaohs. We expect to see the king as always young, always beautiful, always victorious."[30] Akhenaten's agency as a revolutionary was stolen from him by Weigall and others who came after him, who repeatedly tried to explain or blame the circumstances of Akhenaten's reign on an embodied condition.

Later attempts to link or explain Akhenaten's religious revolution and divergent art style have generally fallen into one of three camps, which remain unconvincing. These three main "diagnoses" have included 1) that Akhenaten was a eunuch, 2) Fröhlich's syndrome or another endocrine disorder, or 3) Marfan's syndrome.[31] Donald Redford, another Egyptologist, (1984) describes Akhenaten:

> It may well be that he was intentionally kept in the background because of a congenital ailment which made him hideous to behold. The repertoire of Amarna art has made us familiar with the effeminate appearance of the young man: fleshy lips, slanting eyes, lengthened ear lobes, prominent jaw, narrow shoulders, potbelly, enormous hips and thighs, and spindly legs. Of late the experts have tended to identify his problem with some sort of endocrine disorder in which secondary sex characteristics failed to develop, and eunuchoidism resulted.

Cyril Aldred again links the art to disability in *Akhenaten: King of Egypt* (1988) and uses problematic language that we see repeated in more recent publications:

> It is strange that the 'expressionism'. . . introduced by Akhenaten into Egyptian art should take the form of showing the human figure as though it were exhibiting . . . the abnormalities of an endocrine disorder. As it is the figure of the king which shows these traits . . . there is warrant for thinking that he suffered from Frohlich's Syndrome, and wished to have himself represented with all those deformities which differentiated him from the rest of humanity.[32]

Recent publications, while acknowledging that there is likely little truth to the idea of Akhenaten being congenitally disabled, continue to paint him using problematic terminology. An example is the 2022 publication *Egypt's Golden Couple: When Akhenaten and Nefertiti Were Gods on Earth* by Colleen Darnell and John Coleman Darnell:

> A pale and sickly young man ascends the throne of Egypt. The young king is as mentally robust as he is physically awkward and strangely proportioned. His strong and unyielding will is at odds with the brittle weakness of his spindly limbs . . . Modern authors have offered an impressive array of theories for the unusual features of Akhenaten's images . . . Each proposed condition comes with a host of symptoms and physical effects that conflict with the existing evidence: eunuchs did not exist as a type of court functionary in New Kingdom Egypt; Frohlich's syndrome causes infertility, while Akhenaten fathered six daughters and a son (also an insurmountable problem of the earlier eunuch suggestion); the king's skeleton, an identification made likely through historical and genetic evidence, shows no trace of Marfan syndrome, nor does it provide evidence of any particularly unusual physiognomy. The most reasonable conclusion is that Akhenaten's art was a form of religious and political expression.[33]

The Darnells explicitly state that there is no evidence for disability yet continue to evoke it. Another example is the previously referenced 2022 book by Ronald T. Ridley, which continues to use the well-known 'r' slur for intellectual disability in his description of Fröhlich's syndrome, and additionally states, "[T]he Amarna Letters make no reference to any illness suffered by Akhenaten. None of Akhenaten's siblings, moreover, is known to have had any deformity."[34] The secondary quote takes an explicitly medical model approach describing suffering from illness and continues to use the problematic term "deformity." More shockingly, the second book was published by a university press with accessibility guidelines (including appropriate terminology) in their publication standards. Similarly, historian Guy de la Bedoyere in his 2022 publication *Pharaohs of the Sun: How Egypt's Despots and Dreamers Drove the Rise and Fall of Tutankhamun's Dynasty* continues to describe

Akhenaten using the problematic framing of both disability and mental illness, neither of which has any substantial evidence:

> This was a predictable rhetorical claim substituting the Aten for Amun, but it is also possible that he was unwittingly alluding to hallucinations . . . One could be forgiven for suspecting that Akhenaten was at least a little mad. He was certainly both a narcissist and an obsessive.[35]

We provide these examples to demonstrate that Egyptology, far from having moved beyond its past, still finds itself referencing many of the racist and ableist tropes that formed its foundations.

What entangles Akhenaten in this discourse is that his stark contrast to all those who proceeded and succeeded him meant that his outlying form somehow needed to be rationalised. He could not perfectly fit into the archetype of the dynastic race; therefore his deviance had to be explained by medical imperfection. Petrie already used Egyptian mummified remains – along with his contemporary Francis Galton, the "father of eugenics" – to create his perfect archetype. Therefore, by pinning their theories to the idea of physical perfection, any outlying case also had to be physical in nature. Therefore, Egyptian art – in the absence of bioarchaeological evidence – was also taken quite literally as a representation of these perfect beings. As we see to this day, scholars in both Egyptology and art history continue to sensationalise the Amarna period for its outlying, "deviant" nature.[36]

While contemporary scholarship distances itself from this pseudoscientific analysis, this chapter demonstrates recycling of discussions about Akhenaten embodying comorbidity or expressing some other form of 'deviance.' The portrayal of his actions as 'heresy' – and linking that to his embodiment – undermines any attempt to connect with Akhenaten on his own terms. It denies both his bodily autonomy and agency. That this is repeated as recently as 2022 for a speculative narrative to capitalise on the general public's fascination, to the detriment of that public's understanding of illness and disability, shows how Egyptology is still interested in evoking a sensationalised ancient Egypt rather than a historical one.

This dilemma is most prevalent for Egyptian pharaohs. The discipline has settled upon a universal archetype – a hero – by which all pharaohs are measured and to which they are expected to conform. Egyptology has found itself in a conundrum of its own making: pharaohs must embody these divine, perfect beings while wilfully ignoring the realities of their humanity. Therefore, we are left with a veritable gamut of contradictory and sensationalist accounts: Akhenaten was a "heretic" who made this seismic shift in religious practice, yet he was weak and feeble. He was the indisputable embodiment of his Aten figure, yet dependent on Nefertiti and a few indispensable courtiers to enact his bidding. In all these accounts, Akhenaten's agency is solely responsible, yet also denied. The fact that the Darnells craft their Akhenaten figure as mentally robust in spite of physical awkwardness, which they say could not exist, shows that in this case Egyptology is still utilising an ableist framework. It cannot comprehend the possibility that a person with an impairment could have wielded power in any meaningful way.

There is perhaps no greater victim of this ableism than Akhenaten's son, Tutankhamun.

Tutankhamun

Tutankhamun first came into discussions alongside Akhenaten in the late 1800s and early 1900s. Today, he is believed to have had clubbed foot, Kohler's disease, scoliosis, and a mild cleft palate, amongst other potential physical impairments.[37] Initial theories about him were erroneous, like those about his father. Tutankhamun was described as a usurper to the throne or having achieved the kingship solely through his marriage to one of the Amarna princesses.[38] There was at the time no recognition that Tutankhamun was part of the royal family.[39] Once Tutankhamun's mummified remains were discovered in 1922 and further analysed, the connection to the Amarna royal dynasty was made.[40] From here, two separate dichotomous narratives emerged: that of the frail boy prince, or that of the warrior-hunter-king. Christiane Desrouches-Noblecourt described the last heirs of Thutmosis IV as "physically frail and hence short-lived."[41] Some Egyptologists have also tried to have this both ways. To again quote Desrouches-Noblecourt, "In spite of his apparently delicate health, it was at this time that [Tutankhamun] was taught by his 'master of arms' to hunt . . . according to an ivory bracelet decorated with pictures of an ostrich hunt found in his tomb."[42] It should be noted that many descriptions that follow the Sickly Boy narrative portray Tutankhamun as a child describing him using words like "frail," "sickly," or "weak," but he is never described as disabled. It was not until a reanalysis of the pharaoh's remains in the 2010s that Tutankhamun was labelled as such within Egyptology. Even then, he was instead described as "physically" or "congenitally deformed," and other equally inappropriate terms, rather than using the word "disability."[43] These were accompanied by derogatory reconstructions of the pharaoh in his underwear that seemed designed to exaggerate the physical features of said impairments, rather than offer any scientific value, let alone any humanity or recognition that this historical figure was a man.[44] When compared to reconstructions of other well-known physically impaired figures such as Philip II of Macedonia a stark contrast emerges.[45] Interestingly, historian Paul Doherty did pick up on the possibility of Tutankhamun being disabled over ten years prior in his 2002 biography of the pharaoh but suggested possible intellectual impairment as well as physical impairment.[46] Those who have recently embraced the Warrior King narrative include Bob Brier, Nicholas Reeves, and Marianne Eaton-Krauss, sometimes actively refuting the possibility that Tutankhamun was disabled.[47] Strangely there are also some Egyptologists who seem to accept the idea of disability yet are committed to Tutankhamun dying in a hunting or chariot accident or believe that his canes were purely for status purposes.[48] By perpetuating this idea, Egyptologists reveal their own misunderstandings of physical impairment.[49] Others such as Emily Smith-Sangster have tried to argue against a canonical iconography of disability using Tutankhamun as an example, but in doing so have revealed further weaknesses within the Egyptological field, not the point they were trying to make.[50] These weaknesses include an overreliance on a single data type that has often only been analysed by one person.[51]

To date, the author's (Morris) article remains the only published analysis that considers all evidence in context while using a disabled lens, rather than a single evidence type.[52] As stated by Vogel and Power, "The inclusion of all other evidence however by Morris offers a more rounded and plausible scenario."[53]

What we see is the complete antithesis of Akhenaten's characterisation, yet with the same consequence: whereby Akhenaten's actions and agency are framed as either the direct result of an embodiment, or in spite of one. Tutankhamun's rather clear evidence for the embodiment of multiple impairments is deliberately minimised or sensationalised for the purposes of crafting a dualistic image of the man who must be the hunter-warrior, but equally must be the weak and sickly boy who was subject to the courtly intrigues of Ay and Horemheb. Each seeks to reduce the embodiment of disability to a binary, meaning Tutankhamun's agency is also minimised. Egyptologists want Tutankhamun to be the Warrior King and the Sickly Boy all in one, but what is clear is that the idea of disability can only effectively fall into one of those characterisations.

Discussion

Now that we have examined the literature concerning Akhenaten and Tutankhamun in relation to disability, it is time to consider the implications. To do so, we need to incorporate ideas that have been formulated in the realm of critical Disability Studies. Through this lens, we can grasp the effects of what this framing and language has done to harm our appreciation not only of past lives but also of contemporary ones.

Foremost, it is important to recognise that the inclusion of disability as an identifier – much the same as studies of the previous few decades have grown to include discussions of womanhood, gender identity, sexuality, race, and ethnicity – is in recognition of the more complex nature of these lived embodiments in the past. Our studies must be a continual process of attempting to humanise our past subjects. This affords them the same complexities as our own lives, acknowledging that these factors – while conceived differently in their pasts – nevertheless still existed and were recognised. Therefore, as this volume establishes from the outset, it is important to recognise and define the parameters of disability both in its modern usage and in our analyses.

When the negative image discussed at the start of this chapter becomes the predominant way of seeing disability, we conjure in our minds the disabled person as an inherently passive and ineffective subject. Therefore, the idea of their presence in the ancient past – which we like to see as active and evolving – is seen as antithetical, because only those with agency could effect change. Yet, as was proven by expanding our consideration of the roles of women in antiquity into the socio-economic sphere, we can (and should) involve disability as a lens through which to consider multiple aspects of the ancient world.

These expansions of our studies not only deepen our knowledge but also make the subject more inclusive and inviting to audiences and can have a positive effect on their contemporary view of themselves. As considerations of sexuality and gender fluidity in antiquity have proven to be fruitful for the contemporary LGBTQIA+ movement, so too we ask how interrogating the idea that agency in the ancient world was only afforded to the fit and able could benefit the lives of contemporary disabled people.

Through doing so, we can reckon with the harms this mindset has had on our knowledge of the ancient past, and what it means to contemporary lives – not just for disabled people, but also for the many communities whose agency was denied in the execution of colonial agendas. This includes the extraction of cultural heritage and human remains to be studied abroad, while local people were co-opted for their labour – often to disabling effect – in this enterprise, while simultaneously denying their links to said heritage. This was the very intent behind Petrie's pseudoscientific idea of the "Dynastic Race."[54] Much the same way as the ancient Egyptians, Petrie supposed, were ruled by an Aryan class who were genetically above their African subordinates, so too that equilibrium was recreated by the efforts of British and French colonialism in North Africa. If such a thing is established as historical fact, then contemporary re-enactment is only seen as natural.

This brings us back to Akhenaten and Tutankhamun. Akhenaten's various attributions of impairment were a deliberate attempt to explain his deviance away from this 'racial purity,' which the Pharaonic class had to embody, and thus his Aten "reformation" was – and still is – repeatedly framed within either a narrative of an inherent threat to the established order or an enlightened eventuality of his "genetic" purity.[55] Akhenaten's labelling of possible cognitive impairment is not far removed from the same arguments that were used against Egyptian self-rule during the British colonial administration.[56] Many Egyptologists writing about this today will frame themselves either as defenders of Akhenaten's "revolutionary ideas," or opponents of his "heresy," which is seen to upset the 'canon' of ancient Egyptian belief. In both instances, his divergence away from what came before him is immediately pinned down to his very embodiment, harkening back to eugenicist ideas of the twentieth century that the health of the body was the foundation of the state's own wellbeing. In this way, Akhenaten became something of a cautionary tale: "This is what happens when the weak and feeble-minded take hold." Even when some today disavow any embodiment of disability, it is because they see his innovation as proof that he could *not* have been disabled, because disabled people do not have revolutionary ideas. Both are extremely harmful to the perception of what a disabled person can or could do.

As noted in recent decades, the development of Egyptology is inextricably linked with the growth and expansion of colonial undertakings in Egypt. Colonialism, in turn, is inextricably disabling: the forceful and violent diminishing of another person's capacity in order to subjugate them to your own. It is no surprise then that the foremost minds behind the development of Egyptology continually devalued the bodies and minds of their contemporary help as well as the lives of their ancient interlocutors. The idea of disability is seen as fundamentally incompatible with the idea of wielding absolute authority, and so this helps frame a narrative that sees Akhenaten as a degenerate, and Tutankhamun as something of a reactionary. Therefore, Tutankhamun *could not* have been disabled. His reign restored the "natural order"; how could he possibly be impaired?

Today, continual disagreements over whether Tutankhamun was disabled or not are played out in traditional publishing and the media for the public. This creates a spectacle of freakery to drum up interest in a figure whose lived experience has long since dissolved in favour of a marketability akin to a contemporary pop-culture icon.

Modern discourse and depictions of Tutankhamun regularly fail to humanise him in any measurable way. He can only ever be a fierce and semi-divine warrior who rides his chariot triumphantly, or a sickly young boy caught within the tumult of his father's legacy and in the ensnarement of courtly intrigues. Even attempts that have been made to recognise possible impairment are done in insensitive ways, continuing a long tradition within Egyptology to exploit human remains for prestige and recognition, no matter the human cost. Impairment can only be at the cost of any capacity, rather than reckoned with in its lived reality.

This often leads to excessive leaps in logic to maintain the image of Tutankhamun the pop icon. His tomb contents are regularly taken out of context to construct a fabrication of the same kingly ideal that Petrie and his contemporaries espoused. His chariots are used as a symbol of his warrior nature, despite the fact there's little evidence for their active use in his lifetime.[57] Contrastingly, the overabundance of walking sticks in his tomb – some clearly recognised as his favourites to actively use – are repeatedly dismissed as symbols of status, something that we are told is evident in multiple other tombs yet given no citation. This also deliberately ignores the multifunctionality of an object: functions of authority are seen as antithetical to the varying function of impairments.[58] Most bafflingly of all is the idea that the linen straps found on his throne – which Carter's team discarded – were there to signify to his court not to occupy his chair. Considering that this court society surrounding the pharaoh is constructed around his presence, surely they would not need to be reminded of his seating place amongst them.[59] It makes far more sense for the straps to have been used as stability aids to secure him in his chair.[60]

What this shows is that – as far as Tutankhamun is concerned – the innovativeness of the ancient Egyptians is only recognised when it is convenient to upholding the popular image of the 'Boy' or 'Warrior King.' He is no longer just a historic figure like his father or even his successors; his pop-star status makes him a veritable juggernaut in the sphere of heritage entertainment, which gave rise to the "blockbuster exhibition." The motivation of publications seems to further that image, and thus maintain a multi-million-dollar industry.[61] Disability is seen as a threat to that image, and so all consideration is expunged in the face of overwhelming evidence, often to the detriment of ancient Egyptian agency.

Take for example the attribution of embalming error to explain Tutankhamun's embodiments.[62] What we find most perplexing about this argument is the idea that the royal embalmers – specialised people who were selected for a very significant task – would somehow be in any state of haphazardness when carrying out their duties, to such a violent degree that they harmed his body. This argument is made, despite evidence that mummification is a very deliberate, slow process; while the rushed preparation of his tomb assemblage is one thing, his embalming would still be the same methodically rigorous process. We also see this argument in describing

Tutankhamun's premature daughters, who were buried with him in the tomb.[63] The elder of the foetuses has been described as having "scoliosis (curvature of the spine), spina bifida and Sprengel's deformity (which had affected the baby's left shoulder blade congenitally)."[64] However, recent research has revealed, "CT scans indicate that the alleged pathologies had actually been a result of the embalming process."[65] What is interesting here is that this is the exact same argument used to explain away Tutankhamun's impairments prior: "Full body CT scans . . . indicate that the curved spine resulted not from disease, but from embalming."[66] However, Howard Carter noted in his original object cards which describe both girls that "the wrapping had been carried out in with the XVIIIth Dynasty Method."[67] These cannot both be the case. We must accept that either embalming was a highly skilled profession, or it was an unrefined process, and therefore more mummified human remains would show signs of harm to the body. Both cannot simultaneously be true, or only when it is convenient to fit into preestablished narratives. This example is reflective of the binary thinking when it comes to Akhenaten, Tutankhamun, and the Amarna period in general. It also is another example of denying the deceased agency: both the embalmers as skilled workers, and the care of the royal family in choosing these embalmers to prepare their deceased loved ones. It is more plausible that – if there were any damage to his remains – this was the result of postmortem examinations.[68]

Nefertiti has also been linked to disability, which tells us different things depending upon the context of that link. She was initially given the label by Weigall. In *The Graphic*, Weigall states, "[M]oreover she had suffered the very common Egyptian misfortune of losing the sight of one of her eyes, over which a cataract had formed."[69] He then goes on to theorise:

> The sculptor to whom she sat had been instructed by the King to execute his work always with the greatest realism, and not to hide any defects his patrons might exhibit; and thus he did not shrink from modelling the Queen's blind eye so that it would appear different from the other, and afterwards, in painting the bust, he deliberately blurred the pupil to indicate the greyish film which had grown over the eyeball.[70]

Like his interpretations of Akhenaten, Weigall again bases his theories on a literal reading of evidence. Nefertiti is linked to disability from roughly 1938–1940, with an article appearing in numerous UK newspapers which tells readers about the *Nefertiti Club:*

> There is . . . the Nefertiti Club, perhaps the strangest club in all the world, the members of which are all women suffering from one-eye defects. The club takes its name from the Egyptian Queen Nefertiti, who was known as one of the most beautiful women of her age. Yet, she had one outstanding defect – she was blind in one eye. She succeeded, however, in turning her handicap into an attraction, and captured the heart of every man who saw her. The Nefertiti Club was founded by the young wife of a prominent business

> man of Omaha, Nebraska, who has a defect in her right eye. Though most of the members are good looking, they all possess a defect in one of their eyes. But all like Nefertiti refuse to believe that their disability makes them less attractive, and as they go about their daily tasks none of them shows any signs of self-consciousness or embarrassment.[71]

While this is cited by Egyptologist Joyce Tyldesley in her 2018 book on Nefertiti as fact, this story was only picked up by UK-based newspapers for a brief span of time, with no equivalent coverage in the United States. No one has been named or identified as being part of this club and unfortunately one must question the overall veracity of the article.[72] However, what it posits for the inclusion of disability narratives in ancient Egyptian lives is interesting. If we created our own *Nefertiti Club*, the inclusion of perspectives of disability presents the opportunity for disabled people to see themselves in the extraordinary as well as in the everyday. Though it is unlikely that Weigall's assessment is true, empowering the partially blind to imagine themselves within the partially complete bust of Nefertiti expands the richness of their embodiments. They have always been Nefertiti; as mystical and beautiful as she was.

Conclusion

Egyptologists must recognise that their research has an impact on today's communities. They also must recognise that by continuing to repeat flawed narratives, and using outdated language, they are actively causing harm. We like to believe that as a field we have advanced beyond the eugenics of Petrie, but have we really?

To deny the exploration of Tutankhamun through the lens of disability is to fundamentally prevent us from seeing the pharaoh's life as he likely experienced it. Whether or not one gives Tutankhamun the label of "disabled" is irrelevant. The fact is that analysing his life through the experience of disability provides a much clearer picture of his personhood than the tired trope of Warrior King ever will. By granting him this personhood, we are granting him agency as a man, pharaoh, husband, and father.

The same can be said of his father Akhenaten, but in reverse. We do not see the man if we continue to ascribe his actions to cognitive or physical difference based upon a literal and non-rigorous interpretation of his artistic depictions, as well as questionable skeletal evidence. By doing so, scholars devalue his contributions and feed into societal biases of disability as being associated with negativity, wrongness, and otherness. It also denies the Amarna royal family agency. Instead, they are treated as props for financial gain, which does little to advance our understanding of the ancient world. This negatively impacts the communities of today since these circular arguments deny us the agency to engage with our past. It fails to recognise that we even exist. Disabled people today deserve to see ourselves reflected in history, to engage with that history without encountering demeaning and offensive language and societal tropes, and to know we have always been here, an engaged part of society.

Going forward, we as disabled authors implore our peers within Egyptology to critically reflect on the foundations which underpin our studies, and in the instance of this chapter's discussion, on the biographical nature of our studies of Egyptian pharaohs like Akhenaten and Tutankhamun. Doubtlessly these biographies will remain in popular demand for years to come, and that has as much to do with the industry that demands it as well as those who fuel it. Yet, what we hope is that we can seriously challenge the continued recycling of historical error and dehumanising language in these narratives. It serves our knowledge, and the lives of contemporary disabled people, to consider the nature of impairment in more complex and nuanced ways.

Notes

1 Vogel and Power (2023, 7).
2 Dubourg (2023, 14–15).
3 Ibid.
4 de la Bedoyere (2022, 270).
5 One recent example is Wilkinson (2022, 267–68): "Deformity is not often depicted in Egyptian sculpture and painting – the purpose of art being to portray an ideal state of affairs – but skeletons and remains tell a different story. Several bear the tell-tale signs of hernias and spinal tuberculosis, which left sufferers with hunchbacks and twisted spines . . . two skeletons with the latter disease were uncovered, in each case accompanied by pottery representations of the deformity."
6 National Center on Disability and Journalism (Arizona State University), "Disability Language Style Guide," updated August 2021, https://ncdj.org/style-guide/: Nick Brown, "Ableism/Language," updated September 14, 2022, https://www.autistichoya.com/p/ableist-words-and-terms-to-avoid.html: Alexandra F. Morris and Debby Sneed, "Blog: A Brief Guide to Disability Terminology," *Society for Classical Studies*, August30,2021,https://classicalstudies.org/scs-blog/alexandra-morris/blog-brief-guide-disability-terminology-and-theory-ancient-world-studies.
7 Bosack-Shroeder (2023, 151), Graham (2021, 172).
8 Ibid.
9 Challis (2014, 180–81).
10 Sheppard (2010, 16–29), Ramsey (2004, 15–20).
11 Wilkinson quoted in Ridley (2022, 116).
12 Lepsius quoted in Ridley (2022, 117).
13 Petrie (1894, 38–39).
14 Ibid.
15 Davis (1910, 3)
16 Ibid., xiv.
17 Ibid., 3.
18 Ibid., xxiv.
19 Ridley (2022, 347).
20 Ibid., 353.
21 Ibid., 355–56.
22 Ibid., 361–62.
23 Ibid., 355–56.
24 Ibid.
25 Ibid., 326.
26 , 355).Breasted (1909
27 Weigall (2000, 249–50).

28 Dodson (2009, 40–42), Metcalfe (2016, 408–9).
29 Challis (2013, 149–66).
30 Edwards (2022, 326).
31 Ridley (2022, 105–6).
32 Aldred (1988, 233, 236).
33 Darnell and Darnell (2022, XV, 57).
34 Ridley (2022, 104–6).
35 de la Bedoyere (2022, 244, 270).
36 Laboury (2011, 10–13).
37 Morris (2020, 53).
38 Dodson (2022, 137–44).
39 Ibid.
40 Ibid., 7.
41 Desrouches-Noblecourt (1967, 158).
42 Ibid., 112.
43 Riggs (2021, 285).
44 Morris (2022, 38–40).
45 Ibid.
46 Doherty (2003, 142–88).
47 Brier (2023, 177–92), Reeves (2022, 241, 311–13, 339–40, 357–58), Eaton-Krauss (2016, 104–6).
48 Hawass (2013, 159), Brier (2023, 165–92), Veldmeijer and Ikram (2020, 8–13).
49 Hawass (2013, 159), Brier (2023, 165–92).
50 Smith-Sangster (2021, 247–49).
51 Ibid.
52 Morris (2020, 53–72).
53 Vogel and Power (2023, 9).
54 Petrie spoke about his "Dynastic Race" theory during an address to the International Oriental Congress in 1891, reported by Popular Science Monthly as the "Two Ancient Races." See also: Sheppard (2010, 16–29), Ramsey (2004, 15–20).
55 Challis (2013, 149–66).
56 Take for example the British journal *Outlook*'s characterisation of Egyptians as "hysterical children, who are playing at self-government." As cited in Reid (2015, 162).
57 See "Tutankhamun's Chariots" and "Tutankhamun as Warrior" Brier (2023, 166–91).
58 Aziz (2022, 18–20); Nick Brown, "Tutankhamun's Sticks," accessed August 2023, https://arce.org/resource/tutankhamuns-sticks/: Veldemejer and Ikram (2020, 13).
59 Loeben (1996, 25), Eaton-Krauss (2008, 26).
60 Morris (2020, 54).
61 Alina Cohen, "King Tut Exhibitions," October 30, 2019, https://www.artsy.net/article/artsy-editorial-king-tut-exhibitions-multimillion-dollar-industry:ChristinaRiggs, "Tutankhamun's Afterlife Continues," February 14, 2022, https://www.durham.ac.uk/research/current/research-news/one-hundred-years-after-his-tomb-was-discovered-tutankhamuns-afterlife-continues/.
62 Hawass (2011, 268).
63 Dodson (2022, 41).
64 Filer (1995, 61).
65 Aidan Dodson (2022, 41).
66 Hawass (2011, 268).
67 Photographs of object cards for *Mummy of a Child Ritualistically Wrapped: 317a-07, 317b-07, 317b-08*. Tutankhamun: Anatomy of an Excavation and Griffith Institute, 2000–2004, http://www.griffith.ox.ac.uk/discoveringTut/.
68 Aziz (2022, 18–20).
69 Weigall (1927, 496).
70 Ibid.

71 Published as "Making Affliction Attractive: One Eyed-Women," *The Gloucester Citizen*, July 10, 1939, 7: "Listening in to Town Topics by Man in the Street," *Long Eaton Advertiser*, May 12, 1939, 4: "Making Affliction Attractive: One Eyed-Women," *Dundee Evening Telegraph*, July 10, 1939, 10, "Facing Their Misfortune in Brotherhood: Women Who Have One-Eye Defects," *Newcastle Evening Chronicle,* July 10, 1939, 5: "Afflictions Into Attractions Form a Club And Be Cheerful," *Somerset Guardian and Radstock Observer*, July 14, 1939, 2: "Badge of Distinction: Turning Afflictions into Attractions," *Halifax Evening Courier*, July 10, 1939, 3: "Turning Afflictions into Attractions," *Nottingham Evening Post*, July 10, 1939, 3: "Cheerful Clubs," *Torbay Express and South Devon Echo,* July 11, 1939, 5: "Some Queer Clubs," *Coventry Evening Telegraph*, July 10, 1939, 7: "Founded by Young Wife," *Sunderland Daily Echo and Shipping Gazette*, July 10, 1939, 7: "Eye Affliction Club," *Shields Daily News*, July 10, 1939, 3: "Strangest of All," *Scunthrope Evening Telegraph*, July 10, 1939, 5: "Turning Afflictions into Attractions," *Hartlepool Northern Daily Mail*, July 10, 1939, 3: "Listening in to Town Topics by Man in the Street," *Stapleford & Sandicare News*, May 13, 1939, 4: "Turning Afflictions into Attractions," *Ireland's Saturday Night*, April 20, 1940, 8: "Turning Afflictions into Attractions," *Alderley & Wilmslow Advertiser,* July 14, 1939, 7: "Bad Eyes Form Club," *Birmingham Weekly Mercury*, October 2, 1938, 5.

72 Tyldesley (2018, 115).

Bibliography

"Afflictions Into Attractions Form a Club and Be Cheerful." Somerset Guardia*n and* Radstock Observer, July 14, 1939, 2.

Aldred, Cyril. *Akhenaten: King of Egypt.* New York: Thames & Hudson, 1988.

Aziz, Sophia. "Tutankhamun 100 Years of Forensic Investigation." *NILE Magazine* 33 (2022): 13–23.

"Bad Eyes Form Club." *Birmingham Weekly Mercury,* October 2, 1938, 5.

"Badge of Distinction: Turning Afflictions into Attractions." *Halifax Evening Courier,* July 10, 1939, 3.

Bosack-Shroeder, Clara. "Disability Studies and the Classical Body." Edited by Ellen Adams. *Classical Philology* 118, no. 1 (2023): 146–51.

Breasted, James Henry. *A History of Egypt: From the Earliest Times to The Persian Conquests.* New York: Scribner, 1909.

Brier, Bob. *Tutankhamun and the Tomb that Changed the World.* Oxford: Oxford University Press, 2023.

Brown, Nick. "Tutankhamun's Sticks." Accessed August 2023. https://arce.org/resource/tutankhamuns-sticks/.

Challis, Debbie. "Akhenaten's Bloodline." In *The Archaeology of Race: The Eugenic Ideas of Francis Galton and Flinders Petrie: Bloomsbury Studies in Philosophy*, 149–66. London: Bloomsbury Academic Press, 2013.

Challis, Debbie. *The Archaeology of Race.* London: Bloomsbury, 2014.

"Cheerful Clubs." *Torbay Express and South Devon Echo,* July 11, 1939, 5.

Cohen,Alina."HowKingTutExhibitonsBecameaMultimillionDollarIndustry."*Artsy:ArtMarket,* October 30, 2019. https://www.artsy.net/article/artsy-editorial-king-tut-exhibitions-multimillion-dollar-industry.

Darnell, Colleen, and John Darnell. *Egypt's Golden Couple: When Akhenaten and Nefertiti Were Gods on Earth.* New York: St. Martin's Press, 2022.

Davis, Theodore M. *The Tomb of Queen Tiyi: The Discovery of the Tomb.* London: Constable and Co. Ltd, 1910.

de la Bedoyere, Guy. *Pharaohs of the Sun: How Egypt's Despots and Dreamers Drove the Rise and Fall of Tutankhamun's Dynasty.* London: Little Brown, 2022.

Desrouches-Noblecourt, Christiane. *Tutankhamen: Life and Death of a Pharaoh.* London: World Books and George Rainbird, 1967.

Dodson, Aidan. *Amarna Sunset: Nefertiti, Tutankhamun, Ay, Horemheb, and the Egyptian Counter-Reformation.* New York: The American University in Cairo Press, 2009.
Dodson, Aidan. *Tutankhamun King of Egypt: His Life and Afterlife.* New York: The American University in Cairo Press, 2022.
Doherty, Paul. *The Mysterious Death of Tutankhamun.* London: Robinson, 2003.
Dubourg, Ninon. *Disabled Clerics in the Late Middle Ages: Un/suitable for Divine Service?* Amsterdam: Amsterdam University Press, 2023.
Eaton-Krauss, Marianne. *The Thrones, Chairs, Stools, and Footstools from the Tomb of Tutankhamun.* Oxford: Griffith Institute, 2008.
Eaton-Krauss, Marianne. *The Unknown Tutankhamun: A Biography of the Unknown King.* London: Bloomsbury Academic Press, 2016.
Edwards, Amelia. *A Thousand Miles Up the Nile.* Reprinted London: Egypt Exploration Society, (1877) 2022.
"Eye Affliction Club." *Shields Daily News,* July 10, 1939, 3.
"Facing Their Misfortune in Brotherhood: Women Who Have One-Eye Defects." *Newcastle Evening Chronicle,* July 10, 1939, 5.
Filer, Joyce. *Disease.* Austin: University of Texas Press, 1995.
"Founded by Young Wife." *Sunderland Daily Echo and Shipping Gazette,* July 10, 1939, 7.
Graham, Emma-Jayne. "Interactional Sensibilities: Bringing Ancient Disability Studies to Its Archaeological Senses." In *Disability Studies and the Classical Body: The Forgotten Other,* edited by Ellen Adams. London: Routledge, 2021.
Hawass, Zahi. *Tutankhamun and the Golden Age of the Pharaohs.* Washington, DC: National Geographic, 2011.
Hawass, Zahi. *Discovering Tutankhamun: From Howard Carter to DNA.* New York: The American University in Cairo Press, 2013.
Laboury, Dmitri. "Amarna Art." In *UCLA Encyclopedia of Egyptology,* edited by Kathlyn M. Cooney and Willeke Wendrich. Los Angeles: UCLA Department of Near Eastern Languages and Cultures, 2011. http://digital2.library.ucla.edu/viewItem.do?ark=21198/zz0026vj6m.
"Listening in to Town Topics by Man in the Street." *Long Eaton Advertiser,* May 12, 1939a, 4.
"Listening in to Town Topics by Man in the Street." *Stapleford & Sandicare News,* May 13, 1939b, 4.
Loeben, Christian. "La Fonction Funeraire des Meubles Egyptiens." *Egypte, Afrique & Orient* 3 (1996): 25.
"Making Affliction Attractive: One Eyed-Women." *Dundee Evening Telegraph,* July 10, 1939a, 10.
"Making Affliction Attractive: One Eyed-Women." *The Gloucester Citizen,* July 10, 1939b, 7.
Metcalfe, Ryan. "Recent Identity and Relationship Studies, Including X-rays and DNA." In *The Oxford Handbook of the Valley of the Kings*, edited by Richard H. Wilkinson and Kent Weeks, 401–16. Oxford: Oxford University Press, 2016.
Morris, Alexandra F. "Let that Be Your Last Battlefield: Tutankhamun and Disability." *Athens Journal of History* 6, no. 1 (2020): 53–72.
Morris, Alexandra F. "Plato's Stepchildren: Disability in Ptolemaic Egypt and the Hellenistic World, 332–30 BCE." PhD thesis, Teesside University, 2022.
Petrie, W. M. Flinders. *Tell el Amarna.* London: Methuen & Co, 1894.
Photographs of Object Cards for Mummy of a Child Ritualistically Wrapped: 317a-07, 317b-07, 317b-08. Tutankhamun: Anatomy of an Excavation and Griffith Institute, 2000–2004. http://www.griffith.ox.ac.uk/discoveringTut/.
Ramsey, Jason D. "Petrie and the Intriguing Idiosyncrasies of Racism." *Bulletin of the History of Archaeology* 14, no. 2 (2004): 15–20.
Redford, Donald B. *Akhenaten: The Heretic King.* Princeton: Princeton University Press, 1984.

Reeves, Nicholas. *The Complete Tutankhamun: 100 Years of Discovery.* New York: Thames & Hudson, 2022.
Reid, Donald M. "Remembering and Forgetting Tutankhamun." In *Histories of Egyptology,* edited by William Carruthers, 157–73. Oxford: Routledge, 2015.
Ridley, Ronald T. *Akhenaten: A Historian's View.* New York: The American University in Cairo Press, 2022.
Riggs, Christina. *Treasured: How Tutankhamun Shaped a Century.* London: Atlantic Books, 2021.
Riggs, Christina. "One Hundred Years After His Tomb Was Discovered, Tutankhamun's Afterlife Continues." *Durham University Research News,* February 14, 2022. https://www.durham.ac.uk/research/current/research-news/one-hundred-years-after-his-tomb-was-discovered-tutankhamuns-afterlife-continues/.
Sheppard, Kathleen L. "Flinders-Petrie and Eugenics at UCL." *Bulletin of the History of Archaeology* 20, no. 1 (2010): 16–29.
Smith-Sangster, Emily. "Crutched Pharaoh, Seated Hunter: An Analysis of Artistic Portrayals of Tutankhamun's Disabilities." *Journal of the American Research Center in Egypt* 57 (2021): 235–51.
"Some Queer Clubs." *Coventry Evening Telegraph,* July 10, 1939, 7.
"Strangest of All." *Scunthrope Evening Telegraph,* July 10, 1939, 5.
"Turning Afflictions into Attractions." *Hartlepool Northern Daily Mail,* July 10, 1939a, 3.
"Turning Afflictions into Attractions." *Nottingham Evening Post,* July 10, 1939b, 3.
"Turning Afflictions into Attractions." *Alderley & Wilmslow Advertiser,* July 14, 1939c, 7.
"Turning Afflictions into Attractions." *Ireland's Saturday Night,* April 20, 1940, 8.
Tyldesley, Joyce. *Nefertiti's Face: The Creation of An Icon.* Cambridge: Harvard University Press, 2018.
Veldmeijer, Andre J., and Salima Ikram. "Tutankhamun's Sticks and Staves: The Importance of Deceptively Simple Objects." *Scribe* (2020): 8–13.
Vogel, Hannah, and Ronika K. Power. "Recognising Inequality: Ableism in Egyptological Approaches to Disability and Bodily Differences." *World Archaeology* (2023): 1–14.
Weigall, Arthur. "The Beautiful One-Eyed Nefertiti." *The Graphic,* March 26, 1927, 496.
Weigall, Arthur. *The Life and Times of Akhnaton: Pharaoh of Egypt: A Unabridged Republication of the 1922 Edition.* London: First Cooper Square Press Edition, 2000.
Wilkinson, Toby. *Tutankhamun's Trumpet: The Story of Ancient Egypt in 100 Objects.* London: Pan MacMillan, 2022.

Disability Language Style Guides

Brown, Lydia X. Z. "Ableism/Language." Updated September 14, 2022. https://www.autistichoya.com/p/ableist-words-and-terms-to-avoid.html.
Morris, Alexandra F., and Debby Sneed. "Blog: A Brief Guide to Disability Terminology & Theory in Ancient World Studies." *Society for Classical Studies,* August 30, 2021. https://classicalstudies.org/scs-blog/alexandra-morris/blog-brief-guide-disability-terminology-and-theory-ancient-world-studies.
National Center on Disability and Journalism (Arizona State University). "Disability Language Style Guide." Updated August 2021. https://ncdj.org/style-guide/.

4 *Grande Morbidezza*

The Invention of Akhenaten's Illness

Steven M. Stannish

Introduction

For almost two hundred years, the 18th Dynasty pharaoh Akhenaten has fascinated archaeologists and historians, as well as psychologists and popular audiences.[1] Often regarded as the first monotheist, Akhenaten, together with his wife, Queen Nefertiti, worshipped the Aten or "Solar Disk" to the exclusion of other gods. Near his fifth regnal year, he moved his court to Akhetaten, the "Horizon of the Aten" – modern Amarna – and attacked the cult of Amun at Thebes.[2] Following his twelfth regnal year, which featured a *durbar* at the new residence, the record becomes murky, but the Amarna Letters attest to setbacks in western Asia and plague. After Akhenaten's death, his successors struck his name from king-lists, obliterated his image, and dismantled his temples. His memory only survived, perhaps, in the legend of the renegade priest Osarsêph, until the nineteenth century.[3] Egyptologists have described "storm-clouds . . . gathering" and "terror" during Akhenaten's reign, and have inferred a sense of relief at its end.[4]

Without question, Akhenaten's art arrests the Western gaze. While earlier Egyptian sculptures and paintings might seem formal and rigid, those of the Amarna period exhibit fluidity and motion, and explore new emotive themes like royal domestic life. Particularly striking are the pharaoh's portraits, which show an elongated head with protruding chin, pronounced breasts and belly, wide hips, and spindly arms and legs (Figures 4.1 and 4.2). These features, along with Manetho's record of an 18th Dynasty ruler Akenkherês, who had been a princess, convinced early Egyptologists that Akhenaten was female.[5] Even after they correctly identified him as male, they believed his image revealed an illness, possibly a nervous condition or metabolic disorder. Several, allied with medical professionals, speculated that his affliction resulted in a disability that contributed to his monomania, whether through a feeling of difference, weak eyesight, or sensitivity to cold.

This chapter argues that the story of the sickly fanatic Akhenaten derives from a prevailing discourse.[6] From an early detection of *grande morbidezza* through later diagnoses of Fröhlich's syndrome, Marfan's syndrome, and aromatase excess syndrome, this discourse has incorporated Egyptological values, attitudes, and practices – and constrained them. Schematic elements include a Neo-Classical aesthetic, an

DOI: 10.4324/9781003440369-6

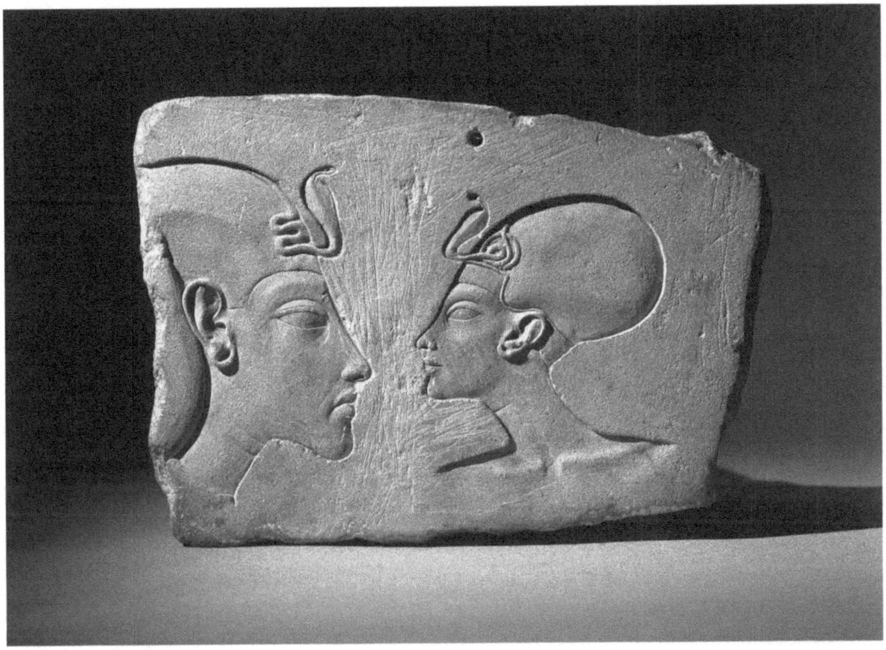

Figure 4.1 *Study of Akhenaten and Nefertiti. The Wilbour Plaque,* c. 1353–1336 BCE or slightly later. Limestone, pigment, 6 3/16 × 8 11/16 × 1 5/8 in (15.7 × 22.1 × 4.1 cm). Brooklyn Museum, Gift of Evangeline Wilbour Blashfield, Theodora Wilbour, and Victor Wilbour honoring the wishes of their mother, Charlotte Beebe Wilbour, as a memorial to their father, Charles Edwin Wilbour, 16.48.

association of reason with health, an application of modern religious categories to antiquity, and a search for breakthroughs at certain sites, such as excavations and forensic labs. Indeed, the conviction that Akhenaten's pathology fostered his zeal has not only been repeated *ad nauseam*, but has also driven conjecture on his childhood, imagination, and singing voice, without weakening until the current millennium. The result is a picture that indicates more about our Enlightenment heritage than about ancient Egypt. This chapter thus has a novel approach. Whereas other studies of disability may focus on overlooked or misunderstood disorders, it examines a physical condition invented to explain a historical phenomenon.

The Emergence of a Discourse

It is well known that modern Egyptology's origins are bound to Napoleon Bonaparte's failed expedition to Egypt in 1798.[7] Accompanying the French army was a contingent of scholars whose task it was, in the spirit of the Enlightenment, to index what the land held. The result of their labor was the monumental *Description de l'Égypte*. Also integral was Jean-François Champollion's decipherment of hieroglyphs in the early nineteenth century. The two events are connected by the

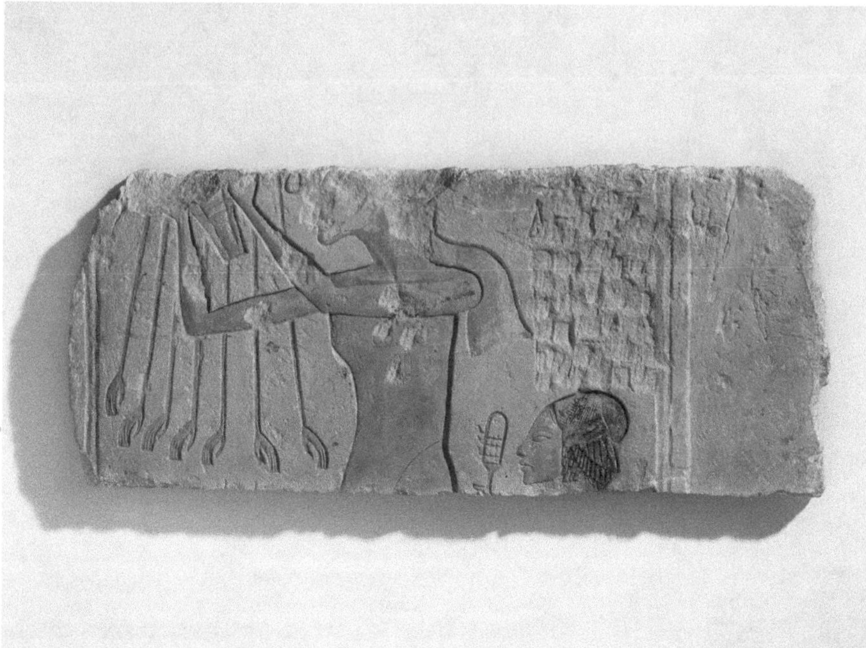

Figure 4.2 *Akhenaten and His Daughter Offering to the Aten,* c. 1353–1336 BCE. Limestone, pigment, 8 15/16 × 20 5/16 × 1 1/4 in, 14.5 lbs (22.7 × 51.6 × 3.2 cm, 6.58 kg). Brooklyn Museum, Charles Edwin Wilbour Fund, 60.197.6.

Rosetta Stone, a trilingual (hieroglyphic, demotic, and Greek) inscription that the expedition discovered and that aided the work of decoding.

During his own travels in Egypt, between 1828 and 1829, Champollion visited Amarna and examined its boundary stelae. Although he was unaware of the site's significance and made only cursory remarks, his reaction stands at the beginning of Western writing about Akhenaten. Reflecting on one monument, Champollion described: "The king, fat, paunchy. Feminine forms . . . *grande morbidezza.*"[8] Besides commenting on Akhenaten's obesity, he detected "great softness," using an expression derived from the Latin *morbidus*, "diseased."

In the early nineteenth century, the imputation of softness, particularly *morbidezza*, evoked the Neo-Classical condemnation of Antonio Correggio, whose paintings featured shimmering flesh-tones, rounded edges, and ecstatic expressions.[9] According to the pioneering art historian Johann Winckelmann, art should instead manifest "noble simplicity and quiet grandeur," and reflect the ideal rather than the natural, like the ancient Greek *Laocoön*, *Niobe*, and *Apollo Belvedere.*[10] The word *morbidezza* thus had a negative charge, implying effeminacy and unwholesomeness, as well as sickness.[11]

Champollion himself did not accept all of Neo-Classicism's judgments, of course. In particular, he rejected the movement's low estimation of the Egyptians, arguing that the Drovetti Collection in Turin proved them to be capable of brilliance.[12] Yet, the great philologist could not escape Neo-Classicism's influence. He said that Egyptian art "is devoted to the notation of ideas rather than the representation of things," just as Winckelmann said the best traditions were, and praised a statue of "Sesostris" (Ramesses II) as "the Egyptian *Apollo Belvedere.*"[13] Clearly then, Champollion's use of *morbidezza* was pejorative, intimating stylistic malaise.

As nineteenth-century Egyptologists reconstructed the Amarna period, Champollion's aesthetic reaction blended with a perception of Akhenaten's fanaticism, based on his exclusive Aten worship and attack on Amun. Decades earlier, the *philosophes* analyzed this *maladie épidémique* from Europe's Age of Religious Wars. The *Encyclopédie* contained an entry on the subject, as did Voltaire's *Dictionnaire philosophique.*[14] The latter even provided a symptomatology, including melancholia, visions, pseudo-prophecy, and lethargy. Following Karl Richard Lepsius, who characterized Akhenaten as a "Puritan,"[15] Auguste Mariette, Heinrich Brugsch, and Gaston Maspero alternately suggested that his appearance revealed Semitic descent, castration, and "blind fanaticism."[16] Indeed, even after criticizing such conjectures as "completely unfounded," Eduard Meyer added that the pharaoh's face "clearly bears the features of a fanatic."[17]

We should not be surprised by Meyer's sudden reversal, for many who dismissed speculation about Akhenaten's ethnicity and mutilation, including eventually Maspero himself,[18] still imagined him gripped by illness and zeal. So Adolf Erman supposed that the "strange eccentric" suffered from poor health and religious enthusiasm.[19] Similarly, Wallis Budge thought the pharaoh's portraits revealed a physical condition and likened him to the caliph al-Ḥākim, "a courageous fanatic" who "suffered from a religious madness at least."[20] Even the whiggish James Henry Breasted and the romantic Arthur Weigall used such language. The former, while extolling Akhenaten's individualism and "simple and beautiful realism," stressed his "fanaticism," which produced "unhealthy symptoms . . . too in the body politic."[21] The latter, like Budge, compared him to al-Ḥākim, suggesting that he suffered from epilepsy and hallucinations, and that he grew up sickly and melancholic, with fits of "holy frenzy."[22]

Needless to say, this tale is better suited to *The Thousand and One Arabian Nights* than to Egyptian history. No doubt, Akhenaten's categorization as a "monotheist," a modern term implying ideas about revelation, orthodoxy and heresy, and iconoclasm contributed to its fabrication. But a distaste for the pharaoh's image was important as well. We have already assayed Champollion's detection of *morbidezza*, and now we find Erman wishing sculptors had spared us Akhenaten's "consumptive face on an overly long neck, . . . fat thighs" and other "unlovely details,"[23] alongside Budge bemoaning his family's "exaggerated . . . undignified caricatures."[24] Even Breasted noted "the strange treatment of the lower limbs by Ikhnaton's artists."[25] An exception was Weigall, who with characteristic breathlessness claimed that Amarna statuary "reached a height of perfection which places it above all but the art of the Greeks."[26]

The Curse of KV55

A scientific assessment of Akhenaten's health requires forensic evidence. Unfortunately, Alessandro Barsanti's partial clearance of the Amarna royal tomb in the early 1890s yielded only a smashed sarcophagus.[27] In 1907, however, an expedition patronized by the millionaire Theodore M. Davis and led by Edward R. Ayrton unearthed a remarkable burial: Tomb 55 in the Valley of Kings (KV55). Davis famously possessed a domineering personality, but few of the complications of professional training, and the excavation was a festival of incompetence that has haunted Egyptology for over a century. Among the tomb's objects, the expedition found a disassembled gilded canopy with images of Akhenaten (excised) and his mother, Queen Tiye, as well as a *rishi*-coffin with a mummified body – whose wrappings and flesh fell to dust in the archaeologists' hands. Two physicians examined the pelvis and determined that it belonged to a female, allowing Davis to announce the discovery of Tiye's remains.[28] Alas, the matter was not so simple, for conditions on site were suboptimal and the millionaire had voiced his opinion on the occupant's sex before the examination. Indeed, Weigall, who was the district's chief inspector, and Maspero, who headed the Service des Antiquités, thought inscriptions pointed to an identification of Akhenaten himself.[29]

After Weigall preserved the KV55 bones in paraffin wax, he sent them to Grafton Elliot Smith, a professor of anatomy at Cairo University. Smith determined that they belonged to a male with a hydrocephalic (enlarged) skull, wide hips, and slender limbs.[30] These conclusions prompted angry letters from Davis and his friend, the Assyriologist Archibald Sayce, but they were potentially important.[31] Presuming the remains were Akhenaten's, they might shed light on his illness. The one problem was the man's age at death, estimated at 25 or 26 years, a decade too young to be the pharaoh.[32] Smith hit upon a medical explanation for the discrepancy, however: Akhenaten could have suffered from adiposogenital dystrophy, or Fröhlich's syndrome.[33] This pituitary condition causes hydrocephalus, a feminine distribution of body fat, atrophied genitalia, sterility, and impaired vision. In addition, Fröhlich's syndrome delays osteogenesis, so that the skeleton might look younger than it actually is. For support, Smith returned to Amarna iconography:

> Forty years ago archaeologists were puzzled by the pictures of [Akhenaten], and it was suggested that he was a woman masquerading as a man. In light of our present knowledge, however, they seem to be quite distinctive of Froehlich's syndrome.[34]

Akhenaten's biography was now complete. His artistic style and fervor, "the eccentricities of his behavior," and "his pathetic failure as a statesman" were all "due to his being subject to a rare disorder."[35] Citing Davis's KV55 publication, Budge declared that if the occupant's identification was correct, "the king suffered from water on the brain."[36]

Of course, complete biographies usually do not last, and in this case, scholars soon pinpointed weaknesses. Smith himself recognized that while Fröhlich's syndrome causes sterility, Akhenaten and Nefertiti often appear with royal daughters.[37] A few years later, Rex Engelbach challenged the identification of KV55's occupant, arguing that his coffin belonged to Akhenaten's successor, Smenkhkare.[38] Most problematic of all, Douglas E. Derry, another professor of anatomy at Cairo

University, determined that the KV55 skull was platycephalic (broad and flat), not hydrocephalic, and dismissed the possibility of Fröhlich's syndrome.[39] He estimated that the subject was at most 20 years old and identified him as Smenkhkare.

Despite these issues, discursive ideas about Akhenaten's infirmity endured. So J. D. S. Pendlebury described one of the pharaoh's Karnak colossi without external genitalia as "a wonderful pathological study," not considering that it might be a representation of Nefertiti, an experiment, or simply unfinished.[40] Some years later, Alan Gardiner characterized Amarna royal portraiture as "frankly hideous," adding that its "general fidelity . . . cannot be doubted,"[41] and Walther Wolf lamented its "enthusiastic asceticism, . . . morbid ugliness, and nervous decadence."[42] Meanwhile, Cyril Aldred, together with the Oxford histopathologist A. T. Sandison, sympathized with Pendlebury's view and took issue with Derry's verdict on the KV55 skull.[43] Arguing that Akhenaten had Fröhlich's syndrome, they suggested that the princesses who accompany him were sired by his father, Amenhotep III. They added that Fröhlich's syndrome might explain the pharaoh's religious revolution, for it tends to produce "introspective depression alternating with euphoria," as well as a scintillating personality and an above-average intelligence.[44]

In 1963, R. G. Harrison, a professor of anatomy at the University of Liverpool, conducted a fresh investigation of the KV55 bones. Harrison determined that they belonged to a male under 25, without hydrocephalus or a pituitary tumor.[45] Based on a reconstruction by medical artist D. J. Kidd, he observed that the subject bore "no resemblance whatsoever" to Akhenaten, but did look like Tutankhamun, as represented by his mummiform coffins.[46] Harrison's investigation was not the last, however. Edward F. Wente, along with James E. Harris, a professor of dentistry at the University of Michigan, estimated KV55's occupant to be 30 or 35, also noting craniofacial similarities to Tutankhamun.[47] Conversely, Joyce Filer favored an age of around 20 and endorsed Derry's description of the skull as platycephalic.[48]

Among major examinations of the KV55 remains, the most recent is that of Zahi Hawass's team between 2005 and 2009. This effort, involving CT scans and DNA testing, aimed to establish the identity and genealogical relationship of eleven mummified bodies from the New Kingdom, and received a Discovery Channel special, *King Tut Unwrapped*. Hawass and company determined that KV55's occupant was between 35 and 45 years old, with no signs of gynecomastia or craniosynostosis, which would have caused a feminine distribution of body fat and a deformed head.[49] They found his skull to be non-pathologically brachycephalic (occipitally flat) and identified him as the father of Tutankhamun, the mother being the "Younger Lady" from the royal cache in Amenhotep II's tomb (KV35).[50]

Unsurprisingly, several Egyptologists and DNA analysts rejected these findings, raising questions about the evidence's contamination, the data's interpretation, and the results' reality.[51] Doubtless, debate on KV55's occupant will continue. Nonetheless, it is useful to highlight some established conclusions about the tomb. The Egyptians sealed KV55 at least twice – archaeologists noted "the original cemented door-blocking . . . partially dismantled" as well as a secondary limestone wall[52] – and they made two burials there. One interment was Tiye, whose remains were later removed to Amenhotep II's tomb,[53] but whose canopy was abandoned.

The other was the man whom Davis and Ayrton found. He was placed in a coffin that was probably made for a woman, but modified for a pharaoh.[54] The man's identity remains uncertain, but two of the tomb's magic bricks bear Akhenaten's name, while no trace of Smenkhkare can be found.[55] Finally – and for us, most importantly – after Smith, few medical professionals have found evidence of a pathology that would have caused KV55's occupant to resemble Akhenaten's portraits.

Akhenaten at the Dawn of the Twenty-First Century

Among the most influential late twentieth-century specialists on the Amarna period are Cyril Aldred, who worked with A. T. Sandison (see previous), and Donald B. Redford. Both mixed careful archaeological study with extravagant speculation. In *The Cambridge Ancient History* in the 1970s, Aldred echoed his forbears, claiming that the "diseased physiques" of Amarna art were redolent of an "inner spiritual malaise," and that Akhenaten was a crazed monotheist who led his iconoclastic followers on a *hijrah*.[56] The revised edition of his biography of Akhenaten, published in 1988, was also striking. Here, Aldred hedged his bet, first remarking on the pharaoh's possible pituitary disorder, then claiming that Amarna notables appear with "peculiar" features because it was "fashionable," and finally acknowledging that his subject "cannot have suffered from an abnormality which was chronic enough to impair seriously his procreative powers."[57]

Redford's biography of Akhenaten, substantially devoted to his own work at East Karnak, bore the subtitle *The Heretic King*, foreshadowing other anachronisms. The author raised the possibility that the "iconoclastic freak" did not father the Amarna princesses, and like Lepsius, described his religion as an austere Protestantism: "Perhaps we moderns might catch the true sense of what was going on were we to imagine a fanatical Christian priest denying Christ, the Trinity, and the saints in favor of the Cross."[58] And while Redford did not offer an aesthetic appraisal of Akhenaten's art, he cited "experts" on his possible illness, "which made him hideous to behold," "some sort of endocrine disorder in which secondary sex characteristics failed to develop, and eunuchoidism resulted."[59] His source for this diagnosis – of Fröhlich's syndrome, of course – was the first edition of Aldred's biography from 1968.

Because Fröhlich's syndrome causes sterility and is acquired, not hereditary, some late twentieth-century scholars did not follow Smith, Aldred, and Redford in detecting it in Akhenaten. Instead of abandoning medical explanations, however, they sought new disorders. Most persuasive was Alwyn Burridge, who argued that the pharaoh had Marfan's syndrome, a genetic condition causing an elongation of the skull and extremities, a protrusion of the breastbone, a widening of the pelvic girdle, and cardio-vascular weakness.[60] Burridge also noted that it results in visual disability and sensitivity to cold, which might explain Akhenaten's solar religion.[61] Indeed, she observed that people with Marfan's syndrome, like Abraham Lincoln and Sergei Rachmaninoff, "are often bright and charismatic," ideal qualities for a revolutionary.[62] Burridge's proposal did not reference KV55 or condemn Amarna art and religion, but it motivated Redford to consider changing his mind.[63]

Yet, around the time Burridge put forward her hypothesis, the idea that Akhenaten's appearance and ideas resulted from illness lost traction. Already in the work of Erik Hornung and Jan Assmann, we find disinterest in the notion. Hornung certainly adopted discursive ideas about the pharaoh, describing his religion as a form of "fundamentalism" and "intolerance" – obvious substitutes for "fanaticism" – but he was not in the thrall of medical explanations.[64] Assmann also drew on earlier motifs, comparing Akhenaten to a Puritan,[65] but he was more interested in the collective memory of the 18th Dynasty. In one study, he traced the tale of Osarsêph and his leper army to a plague during the Amarna period and an allusion to "grave disease" in Tutankhamun's Restoration Edict.[66] This hypothesis, though difficult to verify, had only tenuous connections to the narratives of the past two centuries.

Among recent publications, Aidan Dodson's *Amarna Sunrise* and *Amarna Sunset* were influenced by the prevailing discourse, but avoided the disease theory. The former volume, which chronicled Egyptian history from the beginning of the 18th Dynasty to Akhenaten's *durbar*, referred to "the Age of Heresy," but emphasized the pharaoh's monolatry rather than his "absolute monotheism," and eschewed speculation on his reason and health.[67] The latter, which considered the end of Akhenaten's reign and its aftermath, alluded to an Egyptian "Counter-Reformation" and "orthodoxy," but never invoked pathology.[68] Another example is James K. Hoffmeier's *Akhenaten and the Origins of Monotheism*. Hoffmeier, who studied with Redford at the University of Toronto, compared the pharaoh's Aten worship and iconoclasm to the Desert Faiths.[69] Nonetheless, he offered only limited reflections on Akhenaten's art, and, based on the findings of Hawass's team, doubted medical explanations for his appearance.[70] Finally, Ronald T. Ridley's *Akhenaten: A Historian's View* recognized the limitations of our evidence. Regarding the pharaoh's purported illness, Ridley remarked, "The endless contradictory diagnoses should be enough to convince anyone that this is a false trail."[71] He added that depictions of Akhenaten with normal morphology and of his courtiers with "exaggerated anatomy" support an interpretation of "artistic distortion, or fashion."[72]

It is important to note, however, that the disease theory did not vanish. In 1998, Bob Brier reflected on Akhenaten's condition, having "always been convinced that there was something wrong with [him]," and adopted the diagnosis of Marfan's syndrome.[73] Comparing Akhenaten to a modern patient who accentuated her atypical features, Brier suggested that the pharaoh had colossi made "to validate himself, to assert himself. It would have been a great catharsis after having been shunned and ignored for so long."[74] Shortly thereafter, Nicholas Reeves published *Akhenaten: Egypt's False Prophet*, a different portrayal from the swooning enthusiast of Budge or Weigall, but one still indebted to Enlightenment categorization. The imposter who feigns devotion in order to accumulate power – such is a Western conception of the prophet Muhammad – is another old theme, as Voltaire illustrated.[75] In presenting this cynical interpretation, Reeves endorsed the Marfan's syndrome hypothesis, which he said made Akhenaten susceptible to blindness and sudden death, and somehow gifted him with musical skill.[76] Contemporaneously, Marc Gabolde interpreted Akhenaten's religion as *almost* heretical monotheism. In its exclusivity, it "may be considered impious," but it differed from the Abrahamic traditions in its "absence of revelation."[77] Although Gabolde praised Amarna art's "nonchalant elegance" and "feminine sensuality," he suggested that Akhenaten suffered from acquired partial lipodystrophy, or Barraquer-Simons syndrome.[78] This disorder, especially rare in males, causes adipose tissue loss in the middle and upper body, with fat stored in the hips and legs.

Among recent scientific publications, such conjectures also appear. In 2009, Irwin M. Braverman and Philip A. Mackowiak, of the Yale University and the University of Maryland medical schools, together with Redford, proposed that Akhenaten had aromatase excess syndrome. They observed that this ailment would not only explain the pharaoh's appearance, but also account for his "(potentially) . . . mellifluous (female) voice."[79] A few years later, physicians Jean-Louis Codaccioni, Bernard Conte-Devolx, and Bruno Argémi surveyed other plausible diagnoses, including familial gynecomastia, Kennedy's disease, and fertile eunuch syndrome, but were unable to formulate a working hypothesis.[80]

Notwithstanding exceptions, to what can we ascribe the disease theory's decline, beyond a weariness with shifting medical explanations? Most obviously, postmodernism drew attention to the role of discourses in the production of knowledge and problematized the representation of the past. Already in the 1990s, Hornung appreciated how the opinions of Champollion, Lepsius, and Maspero formed the basis for contemporary views of the Amarna period.[81] Only a few years later, Dominic Montserrat published his *Akhenaten: History, Fantasy and Ancient Egypt*, considering how the pharaoh became a modern "cultural hallucination."[82]

I would also highlight the accumulation of evidence and more careful analysis of past finds. Together, these factors have undermined treatments which conform to Western expectations. An enervated, disabled Akhenaten may appeal to our imaginations, but forensic study has made it nearly impossible to argue for one based on the KV55 remains. Meanwhile, the varying Egyptian portraits of the pharaoh along with depictions of his courtiers in "exaggerated style" have counterbalanced discursive authority.

Here in particular, we must acknowledge a deeper understanding of Amarna art. While some twenty-first-century Egyptologists still characterized Akhenaten as a fanatical monotheist, they were less willing to argue for the realism of his portraits. Of course, in two-dimensional and relief representation, the Egyptians favored what Emma Brunner-Traut called aspective style, representing each element in its ideal form, much as Champollion claimed.[83] This is why a goddess leading a pharaoh might appear with head and torso turned 180 degrees toward him, face in profile, but eye and crown frontal. Even in the round, Egyptian sculptors often increased the relative size of "holy" subjects like deities and rulers. But before the turn of the millennium, Amarna art seemed different. Akhenaten claimed to "live by truth (*mꜣꜥt*)," so his portraits must depict physical features – what Étienne Drioton called "nightmare realism."[84] We have noted how Smith and Gardiner endorsed this view, so we should not be shocked that Breasted and Budge did so as well.[85] Redford conjured a scene – based on the chief sculptor Bek's claim to be an "apprentice whom His Majesty himself taught" – in which the pharaoh directed artists to emphasize his unusual attributes.[86] Burridge cited Akhenaten's devotion to *mꜣʿt*, remarking that "he really was profoundly deformed,"[87] as did Reeves, asserting that the pharaoh stressed "actuality and the here and now."[88] Finally, Gabolde thought royal images reflected physical developments along with "the return of a baroque and unrealistic art."[89] Interestingly, he evoked the European aesthetic heralded by Correggio and epitomized by Winckelmann's *bête noire*, Gian Lorenzo Bernini.[90]

Naturally, not all twentieth-century Egyptologists believed Akhenaten's portraits were true to life. Though involved in the KV55 drama, Weigall suggested that they show an archaizing tendency.[91] Half a century later, Hornung judged the images to be unpleasant, but asked, "[W]hy wander into the distance of medical explanations?"[92] Of paramount importance, however, was the work of Gay Robins in the 1990s and early 2000s. Robins showed that Akhenaten's art not only becomes less "exaggerated" over time, but also changes in terms of its proportional grid.[93] Furthermore, she demonstrated that standing Amarna figures have shorter legs than seated ones, and that royal canons were applied to private individuals. Robins concluded that Akhenaten's appearance, "like the rest of Egyptian art, is conceptual rather than naturalistic,"[94] ruled out Marfan's syndrome,[95] and offered a stylistic explanation for the pharaoh's "asexual" colossus.[96] Her work was consulted by Dodson, Hoffmeier, and Ridley,[97] and it figured prominently in Lise Manniche's study of Akhenaten's Karnak colossi. After citing Robins, Manniche wrote, "It is possible that the king suffered from some affliction that made him stand apart from the rest of the population," but the explanation for his appearance "is rather to be sought in stylistic and ideological criteria."[98]

One other related Egyptological development was the more frequent application of insights from allied fields, such as anthropology and history, contributing to increasingly sophisticated analysis. An example of this trend is the *Encounters with Ancient Egypt* series,[99] featuring essays on subjects ranging from the Nile Valley's evolving view of the past to its broader African context. Naturally, these studies did not ignore previous scholarship – or traditional Western classifications – but they proceeded reflectively, with an appreciation for Egypt's distinctive character.[100] So Robert Morkot, considering archaism in Egyptian art, raised the possibility that Old Kingdom solar temples inspired Akhenaten's natural scenes, and that the king's elongated figures in turn influenced Ramesses II's attenuated ones.[101]

Conclusions

The foregoing analysis indicates that Akhenaten's representation as an ill and disabled ruler, whose condition influenced his revolutionary ideas, derives from an Egyptological discourse grounded in the Enlightenment. This presents certain issues. In the first place, the Egyptological depiction began with an aesthetic reaction, antedating the use of hieroglyphic sources and forensic evidence. It may therefore be thoroughly misguided. Additionally, the depiction has served to confine our perception. As Michel de Certeau observed, all historiography involves conventional attitudes, practices, and sites.[102] When these requisites become entrenched, however, scholarship stagnates and risks becoming farcical. The fact that Nial

Charlton could have a revelation as late as the 1970s – that Akhenaten's "deformities were the thing that mattered: the key fact was that the Eighteenth Dynasty had run out into something physically rotten" – illustrates how unaware Egyptology was of its own ableist predispositions.[103]

Still another problem with Akhenaten's representation is that it has precipitated unlikely associated ideas. Michel Foucault described discourses as "practices that systematically form the objects of which they speak,"[104] and here we witness the range of the dialectical process. Egyptologists have maintained that Akhenaten hallucinated, that he was melancholy-mad, that he was despised as a child, and that he possessed musical talent. The assertion that he had a pleasant, feminine singing voice is most astonishing, since its only conceivable source is Philip Glass's 1983 opera, *Akhnaten*, in which a countertenor performs the title role. It seems as though a professional discourse influenced a popular production – Glass drew on Egyptological literature for his libretto[105] – which in turn shaped that discourse.

A final, related issue is especially intractable: Akhenaten's representation has generated a comfortably familiar story. The Amarna period was a pathology-driven disaster, a time of fanatical heresy or pseudo-prophecy, the sole merit of which was its brief duration. After Akhenaten's death, the Egyptians breathed a sigh of relief and returned as quickly as possible to normal. Such narratives are useful – even inescapable – instruments for understanding the world. But we must recognize that, as Hayden White wrote, "We do not *live* stories." [106] Otherwise, we might confuse mimetic strategies with reality itself.

All of this is not to say that Akhenaten was free of disorders and disabilities, or that he was a successful ruler – or that we might someday look on him in the gray light of objectivity. The analysis of a discourse is not a matter of writing the history of its referent, but of causing it to emerge in its own right and thereby loosening its embrace.[107] Regarding "the heretic pharaoh," this is critical, for as Montserrat observed, both academic and popular treatments of him have been strikingly modern, requiring "a minimum of cultural adjustment."[108] At the very least, I hope this analysis encourages new ideas about Akhenaten, so that future studies will less frequently repeat old motifs.

Notes

1 I would like to thank Stephen Casper, Jason Larson, and Rebekah Vogel for commenting on the draft of this essay.

2 For an overview of the Amarna period, see Gardiner (1961, ch. 9). For an up-to-date discussion of major issues, see Ridley (2019).

3 Assmann (1997, 39–42). The Osarsêph legend is preserved in Manetho's *Aigyptiaka*, fr. 54.

4 Gardiner (1961, 233), Reeves (2001, ch. 7).

5 Baron von Bunsen (1845, 89) still identified Akhenaten as female in the middle of the nineteenth century.

6 Jolliffe (2003, 101–3). My conception of discourse has been influenced by Michel Foucault's (2010), but approaches that of Edward Said, for whom it was ideological, with a "closed, self-evident, self-confirming character." Asad (1980, 648).

7 Said (1979, 80ff.).

8 Champollion (1974, vol. 2, 319).
9 Diderot and d'Alembert (1751–72, *s.v.* "morbidezza").
10 Pratz (1969, 41–69).
11 Imbs (1985, *s.v.* "morbidezza").
12 Lacouture (1988, 332–34).
13 Lacouture (1988, 334, 339–40).
14 Diderot and d'Alembert (1751–72, *s.v.* "fanatisme), Voltaire (1961, *s.v.* "fanatisme"). The expression *maladie épidémique* is Voltaire's.
15 Lepsius (1852, 359).
16 Mariette (1872, 56–57), Brugsch (1877, 419–20), Maspero (1872, 211–12).
17 Meyer (1884, vol. 1, 270–72).
18 Maspero (1909, 64–65).
19 Erman (1885, 44, 74, 1934, 116).
20 Budge (1923, 103, 107).
21 Breasted (1909, 378, 392).
22 Weigall (1923, xix, 51–52).
23 Erman (1885, 541).
24 Budge (1923, 103).
25 Breasted (1909, 378) doubted this representation "could be wholly accounted for by supposing the malformation of the king's own limbs."
26 Weigall (1923, 66).
27 Martin (1974, vol. 1, 5–6, 13–30).
28 Risse (1971, 9–10).
29 Reeves (1990, viii).
30 Smith (1912, 51–56), Reeves (1990, viii).
31 Weigall (1911, 189).
32 Smith (1990, 11–12).
33 Smith (1923, 84).
34 Smith (1926, 37).
35 Smith (1923, 84).
36 Budge (1923, 75).
37 Smith (1928, 28).
38 Engelbach (1931, 115–19).
39 Derry (1931, 15–19).
40 Pendlebury (1935, pl. 6). For the colossus as Nefertiti, see Harris (1977, 5–10), Dodson (2020, 29–30). For the possibility of an experiment, see Tyldesley (1998, 100–2). For an overview, see Manniche (2010, 93ff.).
41 Gardiner (1961, 214).
42 Wolf (1957, 453).
43 Aldred and Sandison (1962, 314–15). Years later, Aldred (1988, pl. 33) admitted other interpretations of the colossus were possible.
44 Aldred and Sandison (1962, 308).
45 Harrison (1966, 111).
46 Harrison (1966, 113–14).
47 Wente and Harris (1992, 5–6, 14).
48 Filer (2000, 13–14).
49 Hawass et al. (2010, 638, 640).
50 Hawass et al. (2010, 638–42).
51 Marchant (2013, 192–95, ch. 15), Dodson (2020, x, 20–22).
52 Reeves (1990, vi), Bell (1990, 133).
53 A KV55 glass fragment from the Harold Jones Collection joins a KV35 vase, linking the tombs. Bell (1990, 108, cf. 109, 136–37). Also, the hair of the "Elder Lady" from KV35 matches a lock in four miniature coffins bearing Tiye's name from Tutankhamun's tomb (KV63). Harris et al. (1978, 1151).

54 Ridley (2019, 307–9).
55 Bell (1990, 135).
56 Aldred (1975, part 2, vol. 2, 94).
57 Aldred (1988, 231–34).
58 Redford (1984, 138, 158, 226).
59 Redford (1984, 58).
60 Burridge (1993, 63–74).
61 Burridge (1993, 66, 70–71).
62 Burridge (1996, 128).
63 Redford (1996, 128).
64 Hornung (1999, 126).
65 Assmann (1998, 28).
66 Assmann (1997, 39–42).
67 Dodson (2014, 129).
68 Dodson (2018, xxiii, 46, 52, 61).
69 Hoffmeier (2015, 203–10).
70 Hoffmeier (2015, 130–34).
71 Ridley (2019, 57).
72 Ridley (2019, 59).
73 Brier (1998, 53).
74 Brier (1998, 55–56).
75 Quinn (2008, 71). Aldred (1975, 246–57) previously suggested that Akhenaten was a pseudo-prophet.
76 Reeves (2001, 150–52).
77 Gabolde (2005, 43, 51).
78 Gabolde (2005, 46–49). Cf. Crubezy (1994, 30–33).
79 Braverman, Redford, and Mackowiak (2009, 558).
80 Codaccioni, Conte-Devolx, and Argémi (2013, 231–33).
81 Hornung (1992, 43–49).
82 Montserrat (2000, 184).
83 Brunner-Traut (1990, ch. 2).
84 Drioton and du Bourguet (1978, 271).
85 Breasted (1909, 378), Budge (1923, 87, 103).
86 Redford (1984, 63). Cf. Sandman (1938: §204).
87 Burridge (1993, 63).
88 Reeves (2001, 139).
89 Gabolde (2005, 49).
90 According to Winckelmann (1972, 94), under Bernini's influence, figures "looked as if they suffered from dropsy."
91 Weigall (1923, 58–66).
92 Hornung (1971, 77).
93 Robins (1993a, 121ff.).
94 Robins (1993a, 121).
95 Robins (2003, 225–29).
96 Robins (1993b, 36–38).
97 Dodson (2014, 231), Hoffmeier (2015, 128, 133–134), Ridley (2019, 47, 270).
98 Manniche (2010, 148).
99 Cf. Ucko (2003, v).
100 Esp. Layton (2011, 203). "Ancient Egypt is itself a somewhat mysterious land for the modern European, posing its own problems of representation and translation in academic discourse."
101 Morkot (2003, 98–99). Ironically, Akhenaten's influence may have been due to the Ramesside dismantling of his structures and re-use of their materials.
102 de Certeau (1998, 56–113).

103 Charlton (1973, 200).
104 Foucault (2010, 48).
105 Liner notes for Philip Glass, *Akhnaten* (1984).
106 White (1978, 90).
107 Foucault (2010, 47).
108 Montserrat (2000, 12).

Bibliography

Aldred, Cyril. "Egypt: The Amarna Period." In *The Cambridge Ancient History*. Vol. 2, Part 2, 49–97. Cambridge: Cambridge University Press, 1975.

Aldred, Cyril. *Akhenaten: King of Egypt*. London: Thames & Hudson, 1988.

Aldred, Cyril, and A. T. Sandison. "The Pharaoh Akhenaten: A Problem in Egyptology and Pathology." *Bulletin of the History of Medicine* 36, no. 4 (1962): 293–316.

Asad, Talal. Review of *Orientalism*. by Edward Said. *EHR* 95, no. 376 (1980): 648–49.

Assmann, Jan. *Moses the Egyptian: The Memory of Egypt in Western Monotheism*. Cambridge: Harvard University Press, 1997.

Assmann, Jan. *Monotheismus und Kosmotheismus: Ägyptische Formen eines "Denkens des Einen" und ihre europäische Rezeptionsgeschichte*. Heidelberg: Winter, 1998.

Bell, Martha R. "An Armchair Investigation of KV 55." *JARCE* 27 (1990): 97–137.

Braverman, Irwin M., Donald B. Redford, and Philip A. Mackowiak. "Akhenaten and the Physiques of Egypt's 18th Dynasty." *Annals of Internal Medicine* 150, no. 8 (2009): 556–60.

Breasted, James Henry. *A History of Egypt: From the Earliest Times to the Persian Conquest*. New York: Scribner's Sons, 1909.

Brier, Bob. *The Murder of Tutankhamen: A True Story*. New York: Putnam's Sons, 1998.

Brugsch, Heinrich Karl. *Geschichte Aegypten's unter den Pharaonen: Nach den Denkmälern*. Leipzig: Hinrichs, 1877.

Brunner-Traut, Emma. *Frühformen des Erkennens: am Beispiel Altägyptens*. Darmstadt: Wissenschaftlich Buchgesellschaft, 1990.

Budge, E. A. Wallis. *Tutānkhàmen: Amenism, Atenism and Egyptian Monotheism*. New York: Dover, 1923.

Burridge, Alwyn. "Akhenaten: A New Perspective, Evidence of a Genetic Disorder in the Royal Family of 18th Dynasty Egypt." *JSSEA* 23 (1993): 63–64.

Burridge, Alwyn. "Did Akhenaten Suffer from Marfan's Syndrome?" *BA* 59, no. 2 (1996): 127.

Champollion, Jean-François. *Notices descriptives*. 5 Vols. 1st ed. 1844–49. Geneva: Éditions de Belles-Lettres, 1974.

Charlton, Nial. "Some Reflections on the History of Pharaonic Egypt." *JEA* 59 (1973): 200–5.

Codaccioni, Jean-Louis, Bernard Conte-Devolx, and Bruno Argémi. "Was Akhenaten Really Sick?" *Annales d'Endocrinologie* 74 (2013): 231–33.

Crubezy, Éric. "Le pharaon Akhenaton: avait-il une maladie auto-immune?" *Synoviale* 28 (1994): 30–33.

de Certeau, Michel. "The Historiographic Operation." In *The Writing of History*, translated by Tom Conley, 56–113. New York: Columbia University Press, 1998.

Derry, Douglas E. "A Note on the Skeleton Hitherto Believed to Be that of King Akhenaten." *ASAÉ* 31 (1931): 15–19.

Diderot, Denis, and Jean le Rond d'Alembert, eds. *L'Encyclopédie, ou dictionnaire raisonné des sciences, des arts et des métiers*. 28 Vols. Paris: Briasson, David, Le Breton, and Durand, 1751–72.

Dodson, Aidan. *Amarna Sunrise: Egypt from the Golden Age to the Age of Heresy*. Cairo: American University in Cairo Press, 2014.

Dodson, Aidan. *Amarna Sunset: Nefertiti, Tutankhamun, Ay, Horemheb, and the Egyptian Counter-Reformation.* New ed. Cairo: American University in Cairo, 2018.
Dodson, Aidan. *Nefertiti: Queen and Pharaoh of Egypt.* Cairo: American University in Cairo Press, 2020.
Drioton, Étienne, and Pierre du Bourguet. *Les Pharaons à la conquête de l'art.* 2nd ed. Paris: Desclée De Brouwer, 1978.
Engelbach, Rex. "The So-Called Coffin of Akhenaten." *ASAÉ* 31 (1931): 98–114.
Erman, Adolf. *Aegypten und aegyptisches Leben im Altertum.* Tübingen: Laupp, 1885.
Erman, Adolf. *Die Religion der Ägypter.* Berlin: de Gruyter & Co., 1934.
Filer, Joyce. "The KV 55 Body: The Facts." *EA* 17 (2000): 13–14.
Foucault, Michel. *The Archaeology of Knowledge and the Discourse on Language.* Translated by A. M. Sheridan Smith. New York: Vintage, 2010.
Gabolde, Marc. *Akhenaton: Du mystère à la lumière.* Paris: Gallimard, 2005.
Gardiner, Alan. *Egypt of the Pharaohs: An Introduction.* Oxford: Oxford University Press, 1961.
Harris, James E., Edward F. Wente, Charles F. Cox, Ibrahim El Nawaway, Charles J. Kowalski, Arthur T. Storey, William R. Russell, Paul V. Ponitz, and Geoffrey F. Walker. "Mummy of the 'Elder Lady' in the Tomb of Amenhotep II: Egyptian Museum Catalog Number 61070." *Science* 200, no. 4346 (1978): 1151.
Harris, J. R. "Akhenaten or Nefertiti." *AO* 38 (1977): 5–10.
Harrison, R. G. "An Anatomical Examination of the Pharaonic Remains Reported to be Akhenaten." *JEA* 52 (1966): 95–119.
Hawass, Zahi, Yehia Z. Gad, Somaia Ismail, Rabab Khairat, Dina Fathalla, Naglaa Hasan, Amal Ahmed, et al. "Ancestry and Pathology in King Tutankhamun's Family." *JAMA* 303, no. 7 (2010): 638–47.
Hoffmeier, James K. *Akhenaten and the Origins of Monotheism.* Oxford: Oxford University Press, 2015.
Hornung, Erik. "Gedanken zur Kunst der Amarnazeit." *ZÄS* 97 (1971): 74–78.
Hornung, Erik. "The Rediscovery of Akhenaten and His Place in Religion." *JARCE* 29 (1992): 43–49.
Hornung, Erik. *Akhenaten and the Religion of Light.* Translated by David Lorton. Ithaca: Cornell University Press, 1999.
Imbs, Paul. *Trésor de la langue française: dictionnaire de la langue du XIXe et du XXe siècle (1789–1960).* 16 Vols. Paris: Gallimard, 1985.
Jolliffe, David. "Discourse." In *Encyclopedia of Postmodernism,* edited by Victor E. Taylor and Charles E. Winquist, 101–3. London: Routledge, 2003.
Lacouture, Jean. *Champollion: une vie des lumières.* Paris: Grasset, 1988.
Layton, Robert. "Mysterious Lands – the Wider Context." In *Mysterious Lands,* edited by David O'Connor and Stephen Quirke, 203–13. London: Routledge, 2011.
Lepsius, Karl Richard. *Briefe aus Aegypten, Aethiopien und der Halbinsel des Sinai.* Berlin: Hertz, 1852.
Liner Notes for Glass, Philip. *Akhnaten.* Paul Esswood, the Stuttgart State Orchestra, Opera & Chorus, Dennis Russel Davies, conductor. CBS Masterworks, 1984.
Manniche, Lise. *The Akhenaten Colossi of Karnak.* Cairo: American University in Cairo Press, 2010.
Marchant, Jo. *The Shadow King: The Bizarre Afterlife of King Tut's Mummy.* Boston: Da Capo, 2013.
Mariette, Auguste. *Aperçu de l'histoire d'Égypte: Depuis les temps les plus reculés jusqu'à la Conquête Musulmane.* 3rd ed. Alexandria: Mourès, 1872.
Martin, Geoffrey T. *The Royal Tomb at El-'Amarna.* 2 Vols. London: Egypt Exploration Society, 1974.
Maspero, Gaston. *Histoire ancienne des peoples de l'Orient.* Paris: Hachette et Cie, 1872.
Maspero, Gaston. *New Light on Ancient Egypt.* Translated by Elizabeth Lee. New York: Appleton and Company, 1909.
Meyer, Eduard. *Geschichte des Altertums.* 5 Vols. Stuttgart: Cotta, 1884–1902.

Montserrat, Dominic. *Akhenaten: History, Fantasy and Ancient Egypt.* London: Routledge, 2000.

Morkot, Robert. "Archaism and Innovation in Art from the New Kingdom to the Twenty-Sixth Dynasty." In *'Never Had the Like Occurred:' Egypt's View of Its Past,* edited by John Tait, 79–99. London: Routledge, 2003.

Pendlebury, J. D. S. *Tell el-Amarna.* London: Dickson & Thompson, 1935.

Pratz, Mario. *On Neo-Classicism.* Translated by Angus Davidson. Evanston: Northwestern University Press, 1969.

Quinn, Frederick. *The Sum of All Heresies: The Image of Islam in Western Thought.* Oxford: Oxford University Press, 2008.

Redford, Donald B. *Akhenaten: The Heretic King.* Princeton: Princeton University Press, 1984.

Redford, Donald B. "Explaining Akhenaten's Physique." *BA* 59, no. 2 (1996): 128.

Reeves, Nicholas. "The Archaeological Analysis of KV 55: 1907–1990." In *The Tomb of Queen Tîyi*, edited by Theodore M. Davis, iv–xiv. 1st ed. 1910. San Francisco: KMT Communications, 1990.

Reeves, Nicholas. *Akhenaten: Egypt's False Prophet.* London: Thames & Hudson, 2001.

Ridley, Ronald T. *Akhenaten: A Historian's View.* Cairo: American University in Cairo Press, 2019.

Risse, Guenter B. "Pharaoh Akhenaton of Ancient Egypt: Controversies among Egyptologists and Physicians Regarding His Postulated Illness." *Journal of the History of Medicine and Allied Sciences* 26, no. 1 (1971): 3–17.

Robins, Gay. *Proportion and Style in Ancient Egyptian Art.* Austin: University of Texas Press, 1993a.

Robins, Gay. "The Representation of Sexual Characteristics in Amarna Art." *JSSEA* 23 (1993b): 29–41.

Robins, Gay. "Image and Reality in Amarna Art." In *Hommages à Fayzal Haikal,* edited by Nicolas Grimal, Amr Kamel, and Cynthia May-Sheikholeslami, 225–29. Paris: Institut française d'archéologie orientale, 2003.

Said, Edward. *Orientalism.* New York: Vintage, 1979.

Sandman, Maj. *Texts from the Time of Akhenaten.* Brussels: Fondation égyptologique Reine Élisabeth, 1938.

Smith, Grafton Elliot. "A Note on the Estimate of the Age Attained by the Person Whose Skeleton Was Found in the Tomb." In *The Tomb of Queen Tiye*, edited by Theodore M. Davis, iv–xiv. 1st ed. 1910. San Francisco: KMT Communications, 1990.

Smith, Grafton Elliot. *The Royal Mummies.* Cairo: Institut française d'archéologie orientale, 1912.

Smith, Grafton Elliot. *Tutankhamen and the Discovery of His Tomb by the Late Earl of Carnarvon and Mr. Howard Carter.* London: Routledge, 1923.

Smith, Grafton Elliot. "The Diversions of an Anatomist in Egypt." *Cambridge University Medical School Magazine* 4 (1926): 34–39.

Smith, Grafton Elliot. "The Pharaoh Akhenaton – A Problem in Medical Diagnosis." *Broadway, Westminster Hospital Gazette* 4 (1928): 25.

Tyldesley, Joyce. *Nefertiti: Egypt's Sun Queen.* New York: Viking, 1998.

Ucko, Peter. Foreward to *'Never Had the Like Occurred:' Egypt's View of Its Past.* Edited by John Tait, v–vi. London: Routledge, 2003.

Voltaire. *Dictionnaire philosophique.* 1st ed. 1764. Paris: Garnier Frères, 1961.

von Bunsen, Christian Karl Josias. *Aegyptens Stelle in der Weltgeschichte, Drittes Buch.* Hamburg: Friedrich Perthes, 1845.

Waddell, W. G. *Manetho.* Cambridge: Harvard University Press, 1940.

Weigall, Arthur. *The Treasury of Ancient Egypt: Miscellaneous Chapters of Ancient Egyptian History and Archaeology.* Edinburgh: Blackwood and Sons, 1911.

Weigall, Arthur. *The Life and Times of Akhnaton: Pharaoh of Egypt.* New York: Putnam's Sons, 1923.

Wente, Edward F., and James E. Harris. "Royal Mummies of the Eighteenth Dynasty: A Biologic and Egyptological Approach." In *After Tut'ankhamūn: Research and Investigation in the Royal Necropolis at Thebes,* edited by C. N. Reeves, 2–20. London: Kegan Paul, 1992.

White, Hayden. "The Historical Text as Literary Artifact." In *Tropics of Discourse: Essays in Cultural Criticism*, 81–100. Baltimore: The Johns Hopkins University Press, 1978.

Winckelmann, Johann. "Essay on the Beautiful in Art." In *Winckelmann: Writings on Art,* translated by David Irwin, 89–103. London: Phaidon, 1972.

Wolf, Walther. *Die Kunst Ägyptens: Gestalt und Geschichte.* Stuttgart: Kohlhammer, 1957.

5 Jaroslav Černý

Working with Disabilities in Egyptology, 1942–1970

Hana Navratilova

Introduction

In the 1940s–1960s, adjustments to accommodate disabled academics were not a common topic of discussion in workplaces. Yet, individually, destigmatisation and adaptation to disability took place. This study analyses the individual experience of a disabled Egyptologist in context of his time, using the methodological framework of disability history studies and biography.[1] In a narrative style, it first introduces the protagonist, adding the context for each episode of ill health and disability. Secondly, it analyses the responses of his epistemic community and social network. The paper contains references to self-harm and suicidal behaviour including paraphrases from primary sources with explicit content.

Jaroslav Černý (1898–1970)[2] experienced two major episodes of mental health difficulty: in the 1940s in Egypt in WWII, and in the 1950s in the UK, at the height of the Cold War. In the 1960s, he also had deteriorating vision while in part-time work as a retired academic. Twice, he experienced the 'total institution' (as E. Goffman described the asylum in 1957; published 1961) first in a military psychiatric unit of the British Army in Egypt in 1942 and then in two major psychiatric hospitals in London in 1951. In 1942, in a military perspective, he could have been easily classified as a man with a 'weak spot' (Roberts-Pedersen 2012) but he was extricated from any possibility of long-term military psychiatric care. In 1951, Černý was exposed to many complex aspects of an asylum life in London hospitals, yet also to the humane response of his psychiatrist, and fellow émigré from Central Europe, Erwin Stengel. Despite the challenges, he had developed a support network during the war, and later, as an employee and later emeritus of two major British universities (UCL, and University of Oxford), he experienced the advantages of the social and cultural capital inherent to his position.[3]

The narrative could easily emphasise Černý's willpower and 'overcoming of the burden of disability': despite systemic pressures, and specific conditions of mental health care in the post-war UK,[4] the protagonist of this paper developed effective coping strategies to maintain his professional and social status. Yet it was precisely this status that helped, as in the cases of other privileged individuals: 'aided by institutional privileges and those around him',[5] he could achieve a destigmatised position. To complicate matters further, Černý also was in an intersectional

DOI: 10.4324/9781003440369-7

position of potentially multiple vulnerabilities: as a stateless émigré, whose first language was not English, and with his status, income and ultimately personal safety entirely dependent on retaining his professional standing. Next to the recognition of a professional with disability, it is his intersectional position that makes his story particularly important.

1942

In late June and early July 1942, many trains from Cairo reached the train station of Qantara in the Eastern Nile Delta. The trains were teeming with people and their anxiety and it was rumoured that the Nazi armies might have overrun the Allied defences in the Western Delta and were ready to capture Egypt – or at least Cairo.[6] The rumours were not detailed, but they were ominous. The people feared Nazi *Einsatzgruppen* ready to destroy people and nations deemed subhuman by the Nazi ideology in Egypt[7] as they did in the *General Gouvernement* in Eastern Europe,[8] and in other regions under their occupation. Among them was a 44-year-old press attaché of the Czechoslovak legation in Cairo, a diplomatic institution entirely dependent on Allied war effort, since it was attached to an exiled Czechoslovak government in London. His name was Jaroslav Černý and like many people he took part in serving the Allied cause and his country of origin. He became known as an Egyptologist and not as a diplomat. Yet, at that point in time, he served in his diplomatic capacity and organised evacuations of Czechoslovak citizens from Cairo. However, he was also on the brink of a major personal crisis. His family was caught in the whirlwind of a Nazi protectorate controlling former Czechoslovakia. His professional, financial and academic standing were vulnerable to the war. His immediate thoughts were divided between the study of the past, the Egyptological work he had done for his internationally networked colleagues in Egypt, Britain, and France, and the mission he had to accomplish in the present: get the evacuees safely from Egypt to Palestine.

However, he could not see a future for himself, for his study, so dependent on the open, transnational lines of communication he had been used to during the years before the war. To the contrary, he could see himself captured by the enemy – the humiliation and death at their hands. He had weeks of reading information about Nazi murders in Bohemia, the monstrous retaliation of the SS after one of their top officers, Reinhard Heydrich, had been successfully assassinated in Prague in a Czech-British operation.

Jaro, as he had been known to his international friends, an affable, calm, self-aware and self-controlled gentleman, suppressed his anxieties for far too long. On the arrival to Qantara, the defences he kept putting up against anxiety, fear and hopelessness broke down. Jaro took a razor out of his travel *necessaire* and slashed his left wrist with deep cuts.

The military hospital in Qantara had a large psychiatric unit.[9] Černý was committed to it, as a 'delusional' patient with a significant physical wound. The Czechoslovak ministry of foreign affairs was informed by its Cairo legation that 'during the evacuation attaché Černý opened his veins'.[10] He stayed there for weeks until he was moved to a sanatorium in Helwan near Cairo. The move was debated, since he would be closer to the frontline in the Western Desert, and one medical opinion suggested this might have prompted further mental instability.[11] Eventually, his Czechoslovak diplomatic network had him moved closer to Cairo; that is closer to his Czechoslovak and international network of professionals and friends. When he was capable of written communication, in early August, he gave laconic references to the major crisis he had just survived. That he was in hospital was referred to briefly, and the reason for being there as an 'accident'. He added a terse footnote: 'I tried to commit suicide cutting my wrist but was saved. My arm is healing in a satisfactory way.'[12] From other records, it is known that this was an inaccurate assessment at best.

To his Egyptological connections, he had presented a clear image focussed on his research and their professional connections and needs. There was no personal space in his narrative. Most of the letter that contained the footnote (it is a footnote in a literal sense, appended to the main body of the text, marked with an asterisk) was dedicated to work on the Late Egyptian grammar. His *front-stage* or *persona* (to use Goffmann's terminology, 1971) was in full operation in the correspondence. This is not unusual for first-person suicide narratives,[13] apart from the fact that his narrative was not concerned with the suicide attempt except as apparent marginalia. A dominant part of that *persona* was Černý as a professional: reliable, hard-working and inventive. The vicissitude of war and its impact on him could not be negated, but it was relegated to a position where it should not be seen as defining him. In his personal narrative, that moment appeared annulled. It might have been Černý's impression management[14] strategy directed at his colleagues and peers, but equally his personal decision to suppress this episode. The impression is intensified by censored correspondence of his professional colleagues and friends, particularly Alan Henderson Gardiner and Herbert Walter Fairman.[15] Yet, next to this enforced silence of the sources, it is Černý's own relegation of a significant crisis point of his life. Irrespective of any specific diagnosis that may be offered or investigated, his self-management of a mental health challenge was that to remove it from the daily *persona,* and make sure it did not interfere with it.

At the time, Černý had support of his peer group in person in Cairo and remotely via correspondence. It is not attested that his work colleagues in the Czechoslovak diplomatic service or his colleagues in Egyptology would have judged him negatively, or attributed some 'lack of moral fibre'[16] to him as a result of his suicidal behaviour. He was often in company, had daily employment and was treated leniently by his employer, the legation, when it came to ringfencing time for his research interests. He might have decided to push the crisis to the background of his mind, as an overcome moment conditioned by one particular wartime setting. A relatively short stay in a psychiatric hospital might have also helped to frame his situation as an acute illness, not a long-term disability.[17]

Whether he spoke to his circle about his crisis or its aftermath at all remains a moot point. The Czechoslovak diplomatic despatches from Cairo to London ceased to mention his personal crisis after he had healed and left the Helwan hospital. In a summary, he lost neither his job nor his professional and personal standing, and he was afforded support at a difficult time. He recovered sufficiently to continue his work portfolio in diplomacy and Egyptology and in late 1943 left Cairo for London where he continued his dual career, eventually settling in London in 1946 as the Edwards Professor of Egyptology at UCL.

1950–1951

In 1950, Černý was again at a breaking point. Ostensibly he was a successful settled professional with a stable occupation in London, and a forthcoming offer of another professorial chair, the professorship of Egyptology at Oxford. Yet, that source of professional prestige was also apparently a source of great anxiety to him. Several factors played a role in his exhaustion, without Černý's articulating them.

At the UCL, he was a respected professional with a professorial chair since 1946, and involved in a teaching as well as research routine. He had not adapted his research workload, formed in the interwar years when he was a freelance, independent scholar, to the routine of the academic year. He might well have underestimated the regularity and time demands of an academic job with the term routine. In the post-war years, his international communication also grew almost exponentially; on most days, there were letters to read and to answer.[18] The workload was one factor.

Despite a privileged academic position, Černý faced a complex degree of uncertainty by 1950. He had lost his Czechoslovak citizenship, becoming a stateless person in the UK. This presented problems regarding his travel pattern (he had a British 'travel document' and later an UNESCO travel document, but not a regular passport). Whenever he left Britain for any of his research trips, easy and customary in his previous freelance interwar Egyptological life,[19] he was questioned by immigration officers upon return to the UK, and had to carry letters from his employer, the UCL, to prove he indeed had a stable employment in Britain. This might have created a low-level, but permanent hassle factor whereby his identity was constantly being destabilised, or so it might have appeared in comparison to his previous life.

He was also concerned about his family, friends and pupils in the Stalinist-controlled state of Czechoslovakia. He could no longer visit them, since any attempt to travel behind the Iron Curtain could have endangered him, and possibly also them. His personal life was, at least where Černý's expectations were concerned, also not stable. He found a partner during the war: a British-Czechoslovak linguist and educator Marie Sargant. They cohabited, but Marie, a divorcée, was not interested in, from her perspective, a precipitous new marriage. Yet this was what Černý preferred, having a very different perspective: that of settling down to create a domestic space in a country where he had become a stateless exile.

During 1950, he had also lost two close friends, people from two different but equally important contexts: from the British academe and from his international circle of expats living in Cairo. The former was Battiscombe 'Jack' Gunn, professor of Egyptology at Oxford. The latter was Bernhard Grdseloff, freelance

Egyptologist based in Cairo. Gunn died unexpectedly, Grdseloff after months of a painful stomach cancer.[20]

The factors combined to destabilise Černý, who had probably not processed his wartime breakdown. This time, Černý's first response, at least the documented one, was not self-harm. He craved attention from his partner and in private became very emotional and unpredictable. For several days in October 1950, he managed a strange balance of a composed public persona and private volatility, before being committed to the Maudsley Hospital. A long period of institutionalisation began, first in the Maudsley Hospital, and later in the Bethlem Royal Hospital. Černý stayed in the hospitals with some breaks from October 1950 to April 1951. During that time, Černý attempted another suicide in early spring 1951, while still in institutional care. Without access to his medical records, the description of his time in the hospital, including care he had been provided, must be approximate. What is undoubted is the level of distress Černý was in, and the anxiety his situation caused to his family, that is mainly Marie Sargant and her daughters, and friends.[21] The response of his mother and brother, cut off from direct contact behind the Iron Curtain in Prague, is unknown. Eventually, Černý recovered during spring 1951, after the crisis in February.

He was in the care of a fellow member of UCL, Aubrey Lewis, and another émigré from Central Europe, Erwin Stengel.[22] In a context of post-war Britain, his case was one among the many men in London statistically captured in the early 1950s. There was a marked rise in suicides and suicide attempts in London in the aftermath of the war, [23] although it had stalled somewhat since 1948 and 1949. Stengel and his colleagues considered the statistics unrepresentative: 'Almost daily, psychiatrists working in hospitals and out-patient clinics, see patients who had made suicidal attempts, often of a serious nature, which had not come to the knowledge of the authorities.'[24]

The immediate medical response was led by Stengel. Stengel's approach to suicide and suicide attempts was open-minded (suicide was technically still criminalised in Britain, and remained so until 1961[25]). 'The suicidal attempt is a complex behaviour pattern based on a variety of motivations: the wish to die, the desire to attack others, the appeal for help, and the urge to challenge fate.'[26] A suicide attempt was understood by Stengel, aware of the developments in sociology and psychiatry,[27] as a message to be interpreted and, once 'the individual significance of the appeal inherent in the suicidal attempt' could be established,[28] to be followed by qualified help and social adjustment. He did not accept a narrative that would see suicide as emotional blackmail, and rather considered them as 'social appeals' to be adequately answered.[29] Stengel's approach contrasted with a coeval search for 'organic aetiology of mental illness and the value of physical therapies, largely dismissing the influence of social and psychological factors in mental distress.'[30] The acute episodes of suicidal ideation and attempts also fitted the pattern of 'a hierarchy of mental disorder in which resources were directed towards 'promising' patients diagnosed with an acute neurotic disorder, at the expense of patients diagnosed with learning disabilities or chronic psychoses.'[31] This context does not lessen the engagement of Stengel with novel approaches, leading away from stigmatisation[32] and potentially damaging interventions, such as lobotomy.[33] The latter's limitations were eventually recognised.[34]

In this context, Černý was not prosecuted, and he was also, with all likelihood, not subject to an often-devastating treatment applied to violent patients, the lobotomy.[35] Instead Stengel treated him civilly, suggested occupational therapy[36] (knitting and light furniture-making), and worked closely with Marie Sargant to support Černý. In Černý's case the target was not to provide him with any alternative qualification that could have helped some patients to enter gainful employment. His own job had a double-edged role: it provided him with a sense of purpose but it could lead to overwork, especially if accompanied by a heightened sense of uncertainty and loss.

Mrs Sargant's role required much understanding and support, but she was also able to communicate her concerns that had led her earlier to some reluctance to commit. Marie Sargant had an interesting career. As one of the few female university graduates from her Moravian market town of Boskovice, she studied linguistics in Prague and then French and later English. She married Thomas Sargant and moved to Britain, losing her Czechoslovak citizenship.[37] As Sargant's wife she had a teaching job in London, and looked after their two daughters. They divorced during the Second World War, when she was working as an educator for the Czechoslovak government in exile in London. There she met Černý. Their relationship moved to cohabitation in 1946, when Černý obtained his UCL professorship of Egyptology. Yet, Černý, a long-time bachelor, was not very open about his previous life, and Sargant, in turn, was concerned about walking into another fully committed relationship and potentially losing a new partner again. In addition, it did not appeal to her to turn into the 'domestic goddess', a sort of motherly figure which Černý seemed to expect[38] (whilst having an undoubted respect for intellectual and professional success of women, shown in his long-term support for his female colleagues in Egyptology and for the ambitions of his stepdaughters). Only during the months of crisis, they learned to communicate their needs and expectations better. It is likely that Erwin Stengel was instrumental in supporting the couple, who eventually married in the summer of 1951. The stabilisation of personal life was probably a vital element in Černý's rehabilitation.

Černý's friends' response to the crisis was predictably uneasy. From early on, Rosalind Moss[39] linked his illness squarely to 'overwork'. Moss noted 'I'm afraid it will be almost impossible to prevent him from overworking when he is out of hospital.'[40] His colleague Eiddon Edwards[41] acted as his research secretary, and his administrative secretary at the UCL, Jean Tudor-Pole, also fielded replies to many letters, institutional and individual. On 6 March, Alan Gardiner, who was in Egypt, wrote a troubled letter that contained a curious mix of concern for Černý and outrage that his valued friend was capable of endangering their shared research mission. There was an element of call-of-duty to Gardiner's appeals, just as there had been during the war, but he exhibited much less understanding of the situation than he had in wartime. Gardiner introduced an element of his own self-interest into the conversation, just as Černý's former student Zbyněk Žába[42] did in his contemporary letters: 'I engaged you to come to England to undertake a very important piece of work which you yourself loved and which you have now tried to leave incomplete.'[43]

Černý's illness also had an institutional framework. UCL was concerned, but along rather different lines. The Provost, Pye, wrote to Dr Lewis on 26 October:

> I have heard with much concern of the illness of Professor J. Černý, our Professor of Egyptology. I do not know whether he will have come under your care. I gather from our lecturer Mr Arkell, who is his assistant, that Professor Černý's diagnosis is being considered by further experts so that presumably no one would wish to express any views at the present time. This note, therefore, is only to let you know of my profound anxiety about the case . . . if the illness is going to be a prolonged one, I shall need to think immediately about providing some alternative teaching for the students who would come under his direct care this term.[44]

In reply to Pye's letter, Lewis tried to reassure him:

> I do not think there are grounds for serious anxiety about Professor Černý's illness. He has had an emotional upset, similar in form to that which occurred in 1942 during the very pathetic circumstances of his departure from Czechoslovakia. His recent visit to Italy revived some of the memories connected with that; some private difficulties also flared up at this time. He has improved greatly, and when I saw him last Saturday, he was free from the more obvious symptoms which had led to his admission to hospital. I do not want to be too sanguine after such a short period of observation, but I would assume that he would certainly be back at University College by next term.[45]

In the same line, when the University of Oxford approached Černý some weeks later with the offer of a professorial chair, Lewis wrote to Douglas Veale, the registrar of University of Oxford, about a delay in recovery brought about by anxiety concerning the new posting. The key observation for Oxford University officials was about:

> A setback, which was to some extent related to his concern about this decision, which he found a very difficult one as he felt he had an obligation towards University College [UCL]. The Provost has recently, however, reassured him on this point, thereby smoothing the way for Professor Černý to accept the Oxford offer with a good conscience.[46]

Lewis helped his patient by highlighting a characteristic that an employer was likely to view as an asset – loyalty. It was a suitable conclusion to the case in the official record. Lewis also came to the conclusion that Černý would be fit to assume his new duties in October 1951, and Veale informed the appropriate academic bodies and the *University Gazette*, which announced a new postholder of the chair of Egyptology.[47]

Černý's healing was conditioned by personal as well as institutional circumstances, yet the personal side proved more decisive. The professorial offer from Oxford was important for his career and for the opportunities he had and also created for others as a high-profile professional in Egyptology. But its immediate impact on him was that of rising anxiety, while he was concerned with a conflict of loyalties, in a tug-of-war, that went three ways: to the UCL and his colleagues there, to Oxford as an institution and to Alan Gardiner, his long-term benefactor, who influenced both his election to the Edwards chair and to the chair at Oxford.

There was no evident ostracism, although his employers wanted to be informed on his suitability for the positions. No doubt, Gardiner's influence in Oxford was important too, yet the university could have decided otherwise, if strong voices prejudiced against the candidate would have been heard. Gardiner himself (see previous quote) may sound indeed not very compassionate at all, and focused largely on his own perspective. Yet, even so, his words also make it clear that he was not stigmatising Černý, and saw him as a high-profile professional. Gardiner's discourse was concerned with the discipline and value both of them had to offer. Although his comment may appear clumsy, Gardiner was also displaying lack of prejudice against mental illness, at least where one individual was concerned. As did other colleagues. Once out of immediate danger, Černý was immediately accepted back into his professional fold. There was no delay in the award of the professorship, and no delay in the outset of his academic duties in Michaelmas term 1951.

His previous professional standing had clearly influenced these views and opportunities. Although the result for him was that of forbearing acceptance, it might have been a case of professional esteem outweighing a potential 'negative', rather than a reflective openness to a psychiatric patient as their future colleague.[48] His social capital might have played a more important role than acceptance of his disability on its own. In other words: Černý was accepted because of *who* he was, not dismissed because of *what* affected him. The usual mechanism of stigma did not apply – the mechanism whereby '[p]eople who are labelled are placed in a distinct category and viewed as separate from the norm (e.g., us vs. them). They are no longer thought of as unique individuals, but as members of a homogeneous group.'[49]

No job is protected from the challenges of mental ill health. 'In the history of medicine, few conditions other than mental illnesses have cast such a pall on an individual, their family, health providers, health systems, and health research.'[50] The levels of stigma surrounding mental ill health and by extension psychiatry[51] spread rapidly. 'Doctors dealing with the insane have long lamented that they get tarred with their patients' brush, and are popularly associated with lunacy itself: words like "shrink" and "trick cyclist" say it all.'[52]

The possibility that mentally ill or disabled academics may and do face discrimination (or at least feel they should not disclose their condition as disadvantaging) has been discussed, although not necessarily comprehensively (e.g., Brown and Leigh 2018, 2020); hence the subject is not only of historical interest, but also still relevant for lived experience today. It is logical that people trying to get on the employment ladder (or indeed just trying to start their career in academia) are substantially concerned about the negative impact of possible or perceived ableism, since they do not yet have a position of esteem and a social network of a calibre seen as sufficient to protect them, as it protected Černý: 'Peer support is a key component of recovery-oriented care because it focuses on strengths, the positive aspects of people, and their ability to function effectively in social roles that are meaningful to them.'[53]

In addition, the framing of a *curable* patient as opposed to a long-term asylum inmate could have played a role again. Since the 1930s, the debate about mental health care included this aspect: 'Supporting the Mental Treatment Bill in the House of Commons, the Minister of Health Arthur Greenwood discussed the plight of "the man broken down by overwork or the woman suffering from puerperal mania", who "ought to receive treatment different from that of the certified lunatic"'.[54]

With his professional identity well managed, and with a social network that ultimately proved supportive, the career of the professor of Egyptology thus continued for Černý at Oxford from the autumn of 1951 onwards. During the early 1960s, he encountered another, physical illness. His eyesight began to deteriorate. In 1961, Černý had a cataract surgery. He continued his pedagogical and research workload until his retirement in 1965, and beyond. He accepted guest professorships and continued his fieldwork in Egypt. The former, it appears, was one adaptation to the fact of his failing eyesight. His teaching engagement, especially discussions with more experienced students, was unaffected.

Fieldwork in the Late 1960s

His fieldwork in Egypt required different adaptations. Between 1925 and 1970, Černý was a member of several fieldwork teams. His first fieldwork engagement was at Deir el-Medina, a settlement of New Kingdom workmen that had been in his research focus since the 1920s. His fieldwork profile was mainly that of an epigrapher, not a field archaeologist, yet he was occasionally responsible for overseeing archaeological work.

His fieldwork in Deir el-Medina continued until the early 1940s, and was briefly revived after the war, only to lapse in the 1950s, due to both personal factors and political factors in Egypt. However, his lifelong work on the texts from Deir el-Medina continued.

Černý undertook an epigraphy mapping project during the war. It was his private initiative mapping mainly Old Kingdom monuments in Abusir and Saqqara. Although he never published his results, it inspired his and his colleagues' thoughts about systematic mapping projects concerned with all Egyptian monuments. When UNESCO and the Egyptian government initiated such a project in 1954, Černý was involved, and continued to be a part of the Egyptian and international effort in the Nubian campaign in the 1960s.[55]

His last major fieldwork project was the graffiti in the Theban Mountain, in which he had an interest since 1925. These carved, scratched or pecked texts and figures in the rocky landscape reflected the community of workmen operating mostly at the royal necropolis of Western Thebes.[56] This project was also the most affected by his visual impairment. However, Černý developed a method of mapping and recording that involved several steps, maximising his potential and that of his team. The mapping of the Theban Mountain began with aerial photography and geographers' work; a detailed map was produced, followed by recording of stone cliffs that were covered by a network of texts and images, sometimes responding to each other, or to their environment. Since the *Graffiti de la Montaigne Thébaine*,[57] our understanding of this meaningful landscape, shaped by generations of literate Egyptians, has developed significantly, but it was the *GMT* project that gave the study of epigraphy in the landscape an important impetus. The team consisted of an international group of Egyptian and European specialists.

The *GMT* team also used legacy records, notes and maps by Wilhelm Spiegelberg or Howard Carter, to review the locations of known inscriptions and search for new ones, since both texts and images in this setting tend to cluster. Černý revisited texts he had mapped and published himself[58] in addition to Spiegelberg.[59] Enlarged copies of texts (less often figures) were made by team members, mostly Aziz Sadek or Hassan Achiry, often with the help of Marie Černá, for Černý to inspect and help with the reading of hieratic. Everyone learned in the process: Černý was an expert in the cursive script, hieratic, which adopted specific forms when applied onto the rock cliff face.[60] He had an uncanny ability to spot the traces of graffiti, either from memory or from traces he could no longer see accurately. But he had to borrow his colleagues' eyes to analyse the details. A cooperative model of work was not new to him, but it acquired a new dimension, with a consistent involvement of his Egyptian colleagues, directly involved in a highly professional recording and reading. They in turn had the openness to accept Černý as a mentor. Personal qualities and political context were both likely to have had a part in this arrangement. His participation in CEDAE and UNESCO operations, and his perception by colleagues, was characteristic of his transnational beliefs. He was suitable, since he was a scholar with international ties but with a suitably non-aligned UNESCO passport.[61]

Defying Stigma: Creating Opportunity Out of Challenge

Černý was ultimately not stigmatised by his professional community or his family. The 1940s wartime trauma may require a specific perspective: as disabled veterans have been treated differently from disabled civilians, so wartime trauma has its own perception, its own social capital, such as within the 'military citizenship'.[62] The 1950s and 1960s responses and adaptations are more relevant for the general experience of disability, but even here the social position of Černý and his social network were decisive in influencing an outcome that many of his coevals could not have taken for granted, with his social position retained and his family network boosted. Stigma survives in professional, personal and public context (Byrne 2001), and it was a pronounced concern for mental health in the 1950s.[63] The reasons for stigmatisation are not simple, and often reflect the observers' practical concerns and personal fears.[64] Černý was treated as a patient in recovery, not as a chronic mental health 'sufferer' for whom rehabilitation and social acceptance would have been more complicated.

In the early 1950s, the institutional responses of Černý's employer, the UCL, and his then prospective employer, the University of Oxford, were also multifaceted. Both institutions sought reassurances from psychiatrists, yet neither rejected Černý. Recognition of his value as a person and a professional appears to have had more validity than complications envisaged as potentially arising from his illness, no doubt deploying the social capital of esteem in which Černý was held by colleagues. Neither intellectually vain nor timid (see Tanesini 2018), his position assured a positive response affirming his competence and ability, even in the moment of potential 'stigmatisation' and loss of his social capital. Arguably at an intersection of vulnerability and privilege, Černý and his peers challenged expectations about capacity of disabled people, but his exceptional status must always be considered. His personal recovery and professional development depended on many factors: his undiminished social capital, as well as the acute character of his illness were most likely in his favour. He achieved this result because his social network was willing to see him as an individual, but also because he was committed to a high work ethic and his professional value might well have overshadowed most other concerns. He was never 'an individual whose status as a citizen had been subsumed and eroded by their diagnosis'.[65] Yet, before we come to judge his peers and institutions as just 'pragmatic', we may want to consider the value of pragmatic evaluations and solutions, alongside an incremental move toward a more permissive society.[66]

Finally, in the 1960s, as an established scholar, Černý had to seek a solution to his increasing vision impairment, whilst leading a significant epigraphy campaign in Western Thebes, Egypt. He found it via inclusive teamwork by an international workgroup, which strengthened the participation of his Egyptian colleagues in recording and processing roles. It was an example of adaptation to disability that at the same time assured a development of the epistemic community of Egyptology.

His case is an example of an Egyptologist with disability living and working at a historical intersection of social and political changes and his own émigré status. It emphasises the impact and value of both systemic patterns and individual agency in the life of disabled researchers, particularly the importance of social interactions and network, which may prove to be more influential in an individual case than a systemic burden of medical limitations or social expectations.

Notes

1 See Nielsen 2018.
2 For an overview of his life and work see Bierbrier 2019, 94–95, for a recent biography Navratilova 2023.
3 His life, its context and archival sources, as well as modern history secondary literature relevant for the era are included in Navratilova 2023.
4 Taylor and Brumby 2020, Long 2014; see also Harrington 2016, a case study regarding the transformation of mental health care from the late 1940s onwards.
5 Nielsen 2018, 23, about F. D. Roosevelt.
6 For the history of this period see Cooper 1995.
7 Kitchen 2009, 278.
8 Snyder 2010, 188–201.

9 The no. 41 Neuropathic Hospital at Qantara, see Harrison 2004, 123.
10 AMZV, Londýnský archiv, File Legation Cairo, report by envoy B. Szalatnay-Stachó.
11 AMZV, Londýnský archiv, File Legation Cairo, dispatch August 13, 1942.
12 GIA, Collection Gardiner, Correspondence, AHG 42.56.29 [should be 29a], August 5, 1942.
13 Bantjes and Swartz 2019.
14 Goffman 1971.
15 Bierbrier et al. 2019, 175–76 (Gardiner), 157 (Fairman).
16 The term was used in the British military, specifically in the Royal Air Force; and it has been perceived as problematic. In recollections of an RAF medical officer: 'One of the most disturbing problems was the psychological trauma of returning aircrew from bombing raids. Some refused to face the ordeal and we had to classify them as showing lack of moral fibre, a diagnosis that resulted in officers and others being demoted to the lowest ranks. Such draconian measures were considered necessary at that time as we were desperately short of aircrew. The medical officer's task was further aggravated by the aircrew taking the view that those who had never experienced the hazards were not competent to make dispassionate judgement' (Trainer 1994, 330).
17 See the differences noted in perception in short-term and long-term mental illness, Long 2014, chapter 3.
18 For the statistics and details see Navratilova 2023.
19 On which see Navratilova 2023 and also Navratilova 2019.
20 See Navratilova 2023 including references to the correspondence in the Griffith Institute Archive, Černý Mss. 21.
21 Information on this episode is largely derived from the diary of Anna Sargant (family archive, courtesy Anna Allott), and from the exchange of letters between Černý and Marie Sargant, as well as Alan Gardiner, Eiddon Edwards and administration at the UCL: the Černý Collection, Griffith Institute Archive, University of Oxford, Černý Mss. 21.
22 On Stengel, and his generation of psychiatrist and neurologist refugees: Loewenau 2016. See also Berrios and Freeman 1991, 436–44.
23 Stengel 1961, 27–28.
24 Stengel 1961, 30.
25 See Neeleman 1996.
26 Stengel 1961, 123.
27 See also Berrios and Porter 1995, 612–32.
28 Stengel 1961, 130.
29 Stengel 1961, 119–20.
30 Long 2014, 112.
31 Long 2014, 123.
32 The term was promoted by Goffman 1963; a recent view on stigma and mental health: Vogel and Wade 2022, including a review of suicide stigma as a specific category not identical with a more general mental health stigma, 143–57.
33 Stengel 1950.
34 Tooth and Newton 1961, 21.
35 Despite a possible misunderstanding by his stepdaughter Naomi Sargant (Lady MacIntosh of Haringey, see Tuckett 2014).
36 For its context, also beyond occupational therapy itself, see Long in Dale and Melling 2006, 179–99.
37 For the life of Marie Sargant see Navratilova 2021.
38 This was also shown in their oral communication, in his appellation 'Mummy', applied to his partner earlier, and changed into Manya, a diminutive of her name, after the crisis. The details in internal family communications pre-1951 were observed in the diary of Anna Sargant, the daughter of Marie. Courtesy family archive of Anna Allott.
39 Bierbrier et al. 2019, 330.

40 GIA, Collection Černý, Černý Mss. 21.1439.
41 Bierbrier et al. 2019, 146–47.
42 Bierbrier et al. 2019, 507.
43 GIA, Collection Černý, Černý Mss. 21.803, March 6, 1951.
44 London, UCL Records Department, File no. 6/1/3 Professor J. Černý, 52; Letter dated October 26, 1950, from D. R. Pye to A. Lewis, carbon copy.
45 London, UCL Records Department, File no. 6/1/3 Professor J. Černý, 55; Letter from A. Lewis to D. R. Pye, November 1, 1950.
46 OUA, Professorship of Egyptology, Shelf Mark WR 6/ER/2 file 1, April 4, 1951, A. Lewis to the University of Oxford; see also UCL Records Department, File no. 6/1/3, Professor J. Černý.
47 The *Oxford University Gazette*, Vol LXXXI, April 12, 1951, 687. For details of the process see Navratilova 2023.
48 Tanesini 2018, 52.
49 Stuart and Sartorius 2022, 2.
50 Stuart and Sartorius 2022, 1, following Goffman 1963.
51 Madness and psychiatry formed a specifically modern historical dialogue developing throughout the nineteenth and twentieth centuries (overview Porter 1987).
52 Berrios and Porter 1995, 238.
53 Stuart and Sartorius 2022, 9.
54 Long 2014, 103.
55 For details see Navratilova 2023.
56 Summary Salmas 2018; Rzepka 2014; series *GMT;* Dorn 2014, 2018.
57 Černý et al. 1969.
58 Černý 1956.
59 Spiegelberg 1921.
60 Ali 2002, the palaeography of the Theban rock inscriptions is currently investigated also by Tabitha Kraus.
61 This was also the view taken by Christiane Desroches-Noblecourt: see 1992, 176, 2003, 32.
62 Compare Gerber 2018.
63 For an outline of the history of mental health stigma see Stuart and Sartorius 2022, chapter 1. Note that Berrios and Porter (1995) consistently included a clinical and a social section for every diagnosis in their *History of Clinical Psychiatry.* The social sections also noted the perception of each disorder in a complex network of patients, physicians and the public. Stigmatising discourses have many roots and agendas (compare also Long 2014, 'Conclusion'), not least 'the sense of the fragility of the self' (Berrios and Porter 1995, 31).
64 Long 2014, 'Conclusion'.
65 Long 2014, 221.
66 Thomson 2006, 250–88.

Bibliography

Ali, Mohamed Sherif. *Hieratische Ritzinschriften Aus Theben: Paläographie Der Graffiti Und Steinbruchinschriften: Göttinger Orientforschungen, 4.* Vol. 34. Reihe: Ägypten, Wiesbaden: Harrassowitz, 2002.

Avison, William R. "Social Networks as Risk and Protective Factors for Onset and Recurrence of Mental Disorders." *Current Opinion in Psychiatry* 9, no. 2 (1996): 149–52. https://doi.org/10.1097/00001504-199603000-00012.

Bantjes, Jason, and Leslie Swartz. " 'What Can We Learn from First-Person Narratives?' The Case of Nonfatal Suicidal Behavior." *Qualitative Health Research* 29, no. 10 (2019): 1497–507. https://doi.org/10.1177/1049732319832869.

Berrios, G. E., and Hugh L. Freeman. *150 Years of British Psychiatry.* Edited by Royal College of Psychiatrists. London: Gaskell: Athlone, 1991.
Berrios, G. E., and Roy Porter. *A History of Clinical Psychiatry: The Origin and History of Psychiatric Disorders.* London: Athlone, 1995.
Bierbrier, M. L., *Who was Who in Egyptology.* 5th rev. ed. London: Egypt Exploration Society, 2019.
Brown, Nicole, and Jennifer Leigh. "Ableism in Academia: Where Are the Disabled and Ill Academics?" *Disability & Society* 33, no. 6 (2018): 985–89. https://doi.org/10.1080/09687599.2018.1455627.
Brown, Nicole, and Jennifer Leigh. *Ableism in Academia: Theorising Experiences of Disabilities and Chronic Illnesses in Higher Education.* UCL Press, 2020. https://doi.org/10.2307/j.ctv13xprjr.
Byrne, Peter. "Psychiatric Stigma." *The British Journal of Psychiatry* 178, no. 3 (2001): 281–84. https://doi.org/10.1192/bjp.178.3.281.
Černý, Jaroslav. *Graffiti Hiéroglyphiques et Hiératiques de La Nécropole Thébaine: Nos 1060 à 1405. Vol. 9: Documents de Fouilles de l'Institut Français d'archéologie Orientale.* Le Caire: L'institut français d'archéologie orientale, 1956.
Černý, Jaroslav, et al. *Graffiti de la montagne thébaine.* Le Caire: Centre de documentation et d'études sur l'ancienne Egypte, Collection scientifique (Markaz Tasjīl al-Āthār al-Miṣrīyah), 1969.
Cooper, Artemis. *Cairo in the war 1939–1945.* London: Penguin, 1995.
Dale, Pamela, and Joseph Melling. *Mental Illness and Learning Disability since 1850: Finding a Place for Mental Disorder in the United Kingdom.* Edited by Pamela Dale and Joseph Melling. London: Routledge, 2006. http://www.loc.gov/catdir/toc/ecip0517/2005022712.html.
Davis, Lennard J. *The Disability Studies Reader.* Florence, United States: Taylor & Francis Group, 2013. http://ebookcentral.proquest.com/lib/oxford/detail.action?docID=1125176.
Desroches-Noblecourt, Christiane. *La Grande Nubiade: Ou Le Parcours d'une Égyptologue.* Paris: Stock and Pernoud, 1992.
Desroches-Noblecourt, Christiane. *Sous le regard des dieux.* Paris: Albin Michel, 2003.
Dorn, Andreas. "Von Graffiti Und Königsgräbern Des Neuen Reiches." In *The Workman's Progress: Studies in the Village of Deir El-Medina and Other Documents from Western Thebes in Honour of Rob Demarée,* edited by B. J. J. Haring, O. E. Kaper, and R. van Walsem, 57–71. Leiden and Leuven: Nederlands Instituut voor het Nabije Oosten; Peeters, 2014.
Dorn, Andreas. "Graffiti de La Montagne Thébaine (GMT) 2012/2013: Old and New Graffiti from Western Thebes. Report of the 1st Campaign of the Graffiti in the Valleys of Western Thebes Project." In *Outside the Box: Selected Papers from the Conference 'Deir El-Medina and the Theban Necropolis in Contact' Liège, 27–29 October 2014,* edited by Andreas Dorn and Stéphane Polis, 141–55. Liège: Presses Universitaires de Liège, 2018.
Gerber, David A. "Disabled Veterans and the Wounds of War." In *The Oxford Handbook of Disability History,* edited by Michael Rembis, Catherine Kudlick, and Kim E. Nielsen. Oxford University Press, 2018. https://doi.org/10.1093/oxfordhb/9780190234959.013.28.
Goffman, Erving. *Asylums: Essays on the Social Situation of Mental Patients and Other Inmates.* 1st ed. Garden City, NY: Anchor Books, 1961.
Goffman, Erving. *Stigma: Notes on the Management of Spoiled Identity. Spectrum Book.* Englewood Cliffs: Prentice-Hall, 1963.
Goffman, Erving. *The Presentation of Self in Everyday Life.* London: Penguin, 1971.
Harrington, Valerie. "Integration in a Divided World: Salford Community Mental Health Services 1948–1974." In *Deinstitutionalisation and After: Post-War Psychiatry in the Western World: Mental Health in Historical Perspective,* edited by Despo Kritsotaki, Vicky Long, and Matthew Smith, 135–54. Cham: Springer International Publishing, 2016. https://doi.org/10.1007/978-3-319-45360-6_7.

Harrison, Mark. *Medicine and Victory: British Military Medicine in the Second World War.* Oxford: University Press, 2004.
Kitchen, Martin. *Rommel's Desert War: Waging World War II in North Africa, 1941–1943. Cambridge Military Histories.* Cambridge: University Press, 2009.
Kritsotaki, Despo, Vicky Long, and Matthew Smith. *Deinstitutionalisation and after: Post-War Psychiatry in the Western World [Electronic Resource]. Mental Health in Historical Perspective.* Cham: Palgrave MacMillan, 2016. https://ezproxy-prd.bodleian.ox.ac.uk/login?url=; https://link.springer.com/10.1007/978-3-319-45360-6.
Kudlick, Catherine, Kim E. Nielsen, and Michael Rembis. *The Oxford Handbook of Disability History: Oxford Handbooks.* 1st ed. Oxford: Oxford University Press, 2018.
Loewenau, Aleksandra. "Between Resentment and Aid: German and Austrian Psychiatrist and Neurologist Refugees in Great Britain since 1933." *Journal of the History of the Neurosciences: New Perspectives on Forced Migration in the History of Twentieth-Century Neuroscience* 25, no. 3 (2016): 348–62. https://doi.org/10.1080/0964704X.2016.1161407.
Long, Vicky. *Destigmatising Mental Illness? Professional Politics and Public Education in Britain, 1870–1970. Disability History.* Manchester: University Press, 2014.
McGeachan, Cheryl. " 'Do You Have a Frog to Guide You?': Exploring the 'Asylum' Spaces of R. D. Laing." In *Deinstitutionalisation and After: Post-War Psychiatry in the Western World: Mental Health in Historical Perspective,* edited by Despo Kritsotaki, Vicky Long, and Matthew Smith, 195–213. Cham: Springer International Publishing, 2016. https://doi.org/10.1007/978-3-319-45360-6_10.
Navratilova, Hana. "Between Patronage and an Egyptological Invisible College: The Early Career of Jaroslav Černý." In *En Détail – Philologie Und Archäologie Im Diskurs: Festschrift Für Hans-Werner Fischer-Elfert.* Vol. 2, edited by Peter Dils, Dietrich Raue, Franziska Naether, Lutz Popko, and Marc Brose, 799–814. Berlin and Boston: De Gruyter, 2019. https://doi.org/10.1515/9783110629705-037.
Navratilova, Hana. "Student, Diplomat, Wife, Traveller: A Transnational Life of Marie Sargant-Černý." In *Thanks for Typing: Remembering Forgotten Women in History,* edited by Juliana Dresvina, 88–101. London: Bloomsbury Academic, 2021.
Navratilova, Hana. *A Citizen of Nowhere.* Leuven: Peeters for Griffith Institute, 2023.
Neeleman, J. "Suicide as a Crime in the UK: Legal History, International Comparisons and Present Implications." *Acta Psychiatrica Scandinavica* 94, no. 4 (1996): 252–57. https://doi.org/10.1111/j.1600-0447.1996.tb09857.x.
Nielsen, Kim E. "The Perils and Promises of Disability Biography." In *The Oxford Handbook of Disability History,* edited by Michael Rembis, Catherine Kudlick, and Kim E. Nielsen, 0. Oxford University Press, 2018. https://doi.org/10.1093/oxfordhb/9780190234959.013.2.
Oosterhuis, Harry, and Cecile Aan de Stegge. "Between Emotional Involvement and Professional Detachment: The Challenges of Nursing in Dutch Mental Institutions (1880–1980)." *Social History of Medicine* 34, no. 4 (2021): 1277–396. https://doi.org/10.1093/shm/hkaa086.
Porter, Roy. *A Social History of Madness: Stories of the Insane.* London: Weidenfeld & Nicolson, 1987.
Porter, Roy. *The Faber Book of Madness.* London: Faber and Faber, 1991.
Ramanathan, Vaidehi. *Bodies and Language: Health, Ailments, Disabilities.* Bristol, United Kingdom: Multilingual Matters, 2009. http://ebookcentral.proquest.com/lib/oxford/detail.action?docID=543910.
Roberts-Pedersen, Elizabeth. "A Weak Spot in the Personality? Conceptualising 'War Neurosis' in British Medical Literature of the Second World War." *The Australian Journal of Politics and History* 58, no. 3 (2012): 408–20. https://doi.org/10.1111/j.1467-8497.2012.01644.x.
Rzepka, Sławomir. *Who, Where and Why: The Rock Graffiti of Members of the Deir El-Medina Community.* Warszawa: Pro-Egipt, 2014.
Salmas, Anne-Claire. "Space and Society at Deir El-Medina: Delineating the Territory of a Specific 'Social Group'." In *Outside the Box: Selected Papers from the Conference 'Deir*

El-Medina and the Theban Necropolis in Contact' Liège, 27–29 October 2014, edited by Andreas Dorn and Stéphane Polis, 421–45. Liège: Presses Universitaires de Liège, 2018.

Schillmeier, Michael. *Rethinking Disability: Bodies, Senses, and Things.* London, United Kingdom: Taylor & Francis Group, 2010. http://ebookcentral.proquest.com/lib/oxford/detail.action?docID=481141.

Sheehan, Lindsay, and Patrick W. Corrigan. "A Critical Review of Approaches to Erasing the Stigma of Mental Illness." In *The Oxford Handbook of the Sociology of Disability*, November 10, 2021. https://doi.org/10.1093/oxfordhb/9780190093167.013.48.

Snyder, Timothy. *Bloodlands: Europe between Hitler and Stalin.* London: Bodley Head, 2010.

Spiegelberg, Wilhelm. *Ägyptische und Andere Graffiti (Inschriften und Zeichnungen) aus der Thebanischen Nekropolis*. Heidelberg: C. Winters Universitätsbuchhandlung, 1921.

Stengel, Erwin. "A Follow-up Investigation of 330 Cases Treated by Prefrontal Leucotomy." *The Journal of Mental Science* 96, no. 404 (1950): 633–62.

Stengel, Erwin. Attempted Suicide: Its Social Significanc*e and* Effects. *Maudsley Monographs, 4.* London: Oxford University Press, 1961.

Stuart, Heather, and Norman Sartorius. *Paradigms Lost, Paradigms Found: Lessons Learned in the Fight Against the Stigma of Mental Illness.* Oxford: University Press, Incorporated, 2022.

Tanesini, Alessandra. "Caring for Esteem and Intellectual Reputation: Some Epistemic Benefits and Harms." *Royal Institute of Philosophy Supplements* 84 (November 2018): 47–67. https://doi.org/10.1017/S1358246118000541.

Taylor, Steven J., and Alice Brumby. *Healthy Minds in the Twentieth Century: In and Beyond the Asylum. Mental Health in Historical Perspective.* Cham: Springer International Publishing AG, 2020.

Thomson, Mathew. *The Problem of Mental Deficiency: Eugenics, Democracy, and Social Policy in Britain, c. 1870–1959. Oxford Historical Monographs.* Oxford: Clarendon Press, 1998.

Thomson, Mathew. *Psychological Subjects.* Oxford: Oxford University Press, 2006.

Tooth, G. C., Mary P. Newton, Great Britain, and Ministry of Health. *Leucotomy in England and Wales, 1942–1954.* London: H.M.S.O, 1961.

Trainer, J. L. "Memoir: Lack of Moral Fibre." *BMJ: British Medical Journal* 308, no. 6924 (1994): 330–30.

Tuckett, Alan. "Sargant, Naomi Ellen, Lady McIntosh of Haringey (1933–2006), Broadcaster and Educationist." In *Oxford Dictionary of National Biography*, 2014. https://doi.org/10.1093/ref:odnb/97390.

Vogel, David L., and Nathaniel G. Wade. *The Cambridge Handbook of Stigma and Mental Health. Cambridge Handbooks in Psychology.* Cambridge: Cambridge University Press, 2022. https://doi.org/10.1017/9781108920995.

6 Overlooked but on Display

Disability and Human Remains in the British Museum

Roisin Mackie

Introduction

There has been a recent increase in research on how museums display disability; however, this has almost entirely focused on material culture[1] with human remains rarely considered. Given the large number of human remains in UK museums, and the immense public favour towards their display, it is logical to consider disabled remains. Many disabled people are strongly against displaying any disabled human remains because there may be no way to display them in a way that provides no possible risk of dehumanisation and voyeurism by inviting the public to stare.[2] However, museums make their curatorial decisions on what they perceive the public expects to see in displays; as such, human remains are commonly displayed in Egyptological exhibitions.

Disability may be seen as a modern term; however, the concept has existed throughout history. When considering disability and what it means for this study, a key factor is the social model of disability, which creates a clear distinction between impairment and disability. Impairment refers to a biomedical condition, and disability refers to the social relationship between the individual with said condition and the society in which they reside.[3] The social model arose through the civil rights movement in the 1960s in the US.[4] This then influenced a reconceptualisation of disability in the UK, rejecting the previously used medical model which views disability as an individual medical tragedy, usually seen as then requiring a cure, control, or segregation,[5] shifting focus to the disabling nature of society. The social model was radical in that it showed that social oppression and the perceived negativity of disability were not inevitable or inherent, thus providing a mechanism for social change.[6] Creating a binary between disability and impairment, as the social model does, can lead to a continuation of binary thinking, in that impairment is purely associated with the body, and disability with society.[7] However, the body is material and will be affected by societal and environmental factors. Bodies are therefore significant[8] and impairment and disability are intrinsically linked. While impairment itself will not make an individual disabled, it is important to consider what it would have meant in the past.

Nothing About Us Without Us

For this study, the researcher's lived experience of disability has impacted their opinion on the curation of disabled remains and how they interpret disability. The

DOI: 10.4324/9781003440369-8

curation of disability in museum spaces will always be the most authentic when done by or with disabled individuals. This is in line with "Nothing about us without us," the phrase which fuels much of the disability rights movement, which "expresses the conviction of people with disabilities that *they* know what is best for them."[9] This will be the case when interpreting disability in the past. Disabled people will have a more nuanced understanding of the disabled experience, even if what they are investigating in the past may not be an identical experience to their own. The investigation of curation of disabled human remains will also benefit from the researcher being disabled, since they are aware of accessibility requirements for disabled visitors and can evaluate successful representation.

Disability Representation in Museums

The disabled community are often underrepresented in museum spaces and can be seen as disenfranchised from traditional heritage due to the denial of their rights as citizens, and the resulting denial of control over the representation of their pasts.[10] What are often seen are depictions that exist to inspire pity and condescending admiration from the non-disabled while reinforcing a sense of superiority, reminding them how 'lucky' they are to not be disabled.[11] This influence of negative representations of disability affects the interactions between disabled and non-disabled people, often providing justification for enduring prejudice and discrimination.[12] However, if representation and curation are done right, it can cause fundamental shifts in perceptions of disabled people.[13]

It is important for disabled people to be able to see themselves in museums. "Rethinking Disability Representation in Museums and Galleries" was a project led by the Research Centre for Museums and Galleries (RCMG).[14] It showed that centring disabled stories in spaces where, historically, they have been overlooked can have a powerful impact on disabled audiences.[15] One of the exhibitions formed for the project was "Talking about . . . Disability and Art," a fine art display showing representations of disability with accessible interpretation by disabled people. One response to the exhibition, from a disabled woman called Elaine, highlights the significance and emotional impact of curating disability. She wrote: "At last . . . I'm here [in the centre] . . . not here [at the margins]."

It is also crucial for museums to be accessible. Not only does accessibility benefit everyone, but often adjustments to museums are inexpensive, with excuses for them not being implemented being awareness and willingness of staff. However, adjustments also need not be made if a display is designed to be accessible from the start. This should especially be a consideration when curating disability-related displays: what is the point of telling disabled stories if disabled people themselves cannot access them?

The Curation of 'Freaks'

Historically, disability in museums was presented through the lens of 'freakery.' From the mid-eighteenth to the late nineteenth century, museums were often allied to freakshows, and collected artefacts related to disabled, often exploited, individuals in the name of curiosity or study.[16] Physical difference was sensationalised and displayed, forcing individuals to exploit themselves through freakshows during their lives and past their death. Many individuals have unwillingly formed large parts of anatomical and pathological collections. Disabled people today still experience the everyday invasion of staring which freakshows exploited. The implications of this permission to stare could then have impacts outside museums.[17]

An example is Charles Byrne. He had pituitary gigantism and displayed himself as "The Irish Giant" in eighteenth-century Ireland. He requested that his body be buried at sea, but after his death, his body was stolen from its coffin by anatomist John Hunter and included in his collection. Hunter secretly dissected Byrne's body and waited four years before displaying it. Byrne's body was displayed in the Hunterian Museum in London until 2017. Since reopening, the museum has removed his body from display; however, he is being kept in their collection, despite calls to bury his remains at sea.[18]

Dehumanisation can also be seen through the presentation of other objects showing disability in the past, such as paintings and images. Gartner and Joe highlighted historic 'disabling images' which contributed to dehumanisation in the past, but also continue to do so in the interpretation of these images:

> Images of the disabled as either less or more than merely human can be found throughout recorded history . . . The disabled are blessed or damned but never quite human.[19]

The 2005 study "In the Shadow of the Freakshow" found that curators were often nervous about deeper interpretation of disability history in freakshow material, treating information with delicacy and without interrogation.[20] There were no deliberate attempts to suppress or distort evidence of disabled people's history in museums; instead, there was a lack of consensus about the importance of these issues, as well as anxiety about how to display and interpret objects related to disability, leading to poor interpretation or a lack of display. There is great potential for the telling of disabled stories through objects already held by museums, but this must be done critically, and should be done by, or with, disabled people. While it may not be deliberate, current museum practice is contributing to the continued cultural invisibility of disabled people in museum spaces.[21]

Human Remains and Disability in Museums

The ethics of displaying human remains is something which has been greatly debated, particularly concerning the remains of Indigenous or colonised peoples.[22] Despite this, surveys conducted by English Heritage[23] and Leeds Museums and Galleries[24] showed public favour for displaying human remains. Interestingly, in the English Heritage survey, 42% of people were in favour of human remains on display only if unnamed, suggesting they were against acknowledging the bones came from a once-living human. However, it is important to recognise this when displaying human remains, since ignoring this continues the historic exploitation and erasure of the individuals whose bones have been commodified and unjustly taken for museum collections.[25] Humanising the individual sheds light on their lived experiences, and while the individual may never have wanted to be on display in this manner, respect for them and their life can, and should, be achieved.

Disability in the Context of the Past

Until recently, most bioarchaeological literature has focused on clinical examinations of pathological lesions on human remains, or the effects of disease on wider society. Focus on diagnosis of palaeopathology, very much in line with the treatment of disabled people under the medical model, has led to an erasure of the nuanced experience of impairment and disability in the past.[26]

Disabled people have been overlooked or been 'hidden from view,' with many impairments not being visible on bones, but also as assemblages only present a relatively small, non-representative, population sample.[27] It is also important to consider the osteological paradox. Individuals showing skeletal changes from disease or stress may be the healthiest in that population, since they survived longer and developed bony changes in response to these factors. Individuals showing no markers may have been most affected, dying quickly as a result.[28] This means that further disabled individuals may be being 'hidden' by the skeletal record, and extra care should be taken when inferring disability from skeletons showing more markers of disease or stress.

In recent years there have been calls for an integration of archaeology with anthropology, history, and critical Disability Studies.[29] Bioarchaeology has seen a shift towards using theories of human behaviour to form frameworks for the data collected from human remains,[30] with examples focusing on structural violence[31] and inequality.[32] Evaluation of human remains within the bioarchaeology of inequality and critical Disability Studies could be used to analyse impairment alongside a critical view of past societies and disabling effects through the social model.

When considering disability in the past through human remains, the focus must be on the lived experience of the individual with the impairment, looking at their social context and how circumstances may have changed over time.[33] Disabled and non-disabled do not exist as mutually exclusive binary concepts, instead being fluid with the possibility to change as time goes on. Analysing skeletal paleopathology and reflecting on both models of disability, the link between impairment and disability, and fluidity across a life course, allow lived experiences to be considered.

The Bioarchaeology of Care

The "Bioarchaeology of Care" methodology aims to interpret health-related care provision through skeletal remains.[34] While this method provides an addition to understanding disability in the past, and the earlier stages provide a useful framework for diagnosis and the consideration of symptoms, the main issue with this method lies in several assumptions that it makes. Mainly, it assumes that an individual must have been reliant on care with no possibility for survival otherwise, care received by an individual must have been from another party and not themselves, and that caregiving is evidence of compassion. Assumptions of dependency are a main point of contention for the disability rights movement and critical disability scholars:[35] not just that an individual is reliant on care, but reliant on another party for care. Dettwyler echoed this,[36] arguing against reading compassion into caregiving and stating that researchers were often making assumptions of compassion given no evidence. Tilley did refute this claim,[37] stating that using the idea of caring for a disabled individual as a proxy for social attitudes towards the "vulnerable and weak" in society should be used with caution, and that evidence of compassion is difficult to quantify or qualify,[38] almost entirely agreeing with Dettwyler's paper.[39]

The Osteobiographical Approach

Osteobiography was initially conceived by Saul,[40] who aimed to recreate individual lived experiences from skeletal remains, then further developed[41] by taking individual experiences and using them to make wider projections about populations. Two key focuses have shaped osteobiography since – acknowledgement of the biosocial nature of the body as a material object shaped by biology and culture,[42] and life course through the exploration of age-related biological development within social contexts.[43] This method has since been further developed to address individual agency and relationships between individuals and populations through the formation of a fleshed-out biography of the individual with the priority lying on social context and intersectionality,[44] humanising past individuals both as a tool for archaeological research, and for communicating the past to wider audiences.[45]

The British Museum, Case 14, Room 63

The consideration of this study was case 14 "Bioarchaeology of the Nile valley" in room 63, "Egyptian funerary archaeology." It is worth noting there is no human remains content warning before entering this gallery. In this case is a display focusing on "Studying ancient diseases," to educate visitors on palaeopathology. This display contains 14 examples of pathology on human bones, all extreme examples. All the bones were isolated, without the rest of the skeleton, with the exception of a juvenile skeleton showing *osteogenesis imperfecta* (brittle bone disease). Space is very limited in the British Museum, especially in the Egypt and Sudan galleries that house an immense amount of material culture. In terms of educating the public, isolated bones make sense to show a wide variety of pathology in a small space; however, what it does lead to is the dehumanisation of the individuals by isolating their bones with demonstrated differences.

All museum curation should ideally be as accessible as possible, but disabled people should especially be able to access stories that reflect their own. While many disabled people, including the author, would prefer disabled remains are not on public display, making these displays accessible contributes to humanising the individuals on display. Providing an equal opportunity for disabled and non-disabled visitors to view them, and learn about the individual, is a step towards moving away from historic freakshow associations and the viewing of disabled people as other. Therefore, this study also assessed the accessibility of the case study display, alongside the curation.

Accessibility

The text panels were limited in the information they could include, like in any museum. However, within both the smaller text panels for each bone and the larger overview panels for the cabinet, there was very little consideration of the individuals on display. There are brief mentions of how impairments seen on the bones may have affected mobility, and some mentions of the causes of diseases such as leprosy, but nothing beyond this. There is no interpretation of lived experience, and no use of the word disability.

The display was at wheelchair-accessible height, with lighting that did not interfere with reading the text, but this is not the case across the museum. The text panels were in a clear font but small and may present a barrier for visually impaired visitors. Large print guides are available but are only downloadable online for mobile phones. There is a sensory map available on the museum's website,[46] as well as information about access to specific parts of the museum. British Sign Language (BSL) and audio descriptive guides are available on YouTube and Soundcloud, and audio tours via an app, and these cover a large range of objects in the museum, though not all. This information is mostly available on the museum's access page;[47] however, it does leave out details such as many galleries not having accessible height displays, and no live information about functioning lifts.

Osteobiographical Profile of 'EA37340'

Skeleton EA37340 was excavated from a site in Abydos, Egypt, and was acquired by the British Museum in 1902 through the Egypt Exploration Fund (EEF). They are likely from the late period, after 664 BCE. There is no further information about the specifics of the site on the museum's online collection,[48] and the EEF conducted several excavations across Abydos in the years leading up to 1902.[49]

No sex or age estimation is given. Only their right femur is on display, making any estimations difficult. The femur has finished epiphyseal fusion across the proximal and distal femur, the femoral head, and the greater and lesser trochanters, giving an age range of 12–20 years old.[50] This individual's femur shows a misaligned fracture, which had healed. Complete healing of a femoral shaft fracture takes around 3 to 6 months, always requiring surgery to heal correctly, and without this, healing time increases significantly.[51] Without surgical intervention over time, healing may never occur.

The misalignment of the femur led to a shortening of the leg compared to the left leg, known as a structural leg length discrepancy (LLD). LLD also causes hip joints to be misaligned, resulting in a lateral pelvic tilt. This can then lead to

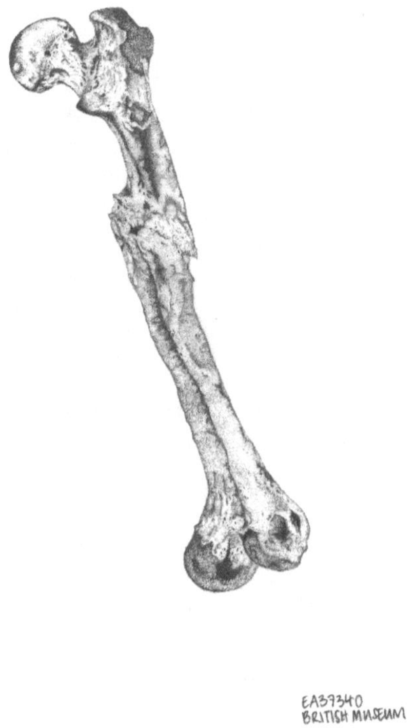

Figure 6.1 Drawing by Alexandra Doubleday of Right femur of 'EA37340' currently displayed in the British Museum. © A. Doubleday.

scoliosis which can lead to further skeletal degeneration, such as changes to the ribs and vertebrae, as well as degeneration of the intervertebral discs.[52] However, since only the femur of this individual has been examined, whether this was the case for them cannot be commented on.

The misalignment led to the distal femora being rotated. This rotation along with the lateral pelvic tilt would have affected the way in which this individual moved and walked. LLD and scoliosis are known to cause difficulty walking, a change in gait, and difficulty with balance.[53] Not only this, but it also would have likely caused this individual chronic pain, especially in the lower back. It also would have caused pain in their hip, knees, and ankles, as well as a hyperextended knee on the shorter leg, and a flexed knee on the longer leg.

Some individuals with leg length discrepancy today use shoe lifts of varying kinds.[54] Adaptive footwear is something which can be seen in ancient Egypt, with the notable case of Tutankhamun, whose tomb was found to contain footwear with an extra strap theorized to help stabilize his club foot when walking.[55] While the adaptations to footwear for LLD would be different, it is worth considering it as a possibility. Additionally, throughout ancient Egypt there is evidence of walking aids.[56] Specifically there is a case of a walking stick being discovered with the body of someone from an earlier period in Egypt who developed a lesion on their left femur causing it to be two inches shorter than the right.[57] It is also possible the individual in case 14 used a mobility aid such as this to support their walking.

Where the fracture healed shows a large amount of new bone growth, not only causing a visible change to the morphology of the bone, but also a visible limb difference. Representations of visibly disabled people are not uncommon in ancient Egyptian art across a wide variety of perceived social classes and time periods.[58] Iconographic representation of visibly disabled individuals may suggest that they "were not regarded as subnormal or in any way socially diminished,"[59] but it is difficult to say whether art accurately reflects the exact societal treatment and mindset towards disability. It is also possible that this individual received forms of external care, such as managing their symptoms, medical treatment, or more general assistance. However, this is not information which can be gathered from the skeletal remains themselves, so external care or compassion of this kind cannot be inferred.

Due to the lack of information about this individual and the fact that their femur appears to be separated from the rest of their skeleton, other facets of this individual's intersectional identity are hard to comment on. It is clear they lived to at least their teen years if not early adulthood, but no more than that is known. The sex of this individual also is unknown, and while this of course does not equate to their gender, we also have no record of any associated grave goods to start to discuss gender ideas from that either – but what may their disability have meant in relation to the societal gender roles at the time? This also directly ties into their position within society; perception and treatment of disability may have differed between people of different social statuses. Unfortunately, intersectional identity for an individual such as this, when a single bone was been displaced and no record exists of the rest of their skeleton, grave goods, or where they were buried, is incredibly difficult to evaluate. However, in terms of using a profile like this in a museum space, posing questions to visitors and asking them to consider facets of intersectional identity in relation to this possible experience of disability would be a powerful tool to get visitors thinking further about the individual, their life, and ancient Egyptian society.

Conclusions

In this case in the British Museum, isolated bones showing impairments are displayed in a 'cabinet of curiosities' style display. A small amount of information is provided for each individual on display, mainly describing the pathological lesion or bony difference that can be seen on the bone. It was clear they were aiming to showcase as many different types of pathological lesions or bony changes in a small space as possible, but this is then one of the main contributing factors to the dehumanisation of these individuals. These types of displays very much continue the freakshow association of museums. They present disabled individuals as something to be commodified through display, reducing them to the visible differences on their bones and using them purely as an educational, medicalised example of what different diseases or impairments can look like. Any trace of lived experience is ignored.

However, colonialism must be considered. There will be gaps in knowledge in the case of human remains excavated by the EEF, who focused on excavating as many objects and remains as possible and then distributing them to subscribing organisations like the British Museum.[60] While this large-scale pillaging was done legally, this was under the context of the inequality that existed between a colonised country and oppressive imperial powers. This commercialised separating of assemblages with little to no context attached to them is a huge barrier to understanding these human remains today. This leaves many bones, such as the femur from "EA37340," separated from the rest of the individual's skeleton, meaning that if the museum is including the femur in a display, it must be isolated, which can then lead to dehumanisation. Displaying complete skeletons is preferable since it further humanises the individual, providing a more immediate representation of a once living individual for visitors. However, despite the limitations of incomplete skeletons or a lack of grave goods or burial information, the osteobiographical profile presented in this study is a testament to just how much information can be extracted purely from publicly available information and the bone itself, and how it can be used to form part of a possible lived experience of an individual.

If complete skeletons are present in collections, and space is a limiting factor, perhaps it is instead better to reduce the number of individuals on display and focus more on humanising curation through interpretive text. When there is not a more complete skeleton to display, providing lived experience allows for visitors to think of the individual, not just the bone. This is something which can be seen to a degree in other museums including the Science Museum (London) and the Mary Rose Museum (Portsmouth). Each displays a complete skeleton of an individual and presents more in depth information about the pathology displayed on their skeleton, as well as a further consideration of their lived experiences, considering sex and possible gender roles, age, occupation, and in the case of the individual at the Science Museum the experience of social isolation due to disability.

They both show the benefit of providing societal and historical context alongside an individual and discussing how this related directly to how they may have lived, with visitors gaining a deeper understanding of life in the past as a disabled individual, and a better understanding of bioarchaeology.

"EA37340" is displayed in a part of the gallery focusing on illness, injury, pathology, and death. This is something which can also be seen in other museums – the author visited multiple museums while researching disability in museums and most human remains were located in sections related to one of these topics or were in specific medical museums. There is a perceived natural link between medicine, illness, and disability due to the medical model, and so it makes sense that this would be seen throughout museum curation, but it is notable that disabled human remains are rarely presented to the public not in a medicalised light. In a case such as the British Museum where there are human remains throughout many of the galleries, why are the disabled remains almost exclusively shown in this one cabinet?

The British Museum never uses the words "disabled" or "disability" in any of the text accompanying the individuals in case 14. Museums should not shy away from being clear that they are telling disabled stories and histories. Explicitly stating that these individuals were disabled people is another way to move away from commodifying them as medical specimens, and another way for visitors to understand and relate them to the modern day and to their own lives.

While the osteobiographical method provides extensive information on an individual, the one formed for this study could be expanded given further research within the British Museum's collection and talking to curatorial staff. This highlights the limitations of looking to create an osteobiography purely from publicly available information. Not all available information can ever be worked into displays; they are curated to include information that is deemed the most interesting and relevant to the public. However, limited information can provide a good foundation from which to extract information for further interpretation based on information the public is already interested in learning.

The osteobiographical method also has applications in any curation of human remains, not just those of disabled individuals. Colonial archaeologists long argued for ancient Egyptians' "whiteness," which was pushed onto the public through museums, seen in the separation of Egypt and Sudan from the rest of the African continent in museum curation.[61] The persistence of white supremacy in museums is interesting given the co-dependence of racism and ableism. White supremacy attempts to maintain a value system about people's bodily worth,[62] with dehumanising displays of disabled people reinforcing this idea even despite the whitewashing of ancient Egypt. Humanising curation using the osteobiographical method can help towards dismantling these ideals, providing human stories of individuals in the past that can work towards reframing these persistent white supremacist perceptions in museums, as well as wider society.

Personal experiences are essential to authentic, humanising curation, especially in conjunction with a method rooted in bioarchaeological analysis which can sometimes present as clinically distanced from the individual. The present study showcases the impact of personal experience of disability on uncovering the possible life of a disabled individual in the past. Consider the osteobiographical method conducted in collaboration with people who share their diverse experiences to help convey authentic and intersectional narratives of the past, not just in ancient Egypt but across global history. Ideally this is how osteobiographies should be formed, since there will always be biases when interpreting as an individual; however, this case study shows what is possible when using this method along with personal lived experience, and the possibilities of its application.

Notes

1 Delin (2002, 84–97), Dodd et al. (2004), Sandell et al. (2005, 4).
2 Isabelle Lawrence, Teams call with author, August 5, 2022.
3 Abberley (1987, 5–21).
4 Pfeiffer (1994, 533–42).
5 Abberley (1987, 5–21), Oliver (1990).
6 Scotch (1988, 159–72).
7 Gowland (2004, 135–46).
8 Gowland (2004, 135–46), Sofaer (2006).
9 Charlton (2000).
10 Scham and Yahya (2003, 399–416).

11 Riley (2005).
12 Sandell and Dodd (2010, 3–22).
13 Dodd et al. (2010, 92–112).
14 Dodd et al. (2008).
15 Dodd et al. (2010, 92–112).
16 Altick (1978, 235–39).
17 Sandell et al. (2005, 39).
18 Devlin (2018).
19 Gartner and Joe (1987).
20 Sandell et al. (2005, 39).
21 Dodd et al. (2004).
22 Fforde, Hubert, and Turnbull (2004), Kreps (2011, 70–84).
23 English Heritage (2009).
24 Leeds Museums and Galleries (2018).
25 Sandell et al. (2005, 39).
26 Southwell-Wright (2013, 67–95), Vogel and Power (2023, 1–14).
27 Waldron (2007, 195–210).
28 Wood et al. (1992, 343–70).
29 Cross (2007, 179–94), Battles (2011, 107–24).
30 Sofaer (2011, 285–311), Martin (2013, 1–21), Zuckerman, Kamnikar, and Mathena (2014, 513–22).
31 Klaus (2012, 29–62).
32 Martin (2013, 1–21).
33 Zakrzewski (2014, 57–68), Zakrzewski (2015, 157–67), Zakrzewski, Evelyn-Wright, and Inskip (2017, 269–90).
34 Tilley and Oxenham (2011, 35–42), Tilley (2012, 39–41).
35 Shuttleworth and Meekosha (2017, 19–38).
36 Dettwyler (1991, 375–83).
37 Tilley (2015, 64–74).
38 Tilley and Schrenk (2017).
39 Dettwyler (1991, 375–83).
40 Saul (1972, 2–123).
41 Saul and Saul (1989, 287–301).
42 Sofaer (2006).
43 Agarwal (2012, 322–35), Agarwal (2016, 130–49).
44 Hosek and Robb (2019, 1–15), Boutin (2016, 17–28), Meskell (2007, 23–43).
45 Boutin (2008), Stojanowski and Duncan (2015, 51–60).
46 The British Museum (2019), accessed August 23, 2022.
47 The British Museum, accessed August 23, 2022.
48 The British Museum, accessed March 10, 2023.
49 Randall-MacIver and Mace (1899–1900, 1–3), Griffith and Mace (1900–1901, 1–3).
50 Scheuer, Black, and Cunningham (2000).
51 Applebaum, Nessim, and Cho (2021, 127–34).
52 Ibid.
53 Ibid.
54 Campbell et al. (2018, 981–93).
55 Collins (2014).
56 Loebl and Nunn (1997, 450–54), Colton (2013).
57 Petrie (1898), Penn Museum, accessed February 9, 2023.
58 Reeves (1992), Dasen (1993), Morris (2020, 53–72).
59 Tait and Jeffreys (2000, 87–95).
60 Stevenson (2019).
61 Stienne (2022).
62 Brown (2022), accessed March 14, 2023.

Bibliography

Abberley, Paul. "The Concept of Oppression and the Development of a Social Theory of Disability." *Disability, Handicap and Society* 2 (1987): 5–21.

Adams, Geraldine Kendall. "Hunterian Museum Defends Decision to Retain Skeleton of 'Irish Giant' Charles Byrne." Last modified January 13, 2023. Accessed January 15, 2023. https://www.museumsassociation.org/museums-journal/news/2023/01/hunterian-museum-defends-decision-to-retain-skeleton-of-irish-giant-charles-byrne/#.

Agarwal, Sabrina C. "The Past of Sex, Gender, and Health: Bioarchaeology of the Aging Skeleton." *American Anthropologist* 114, no. 2 (2012): 322–35.

Agarwal, Sabrina C. "Bone Morphologies and Histories: Life Course Approaches in Bioarchaeology." *American Journal of Physical Anthropology Supplement: Yearbook of Physical Anthropology* 159, no. S61 (2016): 130–49.

Altick, Richard D. *The Shows of London.* Cambridge and London: Harvard University Press, 1978.

Applebaum, Ariella, Adam Nessim, and Woojin Cho. "Overview and Spinal Implications of Leg Length Discrepancy: Narrative Review." *Clinics in Orthopedic Surgery* (2021): 127–34.

Battles, Heather. "Toward Engagement: Exploring the Prospects for an Integrated Anthropology of Disability." *Explorations in Anthropology* 11, no. 1 (2011): 107–24.

Boutin, Alexis T. "Embodying Life and Death: Osteobiographical Narratives from Alalakh." Unpublished PhD diss., University of Pennsylvania: Anthropology, 2008.

Boutin, Alexis T. "Exploring the Social Construction of Disability: An Application of the Bioarchaeology of Personhood Model to a Pathological Skeleton from Ancient Bahrain." *International Journal of Paleopathology* 12 (2016): 17–28.

The British Museum. "Sensory Map." Last modified September 23, 2019. Accessed August 23, 2022. https://www.britishmuseum.org/sites/default/files/2019-11/British-Museum-Sensory-Map-PDF-Download.pdf.

The British Museum. "Accessiblity at the Museum." Accessed August 23, 2022. https://www.britishmuseum.org/visit/accessibility-museum.

The British Museum. "Human Mummy." Accessed March 10, 2023. https://www.britishmuseum.org/collection/object/Y_EA37340.

Brown, Lydia X. Z. "We Can't Address Disability without Addressing Race. Here's Why." Last modified July 6, 2022. Accessed March 14, 2023. https://learnplaythrive.com/we-cant-address-disability-without-addressing-race/.

Campbell, Mark, Bahareh Ghaedi, Elizabeth Ghogomu, and Vivian Welch. "Shoe Lifts for Leg Length Discrepancy in Adults with Common Painful Musculoskeletal Conditions: A Systematic Review of the Literature." *Archives of Physical Medicine and Rehabilitation* (2018): 981–93.

Charlton, James. Nothing About Us Without Us: Disability Oppression and Empowerment. Berkeley, Los Angeles, and London: University of California Press, 2000.

Collins, Paul. *Discovering Tutankhamun.* Oxford: Ashmolean Museum, 2014.

Colton, Chris. "Orthopaedic Challenges in Ancient Egypt." *Bone & Joint* 360, no. 2 (2013).

Cross, Morag. "Accessing the Inaccessible: Disability and Archaeology." In *The Archaeology of Identities: A Reader*, edited by Timothy Insoll, 179–94. London: Routledge, 2007.

Dasen, Veronique. *Dwarfs in Ancient Egypt and Greece.* Oxford: Oxford University Press, 1993.

Delin, Annie. "Buried in the Footnotes: The Absence of Disabled People in the Collective Imagery of Our Past." In *Museums, Society, Inequality*, edited by Ricard Sandell, 84–97. London and New York: Routledge, 2002.

Dettwyler, Katherine A. "Can Paleopathology Provide Evidence for 'Compassion'?" *American Journal of Physical Anthropology* 84 (1991): 375–83.

Devlin, Hannah. "'Irish Giant' May Finally Get Respectful Burial after 200 Years on Display." Last modified June 22, 2018. Accessed July 24, 2022. https://www.

theguardian.com/science/2018/jun/22/irish-giant-may-finally-get-respectful-burial-after-200-years-on-display#:~:text=4%20years%20old-,'Irish%20giant'%20may%20finally%20get%20respectful%20burial,after%20200%20years%20on%20display&text=The%20%E2.

Dodd, Jocelyn, Ceri Jones, Debbie Jolly, and Richard Sandell. "Disability Reframed: Challenging Visitor Perceptions in the Museum." In *Re-Presenting Disability: Activism and Agency in the Museums*, edited by Richard Sandell, Jocelyn Dodd, and Rosemarie Garland-Thomson, 92–112. Abingdon and New York: Routledge, 2010.

Dodd, Jocelyn, Richard Sandell, Annie Delin, and Jackie Gay. *Buried in the Footnotes: The Representation of Disabled People in Museum and Gallery Collections.* Leicester: Research Centre for Museums and Galleries, 2004.

Dodd, Jocelyn, Richard Sandell, Debbie Jolly, and Ceri Jones. *Rethinking Disability Representation in Museums and Galleries.* Leicester: Research Centre for Museums and Galleries, 2008.

English Heritage. *Research into Issues Surrounding Human Bones in Museums.* BDRC, 2009.

Evans, Jessica. "Introduction to Part Three." In *Representing the Nation: A Reader: Histories, Heritage and Museums*, edited by David Boswell and Jessica Evans, 235–39. London and New York: Routledge, 1999.

Fforde, Cressida, Jane Hubert, and Paul Turnbull. *The Dead and Their Possessions: The Repatriation in Principle, Policy, and Practice.* New York: Routledge, 2004.

Gartner, Alan, and Tom Joe. *Images of the Disabled, Disabling Images.* New York: Praeger, 1987.

Gowland, Rebecca. "The Social Identity of Health in Late Roman Britain." In *TRAC 2003: Proceedings of the Thirteenth Annual Theroetical Roman Archaeology Conference which Took Place at the University of Leicester 3rd–6th April 2003*, 135–46. Oxford: Oxbow Books, 2004.

Griffith, F. L., and A. C. Mace. "Excavations at Abydos." *Archaeological Report (Egypt Exploration Fund)* (1900–1901): 1–3.

Hosek, Lauren, and John Robb. "Osteobiography: A Platform for Bioarchaeological Research." *Bioarchaeology International* 3, no. 1 (2019): 1–15.

Klaus, Haagen. "The Bioarchaeology of Structural Violence: A Theoretical Model and a Case Study." In *The Bioarchaeology of Violence*, edited by Debra Martin, Ryan Harrod, and Ventura Perez, 29–62. Gainesville: University Press of Florida, 2012.

Kreps, Christina. "Changing the Rules of the Road: Post-Colonialism and the New Ethics of Museum Anthropology." In *Routledge Companion to Museum Ethics*, edited by Janet Marstine, 70–84. New York: Routledge, 2011.

Leeds Museums & Galleries. *Visitor Responses to Human Remains in Leeds City Museum: Final Report.* Leeds: Leeds Museums & Galleries, 2018.

Loebl, W. Y., and John F. Nunn. "Staffs as Walking Aids in Ancient Egypt and Palestine." *Journal of the Royal Society of Medicine* 90, no. 8 (1997): 450–54.

Martin, Debra. "The Practice of Bioarchaeology." In *Bioarchaeology: An Integrated Approach to Working with Human Remains*, 1–21. New York: Springer, 2013.

Meskell, Lynn M. "Archaeologies of Identity." In *The Archaeology of Identities: A Reader*, edited by Timothy Insoll, 23–43. Abingdon and New York: Routledge, 2007.

Morris, Alexandra F. "Let that Be Your Last Battlefield: Tutankhamun and Disability." *Athens Journal of History* 6 (2020): 53–72.

Oliver, Michael. *The Politics of Disablement.* London: Palgrave Macmillan, 1990.

Penn Museum. "Human Skeleton Man." Accessed Feburary 9, 2023. https://www.penn.museum/collections/object/171752.

Petrie, W. M. Flinders. *Deshasheh, 1897.* London: Egypt Exploration Fund, 1898.

Pfeiffer, David. "The Americans with Disabilities Act: Costly Mandates or Civil Rights?" *Disability and Society* 9 (1994): 533–42.

Randall-MacIver, David, and A. C. Mace. "Excavations at Abydos." *Archaeological Report (Egypt Exploration Fund)* (1899–1900): 1–3.

Reeves, Carole. *Egyptian Medicine.* Princes Risborough: Shire, 1992.

Riley, Charles R. *Disability and the Media: Prescriptions for Change.* Hanover and London: University Press of New England, 2005.
Sandell, Richard, Annie Delin, Jocelyn Dodd, and Jackie Gay. "In The Shadow of the Freak-show: The Impact of Freakshow Tradition on the Display and Understanding of Disability History in Museums." *Disability Studies Quarterly* 25, no. 4 (2005).
Sandell, Richard, and Jocelyn Dodd. "Activist Practice." In *Representing Disability: Activism and Agency in the Museum*, edited by Richard Sandell, Jocelyn Dodd, and Rosemarie Garland-Thomson, 3–22. Abingdon and New York: Routledge, 2010.
Saul, Frank P. "The Human Skeletal Remains of Altar de Sacrificios: An Osteobiographic Analysis." *Papers of the Peabody Museum* 63, no. 2 (1972): 2–123.
Saul, Frank P., and Julie M. Saul. "Osteobiography: A Maya Example." In *Reconstruction of Life from the Skeleton*, edited by M. Y. Iscan and K. A. R. Kennedy, 287–301. New York: Wiley-Blackwell, 1989.
Scham, Sandra A., and Adel Yahya. "Heritage and Reconciliation." *Journal of Social Archaeology* 3, no. 3 (2003): 399–416.
Scheuer, Louise, Sue Black, and Craig Cunningham. *Developmental Juvenile Osteology.* San Diego: Elsevier Academic Press, 2000.
Scotch, Richard K. "Disability as the Basis for a Social Movement: Advocacy and the Politics of Definition." *Journal of Social Issues* 44 (1988): 159–72.
Shuttleworth, Russel, and Helen Meekosha. "Accomodating Critical Disability Studies in Bioarchaeology." In *Bioarchaeology of Impairment and Disability: Theoretical, Ethnohistorical, and Methodological Perspectives*, edited by Jennifer Byrnes and Jennifer Muller, 19–38. Cham: Springer, 2017.
Sofaer, Joanna R. *The Body as Material Culture: A Theoretical Osteoarchaeology.* Cambridge: Cambridge University Press, 2006.
Sofaer, Joanna R. "Towards a Social Bioarchaeology of Age." In *Social Bioarchaeology*, edited by Sabrina C. Agarwal and Bonnie Glencross, 285–311. Chichester: Wiley-Blackwell, 2011.
Southwell-Wright, William. "Past Perspectives: What Can Archaeology Offer Disability Studies." In *Emerging Perspectives on Disability Studies*, edited by Matthew Wappett and Katrina Arndt, 67–95. New York: Palgrave Macmillan, 2013.
Stevenson, Alice. *Scattered Finds: Archaeology, Egyptology and Museums.* London: UCL Press, 2019.
Stienne, Angela. *Mummified: The Stories Behind Egyptian Mummies in Museums.* Manchester: Manchester University Press, 2022.
Stojanowski, Christopher, and William N. Duncan. "Engaging Bodies in the Public Imagination: Bioarchaeology as a Social Science, Science, and Humanities." *American Journal of Human Biology* 27, no. 1 (2015): 51–60.
Tait, John, and David Jeffreys. "Disability, Madness and Social Exclusion in Dynastic Egypt." In *Madness, Disability, and Social Exclusion: The Archaeology and Anthropology of 'Difference'*, edited by Jane Hubert, 87–95. London and New York: Routledge, 2000.
Tilley, Lorna. "The Bioarchaeology of Care." *Society for American Archaeology Special Issue: New Directions in Bioarchaeology* 12 (2012): 39–41.
Tilley, Lorna. "Accomodating Past Difference in the Prehistoric Past: Revisiting the Case of Romito 2 from a Bioarchaeology of Care Perspective." *International Journal of Paleopathology* 8 (2015): 64–74.
Tilley, Lorna, and Marc F. Oxenham. "Survival against the Odds: Modelling the Social Implications of Care Provision to Seriously Disabled Individuals." *International Journal of Paleopathology* 1 (2011): 35–42.
Tilley, Lorna, and Alecia A. Schrenk. *New Developments in the Bioarchaeology of Care: Further Case Studies and Expanded Theory.* Cham: Springer, 2017.
Vogel, Hannah, and Ronika Power. "Recognising Inequality: Ableism in Egyptological Approaches to Disability and Bodily Differences." *World Archaeology* (2023): 1–14.

Waldron, Tony. "Hidden or Overlooked? Where are the Disadvantaged in the Skeletal Record?" In *The Archaeology of Identities: A Reader*, edited by Timothy Insoll, 195–210. Abingdon and New York: Routledge, 2007.

Wood, James W., George R. Milner, Henry C. Harpending, and Kenneth M. Weiss. "The Osteological Paradox: Problems of Inferring Prehistoric Health from Skeletal Samples." *Current Anthropology* 33 (1992): 343–70.

Zakrzewski, Sonia R."Paleopathology, Disability and Bodily Impairments." In *Palaeopathology in Egypt and Nubia: A Century in Review,* edited by Ryan Metcalfe, Jenefer Cockitt, and Rosalie David, 57–68. Oxford: Archaeopress, 2014.

Zakrzewski, Sonia R. "Behind Every Mask there is a Face, and Behind that a Story. Egyptian Bioarchaeology and Ancient Identities." In *Egyptian Bioarchaeology: Humans, Animals, and the Environment*, edited by Salima Ikram, Jessica Kaiser, and Roxie Walker, 157–67. Havertown: Sidestone Press, 2015.

Zakrzewski, Sonia R., Stephanie Evelyn-Wright, and Sarah Inskip. "Anglo-Saxon Concepts of Dis/Ability: Placing Disease at Great Chesterford in Its Wider Context." In *Bioarchaeology of Impairment and Disability: Theoretical, Ethnohistorical, and Methodological Perspectives,* edited by Jennifer Byrnes and Jennifer Muller, 269–90. Cham: Springer, 2017.

Zuckerman, Molly K., Kelly R. Kamnikar, and Sarah Mathena. "Recovering the 'Body Politic': A Relational Ethics of Meaning for Bioarchaeology." *Cambridge Archaeological Journal* 24, no. 3 (2014): 513–22.

7 Accessibility and Disability Representation in Ancient Egyptian Exhibits

Considerations for Planning a Classroom Field Trip

Karen L. Kobylarz

Introduction

When studying ancient cultures such as Egypt, museum visits can enrich the learning experience in many ways. According to Marc Behrendt and Teresa Franklin of the education department of Ohio University, "Field trips offer an opportunity to motivate and connect students to appreciate and understand classroom concepts, which increase a student's knowledge foundation, promoting further learning and higher level thinking strategies." [1] In the context of studying ancient Egypt, such experiences give students the opportunity to interact with artefacts and replicas that bring that culture to life. It is essential for educators to ensure such field trips are successful and meet students' educational needs.

However, not all students have the same needs. According to the Learning Disabilities Association of America, approximately 11.2 million US students have learning and attention disabilities. Likewise, in 2019, a UNICEF report estimated a total of 5.1 million school-age children with disabilities live in eastern and central Europe and central Asia. When planning a museum visit, educators must keep the needs of their students with disabilities in mind to ensure the learning experience is accessible to everyone. Also, students who see themselves reflected in the school curriculum "construct a deeper understanding of their personal identities . . . develop empathy, understanding, and respect for others; and [are] empower[ed]. . . to redress inequities and improve the world."[2] Therefore, teachers must consider more than just the accessibility of the museum and its Egyptian exhibit. They need to examine the displays, looking for objects that represent disability.

With this, as with all field trips, preplanning is required for a successful experience.[3] The educator must be aware of the different ways the ancient Egyptians discussed and portrayed disability. Some examples are straight-forward, such as the mummified remains of Siptah, whose left foot is angled with the heel raised,[4] or the image of Roma the doorman, depicted with a cane and one leg less muscular than the other.[5] Others require expert analysis, which can be gained through lectures and articles. Much of the criteria used in this paper to determine whether an artefact on display represents disability comes from Alexandra F. Morris's lecture, "And the Children Shall Lead: Harpocrates & Other Representations of Cerebral Palsy from the Ptolemaic Period," at ARCE's 2021 virtual annual meeting, which noted that

DOI: 10.4324/9781003440369-9

representations of Horus/Harpocrates suggest floppy musculature, possibly indicative of cerebral palsy. Works such as Emily Smith-Sangster's "Personal Experience or Royal Canon?" in *KMT: A Modern Journal of Egyptology* were also helpful for determining the difference between canes used to assist walking and staffs and staves used to denote authority.

In addition to background knowledge of disability in ancient Egypt, familiarity with the museum and its collection is also required. As Behrendt and Franklin note, "The teacher should visit the venue prior to the field trip, to learn the layout of the venue and determine whether the venue is suitable for all students."[6] For the purpose of studying disability in the ancient world, preplanning should also include an examination of the artefacts on display.

This paper uses the three major Egyptian collections in Chicago – the Field Museum of Natural History, the Institute for the Study of Ancient Cultures, West Asia, and North Africa (formerly the Oriental Institute), and the Art Institute of Chicago – to illustrate the type of preplanning required.

Planning the Visit: Case Studies at the Field Museum of Natural History, the Institute for the Study of Ancient Cultures, West Asia, and North Africa, and the Art Institute of Chicago

When planning to visit these institutions, explore their websites first to gather information about the exhibits and the accommodations each museum offers for people with disabilities. While researching and on the days of the planning visits, keep the following questions in mind: How does the museum make its exhibit accessible for students/visitors with mobility needs; visual impairment; hard of hearing; and learning, developmental, intellectual, or mental health disabilities? Does the Egyptian exhibit include artefacts representing disability in the ancient world, and if so, how are the artefacts presented? From August 2022 to April 2023, the author went to each museum and explored their Egyptian exhibits with these questions in mind. Here are the results from each visit.

The Field Museum of Natural History

The Field Museum of Natural History along Chicago's lakefront is very accessible for those with mobility needs. There is a ground level entrance on the east side of the museum, which includes automatic doors. All inside doors are also automated by the press of a button. The museum has two elevators, one on the east side and one on the west, and wheelchair rental is available on a first-come/first-served basis.

The exhibit *Inside Ancient Egypt* begins with the reconstructed mastaba of the Old Kingdom courtier Unas-ankh, which includes some of the original blocks from the tomb. Level flooring makes for easy/safe walking and wheelchair use. Unlike other, newer exhibits in the museum, *Inside Ancient Egypt* offers no benches for visitors who need rest breaks. This exhibit is the only bi-level one, beginning on the main floor and continuing down to the ground level. Although there are many stairs, an elevator located near the staircase provides an accessible alternative. This solution is imperfect because taking the elevator means missing a portion of the exhibit – a view of the tomb's courtyard from the roof of the mastaba. Also, when reaching the ground level, the elevator does not open in the exhibit. There is a short walk to where the exhibit continues, and the ground-level portion of the exhibit has multiple entrances, so visitors using the elevator may have difficulty finding where they left off. The portion of the exhibit displaying mummified human remains and funerary objects has some narrow areas where passage might be difficult in crowded conditions.

Visitors with visual impairments may have the most difficulty navigating the museum. While guide dogs are allowed, currently, the museum does not offer a visually impaired tour or verbal imaging tour. If visitors access the Field for All app, they will find a short verbal description of the highlights of major exhibits, including this one. Display labels are not in braille, and while newer exhibits include many tactile objects, *Inside Ancient Egypt*, which opened in 1988, has very few. Located on the ground-floor level, these tactile objects include a model of an ancient Egyptian bed and two model funerary stelae, which have an audio description when a button is pressed. Lighting in the funerary section of the exhibit is poor, which may cause difficulties for those with limited vision.

For visitors who are hard of hearing, sign language interpreters and assistive listening devices are not available. Videos in exhibits are always closed-captioned in both English and Spanish; however, *Inside Ancient Egypt* does not include videos.

The museum offers accommodations for those with learning, developmental, intellectual, and mental health disabilities. As noted earlier, the Field Museum permits service animals on the premises. Its app provides a sensory-friendly map, which designates areas that are normally loud or quiet. Also, it denotes areas with bright lighting and spaces offering the most opportunity for movement. The map marks *Inside Ancient Egypt* as an exhibit which allows opportunity for movement, especially outside the mastaba on the main level and in the ancient Egyptian marketplace section of the ground level.

Despite the museum's numerous accommodations, visitors travel through most of *Inside Ancient Egypt* without encountering any representations of disability. Only when reaching the final section of the exhibit, the marketplace, does one find objects depicting disability, and significant searching is required to locate them. In one case, a tiny amulet of the dwarf god Bes from the Ptolemaic-Roman period sits on the floor of the case. In another higher and easier-to-view display are three larger Bes amulets, one dating to the New Kingdom and two to Ptolemaic-Roman times. There are also two Bes moulds from the Late period. This second case also includes two statues featuring the god Horus. In the larger statue, Horus sits on Isis' lap. He leans back, suggesting floppy musculature. Isis supports him with one hand on his back. The second smaller statue depicts Horus as a child sitting on a chair. As in the statue with Isis, Horus leans back as if sitting upright is difficult, which suggests representation of cerebral palsy.[7] The labels in this case lack numbers to match descriptions with objects. They seem to date from the Late period.

In addition to the objects on display, two plaques along the replica of the Nile marsh include sketches of tomb scenes. One scene depicts men fishing in the marsh and features a man with a cane waiting on the shore. The other scene has three registers showing the process of making papyrus. To the right on the second register, a man leans on a cane, suggesting he needs it for support.

In total, the exhibit contains ten representations of disability in ancient Egypt. Of the various types of disability, only three are represented: dwarfism, mobility impairment, and cerebral palsy.

The Institute for the Study of Ancient Cultures, West Asia, and North Africa

The Institute for the Study of Ancient Cultures, West Asia, and North Africa (ISAC) on the University of Chicago campus somewhat addresses the needs of those with mobility impairments. The museum has a wheelchair-accessible entrance on the west side of the building and a nearby drop-off point for busses. The entrance door is automated.

The museum is all on one level, but there is an elevator for access to the washrooms in the basement. The washrooms also have automated doors and wheelchair-accessible stalls. The only doors that are not automated are those leading into and out of the exhibits. According to their website, ISAC has a limited number of wheelchairs for rent.

ISAC's galleries are connected, and the Egyptian one is located about halfway through. The floor is level, but while there are several benches for resting located in the other galleries, the Egyptian exhibit has none. Signage indicates the museum is renovating parts of the exhibit, so perhaps benches will be installed in the future.

Currently, ISAC does not offer a visually impaired tour or verbal imaging tour for those with visual impairments. No signs were in braille; however, the museum does allow service animals. There is no specific audio tour available for the Egyptian gallery, and there are no tactile representations of any objects.

For those hard of hearing, ISAC does offer assisted listening devices for lectures and gallery talks. They do not have sign language interpreters. There are several audio guides on ISAC's mobile app, but these only highlight certain items and apply to the museum as a whole – nothing specific to the Egyptian gallery.

To address the needs of those with learning, developmental, intellectual, and mental health disabilities, the museum allows service animals. There are no accommodations to make the exhibits sensory friendly.

As for the artefacts, ISAC has several showing disability representation. There are two small statues of Horus seated on Isis' lap with the leaned-back posture indicative of floppy musculature.[8] The most common disability shown is dwarfism due to the popularity of the god Bes. ISAC has nine Bes images on display and four other images depicting individuals with dwarfism, one being a harpist. Two other harpist images may depict individuals with dwarfism as well, the rough carving making it difficult to tell. There is also a plaque from the early dynastic period on display, which may depict a man with disabilities. His head appears overly large for his body, his legs are spindly, and he walks with a staff.

In addition to these objects, the display case for the mummified remains of Petosiris acknowledges disabilities this individual had in life. Based on CT scans, Petosiris' spine had degenerated and he experienced bone loss in his jaw due to abscessed teeth.

The Art Institute of Chicago

The Art Institute of Chicago, located in the downtown area, has two accessible entrances with ramps, one by its main Michigan Avenue entrance and the other by its Modern Wing on Monroe Street. Only the Modern Wing entrance, however, has a drop-off lane. While the entry door at the Modern Wing entrance is automatic, not all inner doors are. The museum has multiple elevators and ramps and offers wheelchair rentals to make exhibits accessible to those with mobility difficulties.

Visitors can reach *Life and Afterlife in Ancient Egypt*, located in the museum's lower level, by elevator. The flooring is level, except for a raised viewing area by the coffin of Nesi-pa-her-hat. This is only accessible by stairs, which prevents those using wheelchairs or walkers from getting a better view of the inside of the coffin. There are two benches in the exhibit, and an additional rest area is available near the elevator and restrooms.

For the visually impaired the Art Institute used to offer tours with sighted guides, but these went on hiatus during the 2020 COVID-19 pandemic and have yet to be resumed. A verbal description tour of exhibit highlights is available through the museum's app. Signs are not in braille, but guide dogs are permitted. In the past, tactile representations of some of the museum's objects were available, but these, too, have been placed on hiatus since the pandemic. Because the Egyptian exhibit is a newer installation, opening in February 2022, the museum's collection of tactile representations does not include representations of any of its objects.

Visitors who are hard of hearing will need to bring their own sign language interpreter if needed since the museum does not offer this service. Assistive listening devices are not available for gallery talks, and the exhibit does not have any videos that would require closed captioning. The Art Institute does have an audio guide compatible with t-coil hearing aids. The guide for this exhibit highlights five objects: the model of a river boat, a canopic jar, a lintel fragment showing a man and his wife worshipping the gods, the statuette of a sphinx, and a relief fragment depicting fowling in the marshes. Transcripts of the guide, which features commentary by assistant curator Ashley Arico and Egyptologist Emily Teeter, are available through their mobile app by pressing play, tapping the name of the object in the black bar at the bottom of the screen, and scrolling down.

For those with learning, developmental, intellectual, and mental health disabilities as noted earlier, the Art Institute welcomes service animals. A downloadable sensory map, posted in 2021, is available on the website. Since *Life and Afterlife in Ancient Egypt* opened after the map's publication, visitors need to locate the exhibit by gallery number. Marked on the sensory map in grey, gallery 50 is normally a quieter area. Unavailable on the mobile app, the sensory map needs to be accessed through the website.

The Art Institute's collection is smaller than those of the Field Museum and ISAC. Of its nearly 1,000 objects, only about 80 are on display. Of these, three represent disability in ancient Egypt: a copper alloy statue of Isis supporting Horus, a faience amulet of the dwarf god Bes, and another amulet of Isis and Nephthys with Horus the Child between them; Horus's left leg is more muscular than his right.

Virtual Field Trips

If a local ancient Egyptian collection is not available or if the exhibit does not include artefacts representing disability, virtual field trips provide another option. These provide learning experiences without leaving the classroom, but drawbacks exist as well. Virtual trips can be more time consuming to find and arrange than in-person trips. For example, among the three Chicago museums with Egyptian collections, neither the Field Museum nor the ISAC offers virtual field trips on their websites. The Art Institute's website includes a virtual section, but the only content pertaining to ancient Egypt are four interactive features. Three of them give detailed views of a coffin, a cartonnage mask, and a jackal statuette, while the fourth gives viewers insight into coffin preservation. All of these interactives present images and text; no audio is provided, which makes these presentations inaccessible to partially sighted students.

Beyond local museums, an internet search of virtual field trips provides another option. The search term *ancient Egypt virtual field trip* provided multiple results, including *smithsonianjourneys.org*, *virtualfieldtrips.org*, and *exploremorefamilytravel.com*. All of these websites offer content focusing on the highlights of ancient Egyptian culture rather than information specific to disability. *Smithsonianjourneys.org* has several videos with closed captioning, a photo gallery of major sites, a 360 VR tour of Egypt and the Nile, and a link to the Smithsonian's database of Egyptian artefacts – useful for finding images of objects representing disability.

Virtualfieldtrips.org offers a 19-minute video with accompanying learning resources (quizzes, graphic organisers, hands-on activities, etc.) linked to national and state standards. However, the resources lack differentiation and may need modification to meet student needs. Also, *virtualfieldtrips.org* requires a paid yearly subscription, which can range from $6.00 – $10.00 a year for individual access to one video to $350 on up for schoolwide access to their entire collection.

Exploremorefamilytravel.com is a virtual field trip geared toward elementary students. It offers a variety of content, including an overview, literature read-alouds, a podcast, colouring pages, music, crafts, S.T.E.M. (science, technology, engineering, and maths) and movement activities, and videos.

As noted earlier, most virtual field trips comprise audio and visual components, which may not meet the needs of all students, especially those who would benefit from tactile experience. Also, content and links on the virtual field trip websites are not always up to date. For example, *smithsonianjourneys.org*'s link to the 360 VR tour of Queen Meresankh's tomb is no longer valid and one of the linked videos, "Mummies: Secrets of the Pharaohs," is over a decade old. The *exploremorefamilytravel.com* is also in need of some updating since their "Journey down the Nile River" video is no longer available.

Because virtual field trips lack a specific focus on disability in ancient Egypt, supplementing them or creating original content may be necessary. Internet searches for articles, images, and videos produce mixed results. A search for *representations of disability in ancient Egypt* includes links to sources specific to disability in ancient Egypt, but others related to disability in other ancient cultures and disability in general also appeared.

Combining *ancient Egypt* and the name of a specific disability in the search brings more specific results; however, this is not successful for all disabilities. Evidence for learning and intellectual disabilities proves more difficult to find, and such searches often produce information on physical disabilities instead.

Knowing what types of artefacts to look for makes searching a museum's database more fruitful than a general internet search. As with a general search, specific terms such as *Bes* and *Isis and Horus* produce more accurate results. A downside to this is difficulty finding the database, especially on websites of larger institutions. Of the Chicago museums discussed here, ISAC, the smallest of the three, has the easiest online database to locate and navigate. The various pages on the Field Museum's and Art Institute's sites led to longer searches to locate their complete collections. Another downside is that not all objects may be photographed. The Field Museum's database frequently provided only catalogue card information about the object, but no image. However, the database grants access to items not on display, offering a larger selection of objects representing disability.

Other points to consider, whether finding material from a museum database or through general internet search, are checking that the source is reliable, accurate, up to date, and grade-level appropriate. Regardless if the field trip is virtual or in person, a post-experience activity should follow. Behrendt and Franklin state that students need the opportunity to reflect on what they have learned so they can make connections and gain a greater understanding of the material.[9] Possible post-visit activities could include writing to the museum about making the exhibit more accessible and/or how to increase disability representation in the displays. Students could also compare and contrast ancient Egyptian attitudes toward and representations of disability with those of other societies and cultures.

Conclusion

Field trips provide an opportunity to include disability representation in the curriculum. This type of experience requires significant effort – familiarising oneself with the subject matter, visiting sites to evaluate accessibility and the amount of disability representation in the exhibit, and creating post-visit activities to extend the learning experience. Studying disability not only allows students with disabilities to see themselves in history, but it helps their non-disabled peers shift their perspective of disability from negative to positive.[10] Despite the amount of work required to create these experiences, the overall impact on students is worth the extra effort.

Notes

1 Behrandt and Franklin (2014, 242).
2 Kishor and Cooper (2022).
3 Behrandt and Franklin (2014, 240).
4 Partridge (1994, 169).
5 Smith-Sangster (2021, 42).
6 Behrandt and Franklin (2014, 240).
7 Morris (2021).
8 Ibid.
9 Behrandt and Franklin (2014, 241).
10 Minarik and Lintner (2013, 15–16).

Bibliography

"75 Per Cent of Children with Disabilities in Eastern and Central Europe and Central Asia Left out of Inclusive, Quality Education." *UNICEF.* https://www.unicef.org/press-releases/75-cent-children-disabilities-eastern-and-central-europe-and-central-asia-left-out.

"Ancient Egypt: Land of the Pyramids." *Virtual Field Trips,* July 24, 2022. https://virtualfieldtrips.org/ancient-egypt-land-of-the-pyramids/.

Behrandt, Marc, and Teresa Franklin. "A Review of Research on School Field Trips and Their Value in Education." *International Journal of Environmental and Science Education* 9, no. 3 (2014): 235–45. https://doi.org/10.12973/ijese.2014.213a.

"Downtown Chicago's #1 Museum." *The Art Institute of Chicago.* https://www.artic.edu/

"Field Museum." https://www.fieldmuseum.org/.

Journeys, Smithsonian. "Virtual Journey: Ancient Egypt and the Nile." *Ancient Egypt and the Nile Virtual Tour | Smithsonian Journeys.* https://www.smithsonianjourneys.org/virtual-journeys/egypt-virtual-tour/.

Kishore, Nikhil, and Carl Cooper. "Setting up a Disability-Inclusive Curriculum." *Edutopia, George Lucas Educational Foundation,* January 20, 2022. https://www.edutopia.org/article/setting-disability-inclusive-curriculum/.

MacMillan, Kyle. "Jewels of the Nile: 'Ancient Egypt' Exhibit at Art Institute Showcases Museum's Collection in Whole New Light." Chicago Sun-Times, February 11, 2022.

Minarik, Darren W., and Timothy Lintner. "Disability History: Humanity Worth Defending." *The Ohio Social Studies Review* 50, no. 2 (2013): 15–21. https://scholarcommons.sc.edu/aiken_education_facpub/1/.

Morris, Alexandra F. "And the Children Shall Lead: Harpocrates & Other Representations of Cerebral Palsy from the Ptolemaic Period." Online Lecture, The American Research Center in Egypt Virtual Meeting, April 25, 2021.

Partridge, Robert. *Faces of Pharaohs: Royal Mummies and Coffins from Ancient Thebes.* London: The Rubicon Press, 1994.

Smith-Sangster, Emily. "Personal Experience or Royal Canon?" *KMT: A Modern Journal of Egyptology* 32, no. 3 (2021): 40–49.

"The State of Learning Disabilities Today." *Learning Disabilities Association of America.* https://ldaamerica.org/lda_today/the-state-of-learning-disabilities-today/.

The University of Chicago Institute for the Study of Ancient Cultures, West Asia & North Africa. https://isac.uchicago.edu/.

"What Does Stem Stand for?" *Homepage.* https://studyinthestates.dhs.gov/2011/09/what-does-stem-stand.

wpx_explorem. "Explore More Virtual Tours – Egypt." *Family Travel Agency Home – Explore More Family Travel,* October 26, 2020. https://exploremorefamilytravel.com/egypt-virtual-tour/.

Part Two

Disability in Ancient Egypt and Nubia

8 What Was the Occupation of Disabled People in Ancient Egypt?

Samar Kamal

Introduction

The present author argues that ancient Egyptians widely accepted disabled people as suggested in artistic portrayals, tomb wall scenes, or sculptured artefacts, which depicted disabled people engaging in daily life activities. Egyptian art adopted certain rules among which was the representation of the kings and tomb owners in an idealistic body. One could argue that the strict rules of decorum were not applied in the same way when dealing with minor figures and some elite depictions. I argue that some of these figures were probably real disabled people. The inclusion and apparent absence of discriminatory exclusion can be viewed as an expression of cultural and social acceptance of the disabled people.[1] In Egyptian art, human figures were modelled in their most characteristic view; the head and neck are in profile; the eyes are in frontal view and the shoulders from the front. The breast, the arms, the pelvis, and the legs are shown from the side. The orientation of the face, nose, and lips was determined by that of the head, while the back and abdomen were represented as the back and front lines portraying the torso, respectively. People were very occasionally depicted with individual features since they were often portrayed as standardized or idealized figures in the structured decorum associated with the person's position and gender.[2]

Royal and elite representations were almost always represented with youthful body and features. This attitude was reflected above all in the treatment of facial features, which were not commonly individualized. The uncommon visage of Akhenaten in the Amarna style of art is considered an exceptional case. For further discussions on Akhenaten and Tutankhamun please see chapters three, four, and fourteen in the present volume. Minor figures, however, appear to have been represented with greater individualism and not regulated by the same royal proportional standards.[3] Minor figure representations followed a more naturalistic tendency, especially regarding their physical features or even disabilities.[4]

Aims and Scope

This chapter is a descriptive study of the modes of representation related to disabled figures in ancient Egyptian private tombs. I will explore the relationship between disability and occupation and/or social class in ancient Egyptian private

DOI: 10.4324/9781003440369-11

Table 8.1 Disabled People and Source Type

Type of source	*Dwarf persons*	*Leg impairments*	*Spinal conditions*	*Blindness*	*Total*
Wall scene *Note: 4 depict more than one dwarf person.* 1 scene has 3 dwarf people 3 scenes have 2 people	25	28	11	7	71 (total of 66 wall scenes)
Artefact	4	0	0	0	4
Statue	3	0	0	0	3
Mummified remains	0	2	0	0	2
Stelae	0	1	0	1	2
Sarcophagus	1	0	0	0	1
Total	33	31	11	8	83

tomb scenes and a selection of artefacts. This chapter is an overview of artistic evidence for disabilities, and as such it does not aim to provide a comprehensive review of the experience of each person, nor argue that such a thing is possible given the mortuary nature of artistic representations and contextual limitations of textual references. It is hoped that the collation of evidence in this chapter will be an avenue for future research. Given the chapter's aims of presenting a broad overview, it must be acknowledged that an in-depth analysis of the social implications of these individuals (should the depictions represent daily life at all) is beyond the scope of this chapter.

The data for this chapter includes **66** wall scenes, **four** artefacts, **three** statues, **two** mummified individuals, **two** stelae and **one** sarcophagus (see Table 8.1). These portrayals were collected by the author in the private tombs from the Old to the New Kingdoms at Giza, Saqqara, Abusir, Meidum, Deshasha, Beni Hassan, Bersha, El-Amarna, El-Sheikh Said, Meir, Deir el-Gabrawy, Deir Rifeh, Hawawish, Hammamiya, Naga ed-Dier, Abydos, Sheikh Abd el-Qurna, Deir el-Medina, El-Khokha, Moalla, Thebes, and Qubbet el-Hawa, West Aswan.

Results and Discussion

Visual sources provide rich evidence of physically disabled people's position and engagement in the context of 'daily life' activities in ancient Egypt. According to the visual representations collected here, all social classes of physically disabled people were given a visible role in the society. The Egyptian artist does not attempt to 'beautify' or 'hide' disability, which suggests that there was a prevailing attitude of cultural acceptance. Physical disability may have even been received as a positive mark of divinity.[5]

Dwarfism is the most famous bodily difference represented in ancient Egyptian portrayals. The ancient Egyptian designations for the word dwarf were *dng*, *nmw*, and *ḥwꜥ*, and followed by a determinative depicting a disproportionate dwarf person with a long trunk and short limbs.[6] The artistic evidence of dwarf peoples from ancient Egypt includes tomb wall scenes depictions, statuettes, and other minor arts.

Artistic, biological, and written resources suggest that dwarf people were highly integrated in ancient Egyptian society.[7] They were likely employed in many roles were represented performing roles such as jewellers, domestic servants, nurses, entertainers, or animal tenders.[8] The investigated data dealt with **33** dwarf peoples' portrayals. Their occupations varied: **five** herdsmen, **four** musicians, **two** leather makers, **ten** pet-keepers, **one** baker, and **seven** serving staff. Moreover, **four** were elite.

Leg Impairments

This study collected **31** leg impairment representations; **17** cases belong to elite occupations. Others were **12** herdsmen and **two** farmers. From the examined **31** leg impairment portrayals, **13** have been argued to be representations of polio or other diseases, and **five** were depicted with backwards knee impairments. This is where a person's knee was depicted facing the back part of their body. Some leg impairments could be due to old age, or could be poorly healed broken legs.

Pictorial and palaeopathological evidence suggest that polio (poliomyelitis) might have been common in ancient Egypt. Polio is caused by a virus that infects cells of the central nervous system causing paralysis of one or more limbs. The most common activities for people with these leg impairment examples were high-ranking occupations, as priests, local governors or tomb owners, or herdsmen.

Among the prominent examples, is on the Stela of Roma, the door-keeper and priest in the 18th and 19th Dynasties exhibited in Carlsberg Museum, Copenhagen. He was depicted with an impaired leg possibly due to poliomyelitis.[9] One of the most elite examples of a disabled individuals pharaoh Siptaḥ, of the 19th Dynasty (1205–1187 BCE), whose mummified remains are now in the National Museum of Egyptian Civilization at Cairo (CG 61080). Examination revealed a deformed *pes equinovarus*-like left foot and a shortened left leg.[10] The impairment of the left lower extremity of Siptah has been described as clubfoot or *talipes equinovarus*. Alternatively, some studies argue for polio or spastic cerebral palsy (CP).[11]

The Backwards Knee

The backwards knee is medically known as *genu recurvatum*. It is one of the conditions which cause the leg to be concave, and the knee joint to bend backward. The backwards knee may occur as a result of poor bone structure, fractures in the bones of the joints, or weakness of the knee muscles possibly due to poliomyelitis.[12] The medical *Ebers Papyrus* might have recognized this disease, since a statement refers to a prescription to treat it: '*kt nt rd-ḥm.s*', which could be translated as "another for knee which swings backward".[13] The word *ḥm* is generally accepted to be designated as a "knee disease" rather than the back knee.[14] This study collects representations in which **five** backwards knee disabled people were **four** herdsmen, and **one** case was of high-ranking occupation, a supervisor in the tomb of Ty at Saqqara.

Kyphosis (Spinal Curvatures or Pott's Disease)

Kyphosis is derived from the Greek term *kyohos*, meaning hump. It is an impairment that causes an over-curvature of the upper back, making a protuberance which causes a distortion in the bones of the ribcage causing them to come close together. This condition could be accompanied by a side curve of the spine known as kypho-scoliosis.[15]

In ancient Egypt, a person with spinal impairment was known as *iw* and the word has a determinative of a man with a hump. DNA tests from ancient Egyptian mummified and skeletal remains earliest detection of spinal tuberculosis is from the Predynastic period. Statues and wall scenes depict humped backs and curved spines. The oldest surviving material is a wooden statue of a male figure with spinal impairment, found at Saqqara, dating back to the Old Kingdom 3000–2001 BCE.[16]

Kyphosis or a spinal curvature could be a result of structural distortion, or due to osteomalacia (weakening of the muscles and ligaments in the back during adolescence). The hump in this case is round. Kyphosis may be also attested because of certain occupations, as in the case of jewellery makers and fish gutters. Sitting for long hours affects the longitudinal muscles around the spine. Carrying heavy loads may also affect the shoulders and the back. Old age may possibly be one of the factors leading to kyphosis: in this case the whole back becomes round.[17]

In the collected sample there were **11** depictions of people with spinal curvatures: **10** male figures and **one** female figure. Traditional occupations included three pet-keepers with round humps. There are three farmers, one of them with a round hump, one with a pointed hump, and the third with a regular small hump. There is one herder with a round hump, one rope maker with a round hump, and one fish gutter with a round hump. There is one member of serving staff, an offering bearer, with an angular hump, and one unique case of a tomb owner with a spinal curvature, Ankhwedjes, who was an elite person, compared to the others working in manual occupations.

Blindness

Blindness was referred to in various texts. Blindness in ancient Egyptian was known as *ỉrt*, *dgỉ*, *šp*, or *bꜣẖ* with the determinative of a painted upper eyelid.[18] The majority of assumed representations of blindness are as members of musical groups, mostly harpists or singers. The 'blind musician' was called *ḥsw* in ancient Egyptian and was a common theme in New Kingdom art. Blind musicians were frequently depicted as favourable participants in royal banquets.[19] At least 47 tombs in the Theban necropolis depict potentially blind harpists. This motif decorated tombs of nobles and royalty. The blind harp player was perhaps a stereotypical depiction, which was commonly associated with a poetic text about death and the usefulness of the tomb and its funerary rituals.[20] The data collected for this chapter includes **seven** scenes and **one** stela featuring blind musicians, who were occupied as harpists, accompanied by several singers, flute players, and clappers.

The oldest surviving portrayal was the musical ensemble in the tomb of the local governor Ukh-ḥotep at Meir (12th Dynasty). The band consisted of a harpist, singer, and flute player in a banquet context.[21] Some 18th Dynasty private wall scenes included blind persons represented with some examples found at Amarna and Saqqara, like the harpist in the tomb of Paatonemḥeb.[22]

The eye of the blind musician is commonly depicted with no pupil, sometimes half-closed, completely closed, or empty. It is difficult to determine if these portrayals were of blind people, or if this were an artistic convention, since these specific individuals are represented on the same walls alongside other stereotypical themes.[23]

Roles and Responsibilities: A Visual Indication of Potential Real-life Social Roles?

Disabled Herdsmen (Table 2)

Herdsmen depictions in tomb wall scenes are commonly minor figures and represented in a realistic manner. They were generally thin, maybe because of their hard labour. Age varied with some depictions with specific impairments.[24]

The examined data revealed that a great number of disabled people in representations were herdsmen (**17**) and the oldest depiction dated back to the 4th Dynasty. Most disabled herdsmen portrayals (**11**) had a leg impairment of either backwards knee **(four cases)**, polio disease (**three cases**), or disability due to age (**four cases**). They appeared leaning against long sticks (walking aids), either with short hair or as half-bald.[25]

One unique scene of a herder who has a rounded spinal impairment is in the tomb of Ptaḥḥotep at Saqqara.[26] This is the only example of a herder with rounded spinal impairment represented in ancient Egyptian portrayals. The tomb of Ptaḥḥotep at Saqqara (5th Dynasty) has unique depictions of four disabled figures in different daily life contexts: one with leg impairment and three workmen with a spinal hump.[27]

The most common scene context for herders was animal husbandry, occasionally the funeral procession or offering parade, and one rare war siege context (tomb of Kaiemheset at Saqqara).

It is noteworthy that dwarf persons were also occupied with herding animals much larger than themselves. The investigated data includes **five** tomb wall scenes depicting dwarf people leading a young ox or a cow in a procession of these animals, using a leash. In **four** scenes, the dwarf person holds the leash with both hands (tomb of Kai-khent, tomb of Ireru at Giza).

Disabled Musicians and Dancers (Table 3)

The representations attest that disabled people in ancient Egypt could be occupied as musicians in **12** cases. There were **seven** wall tomb scenes, **three** statuettes, and

one stela. The majority were blind figures (**eight cases**) and the others were dwarf people (**four cases**), males and females. They were most commonly depicted in specific roles, such as harpists, singers, flute players, clappers, or even dancers. The oldest surviving material, dated back to the 4th Dynasty, was the scene of the female dancing dwarf person in the tomb of Nuntjer at Giza.[28]

Al-Aboudy argues dwarf titles suggest roles associated with entertainment or ritual, such as 'god's dancers, *dng jbꜣw nṯr*'.[29] They participated in religious rituals, likely because magico-religious significance was attributed to them.[30]

The image of blind (or visually impaired) musicians was iconic and recognizable. The harpist, a symbol of a wise man, likely represents the wisdom of the song he performed. Blind musicians were traditionally portrayed seated cross-legged, usually with their cropped short hair, clean-shaven, or even bald.[31] Their facial features commonly were wrinkled, to indicate their seniority. The eyes were modelled as a split under the heavy eyelids to suggest blindness. Most of these figures were represented as overweight with heavy folds and dressed in a pleated tunic.

Disabled Rope Makers (Table 4)

Portrayals of rope makers in ancient Egypt were very limited. **Eleven** scenes are examined for rope makers.[32] Only **one** scene was found to represent a bald disabled worker with a round spinal impairment, which could be explained as back curvature that was a result of the long-exhausted seating position of this kind of occupation.[33]

Disabled Fish Gutters (Table 5)

Very few depictions represented fish gutters in ancient Egyptian art. Investigating about **20** wall scenes of fish gutters in private tombs from Old to New Kingdom revealed only **one** case of a bald disabled fish gutter with a round spinal impairment.[34] The aforementioned disabled rope maker and the fish gutter both have spinal impairments, and are depicted on the wall scenes of Ptaḥḥotep's tomb, which includes representations of two other disabled workmen. If the back curvature was not congenital or pathological, this could be explained as a possible result of the long hard-working hours while in a back-bending position. Alternatively, the artist may have portrayed the same person in different activities.

Disabled Leather Makers (Table 6)

Dwarf people in ancient Egypt are especially represented in certain occupations that needed high degree of technical skill and hand-eye coordination, such as goldsmiths and leather makers. Leather makers were among the handcrafts which needed a prolonged length of time and repeated actions in specific environments and raises their susceptibility to the acquirement of occupation-related diseases. Occupations can impact health in a direct or indirect manner.[35]

Disabled Pet Keepers (Table 7)

Taking care of animals was the most represented occupation of dwarf people.[36] Dwarf people were shown taking care of domestic animals such as dogs, monkeys, and, rarely, wild animals. They were commonly depicted close to the tomb owner, as favourable attendants, such as the dwarf dog-keeper Ipy. They were occasionally identified by their own names and titles.[37]

The investigated data revealed that animal keeping was a commonly represented occupation for disabled people in ancient Egypt. The total number in the collected sample is **12**: there were **eight** male dwarf persons and **two** of female dwarf persons (Figure 5), and **three** male pet keepers with round spinal curvatures; **two** examples also had physically impaired chests.

The scenes of the animal keepers' occupation usually depicted funeral processions, offering parades, and rarely marshland contexts. The animals illustrated in the examined scenes were **11** dogs, **eight** monkeys, **one** unique example of a leopard, and **one** gazelle. The animals were being led by a leashed rope in the keeper's hands, while in certain rare cases the keepers carried the animal over their heads.[38]

Disabled Farmers (Table 8)

Farming was among the most essential occupations in ancient Egypt. The studied data confirmed that disabled farmers' portrayals were present in **five** wall scenes of private tombs from Old to New Kingdom. The oldest one dated back to the 4th Dynasty, in the tomb of Khafraankh at Giza. The five disabled farmers varied, with **three** spinal impairment cases: **two** rounded shape and **one** pointed shape. The **two** others had leg impairment, possibly because of age. The most common context for disabled farmer scenes was harvesting agricultural crops, especially grain and animal husbandry. See Table 9 for the only representation of a disabled baker (a dwarf person).

Disabled Serving Staff (Table 10)

The investigated data revealed that ancient Egyptian disabled people were engaged in different serving occupations. There are **eight** portrayals, of which **one** female offering bearer has an angular spinal impairment.[39] The remaining **seven** scenes are representing male dwarf people depicting sandal or offering bearers accompanying their masters in funeral or offering parades.[40]

Disabled Elite (Table 11)

The investigated data includes a total **22** representations of elite occupation including **10** scenes, **three** statues, **two** mummified remains, **one** sarcophagus, and **one** stela. These occupations were of high social status in ancient Egypt. The others were **three** priests, **five** local governors, **two** tomb owners, **two** overseers, **eight** supervisors, **one** elite dancer, and **one** pharaoh.

The disabled elite include **four** dwarf people, **one** person with a spinal impairment, and **17** people represented with leg impairment (backwards knee, polio, or impairments associated with age). Potentially disabled people with leg impairments were depicted leaning against a long cane as a walking aid, supporting one leg and leaving the other one free. However, Egyptologists do not all agree that this is a representation of disability, with some arguing that the staff is used iconographically rather than literally.[41]

Conclusion

The investigated data relied on the interpretation of disability based on my visual analysis. The examined portrayals indicated that the artists were observant of the physical differences of people in their communities. Certain variations in physical features, disability type, and meaning actions were observed, whether they depict stereotyped themes or specific figural art. These observations may serve to weaken the assumption that the ancient Egyptian art in general adopted idealistic principles. This chapter found **83** likely disabled people represented in examined **66** wall scenes and **four** artefacts, **three** statues, **two** mummified remains, **two** stelae, and **one** sarcophagus. These portrayals were collected from the private tombs in ancient Egypt from the Old to the New Kingdoms. The elite portrayals numbered **22**, shown performing different high-status occupations, regardless of their disabilities. These occupations were on the top of the hierarchy social status in ancient Egypt and included the pharaoh.

The multi-perspective technique of representing minor figures makes these figures appear somewhat stylized. However, after investigation, one can distinguish certain differences. Minor figures' posture was far from static, since they were shown in some examples swaying to the rhythm produced by musicians in a very dynamic way.

So, what was the occupation of disabled people in ancient Egypt? At least in tomb scenes, they were employed in a range of roles; they were herdsmen, musical band members, rope makers, fish gutters, skilful craftsmen, and animal keepers. The most common occupations in wall scenes for disabled people (including dwarf people, people with leg and/or back impairments), were herdsmen and animal keepers. It is possible that a favourable position for dwarf people and other individuals with disabilities was emphasized by depicting them close to tomb owners, dressed in appropriate garments and sometimes accessories, and occasionally accompanied with their own names and titles. These portrayals were not standardized or repetitive. It may be that these stylistic choices are an insight to specific disabled people in ancient Egypt.

Appendix

Table 8.2 Disabled Herdsmen in Ancient Egyptian Portrayals

Scene and context	*Tomb owner*	*Tomb location and date*	*Disability type*
A bald herdsman leaning against a long stick in an animal husbandry context (Shehab 2022).	The mastaba (G2196) of Iasen	Saqqara, 4th – 6th Dynasties	Probably a leg impairment
A bald herdsman catching an ox by a rope in his right hand, with the other holding a stalk in an animal husbandry context (Mahran and Kamal 2016).	Ptaḥḥotep	Saqqara, 5th Dynasty	Leg impairment (backwards knee)
A squatting man with a round spinal curvature, while feeding a bull (Harpur and Scremin 2008).	Ptaḥḥotep	Saqqara, 5th Dynasty	Spinal curvature with round hump
A bald herdsman pulling an ox by a rope in an animal husbandry context (Evans and Woods 2016).	Niankh-amun and Khnum-hotep	Saqqara, 5th Dynasty	Leg impairment (backwards knee)
A bald herdsman catching an ox by a rope in his left hand in an animal husbandry context (Mahran and Kamal 2016).	Iḥy	Saqqara, 5th Dynasty	Leg impairment (backwards knee)
An aged man leaning against a long staff and holding something bag(?) on his shoulder, in an animal husbandry context (Mahran and Kamal 2016).	Niankh-amun and Khnum-hotep	Saqqara, 5th Dynasty	Leg impairment
A herdsman as pulling an ox with a rope in one hand, and with the other carrying a bag in an animal husbandry context (Mahran and Kamal 2016).	Idut	Saqqara, 5th Dynasty	Leg impairment (backwards knee)
A herdsman with an impairment in his left leg leaning against a long cane as physical support, in a funeral procession (Mahran and Kamal 2016).	Iymery, G 6000	Giza, 5th Dynasty	Leg impairment (possibly polio)

(*Continued*)

Table 8.2 (Continued)

Scene and context	*Tomb owner*	*Tomb location and date*	*Disability type*
A scene of a dwarf person pulling an ox by a rope with two hands, in an animal husbandry context (Kanawati, El-Khouli, and El-Khouli 1990).	Kai-khent	Hammamiya at Sohag, 5th Dynasty	Dwarfism
Scene of a dwarf person pulling an ox by a rope with the assistance of another herdsman, in an animal husbandry context (Kanawati and Mcfarlane 1993).	Inti	Deshasha, 5th Dynasty	Dwarfism
Scene of **two** men with leg impairments, leaning against a long cane as a walking aide, in a war siege context (Mourad 2011).	Kaiemheset	Saqqara, 5th Dynasty	Leg impairments
A third scene of a dwarf person pulling an ox by a rope in his two hands, in an animal husbandry context (El-Aboudy 2021).	Ireru	Giza 8698, 5th – 6th Dynasties	Dwarfism
An elderly herdsman leaning against a sceptre and holding a bag on his shoulder, in animal husbandry context (Walsem 2005).	Kagemni	Saqqara, 6th Dynasty	Polio
An interesting scene of a dwarf person taking care of a gazelle in a wild repertoire (El-Aboudy 2021).	Merw	Naga ed-Dier, 1st Intermediate period	Dwarfism
A herdsman leaning against a sceptre in animal husbandry context (Shafik 2020).	Khety, BH No. 17	Beni Hassan, 11th Dynasty	Possible polio
Scene of a dwarf person pulling an ox by a rope in one hand in an animal procession (Kanawati 2005).	Zau	Dier el Gebrawy at Asiut, 12th Dynasty	Dwarfism
Two or more herders leading groups of cattle in an offering context (Middleton 1999).	Geḥwty-ḥotep	Bersha at Minia, 12th Dynasty	Leg impairments

Table 8.3 Disabled Musicians and Dancers in Ancient Egyptian Portrayals

Scene and context/Artefact	*Tomb owner*	*Tomb location and date*	*Disability type*
A scene of a dwarf woman is in the middle of two groups of women in a dancing context; she wears a floral tiara on her head and wears a belt with strips (Arnold 1999).	Nuntjer	Giza, 4th Dynasty	Dwarfism
Two painted limestone statuettes of dwarf people playing harps, the Oriental Institute of the University of Chicago, Chicago, Illinois (Dasen 1993).	Ni-kau-inpu and his wife, Hemet-re	Giza, Western Cemetery, 5th Dynasty	Dwarfism
A painted limestone statuette of a female harpist, the Oriental Institute of the University of Chicago, Chicago, Illinois (Porter and Moss 1974).	Ni-kau-inpu and his wife, Hemet-re	Giza, Western Cemetery, 5th Dynasty	Dwarfism
The blind harpist Nefer-ḥotep squatting on the ground as an overweight figure while playing music to the tomb owner and his wife, in a funeral context (the Metropolitan Museum, not on display).	A limestone stela of Iki and his wife Renesankh	Provenance is not confirmed, possibly Abydos (now kept in the Metropolitan Museum), 12th Dynasty	Blindness
A painted scene of a blind musical group, a harpist and a singer, in banquet scene (Shafik 2020).	Ukh-ḥotep	Meir at Asiut, 12th Dynasty	Blindness
A scene of a blind musician playing a harp (Menéndez 2011).	Djehuty (TT11)	Dra' Abu el-Naga, Thebes, 18th Dynasty	Blindness
A blind harpist squatting on the ground, resting on his right knee with the other foot in front of him. His eye is reduced to a line, in an offering context (Porter and Moss 1994).	Nefersekheru (TT296)	Khokha, Thebes, 18th Dynasty	Blindness
A scene of a blind musician playing a harp in a banquet scene (Dasen 1993).	Nakht (TT52)	Sheikh Abd el-Qurna, part of Thebes, 18th Dynasty	Blindness
A scene of bald blind musicians who were sitting on the ground, while and clapping on the harp's rhythm (Kemp 1989).	Merire I (No.4)	El-Amarna, 18th Dynasty	Blindness
A limestone scene of a bald and blind harpist in a banquet context, now in Museum van Oudheden, Leiden (Manniche 1991).	Paätenemheb	Saqqara, 18th Dynasty (Amarna period)	Blindness
A scene depicting Raia as a blind harpist playing music before the Memphite gods, Ptah and Hathor, in a funeral procession (Martin et al. 1985).	Raia, Chief of Singers, temple of Ptah at Memphis	Saqqara, 19th Dynasty (Ramesside period)	Blindness

Table 8.4 Disabled Rope Makers in Ancient Egyptian Portrayals

Scene and context	*Tomb owner*	*Tomb location and date*	*Disability type*
A bald man sitting on the ground making ropes in a workshop (Mahran and Kamal 2016)	Ptaḥḥotep	Saqqara, 5th Dynasty	A round spinal impairment

Table 8.5 Disabled Fish Gutters in Ancient Egyptian Portrayals

Scene and context	*Tomb owner*	*Tomb location and date*	*Disability type*
A bald fish gutter sitting on the ground in a market context (Mahran and Kamal 2016).	Ptaḥḥotep	Saqqara, 5th Dynasty	A round spinal impairment

Table 8.6 Disabled Leather Makers in Ancient Egyptian Portrayals

Scene and context	*Tomb owner*	*Tomb location and date*	*Disability type*
Two bald dwarf people making leather belts in a leather-working workshop context (Kanawati and Woods 2009).	Mereruka	Saqqara, 6th Dynasty	Dwarfism

Table 8.7 Disabled Pet Keepers in Ancient Egyptian Portrayals

Scene and context	*Tomb owner*	*Tomb location and date*	*Disability type*
A dwarf woman carrying a monkey over her head; they are under the chair of the tomb owner (Figure 5) (El-Kilany and Rady 2021).	Princess Idut	Saqqara, 5th Dynasty	Dwarfism
A scene of a dwarf person catching a leash of a monkey under the chair of the tomb owner. The monkey is depicted seated on his legs, eating from a basket of fruits (Al-Aboudy 2021).	wr-iri-ny	Sheikh Saied at Minia, 5th Dynasty	Dwarfism
A scene of a dwarf person leading a leashed monkey with one hand while with the other holds a stick which ends with a human hand shape, in a funeral procession (El-Kilany and Rady 2021).	Ty	Saqqara, 5th Dynasty	Dwarfism

(*Continued*)

Table 8.7 (Continued)

Scene and context	*Tomb owner*	*Tomb location and date*	*Disability type*
A scene of two hounds with pointed ears and curly tails, on leashes, being led by a naked young man, in a funeral procession (Mahran and Kamal 2016).	Ty	Saqqara, 5th Dynasty	A round spinal impairment
A scene of disabled dog keeper leading a dog with one hand, while catching a long top curved cane with the other, in a funeral procession (Figure 7) (Mahran and Kamal 2016).	Nykahem and Sekhemen-Hathor	Saqqara, 5th Dynasty	A round curvature on his back and a physically impaired chest
A male servant, named *iri*, is standing next to the tomb owner's chair, while holding a dog by a rope (Mahran and Kamal 2016).	Nikausesi	Saqqara, 6th Dynasty	A round curvature on his back and a physically impaired chest
A dog keeper standing under the chair of the tomb owner while holding his favourite dog (Barta 2006).	Inti (judge)	Abusir, 6th Dynasty	Dwarfism
A scene of **two** naked dwarf persons with a pet monkey and three dogs in the context of the tomb owner funeral procession (Kanawati et al. 2010).	Mereruka	Saqqara, 6th Dynasty	Dwarfism
A dwarf person holding leashes of two dogs and a monkey (El-Kilany and Rady 2021).	Kagemni	Saqqara, 6th Dynasty	Dwarfism
A dwarf person carrying a monkey on his head by a leash in his right hand, while he holds a fruit basket (Figure 6) (Daoud 2004).[42]	Ankhmaḥour	Saqqara, 6th Dynasty	Dwarfism
A scene of a monkey and a leashed leopard led by a dwarf person (El-Aboudy 2021).	Ni-ankh-nswt	Saqqara, 6th Dynasty	Dwarfism
A scene of a dwarf person leading a leashed dog and monkey by one hand, while following tomb owner in a marshland fowling scene (El-Aboudy 2021).	Ni-ankh-nswt	Saqqara, 6th Dynasty	Dwarfism

Table 8.8 Disabled Farmers in Ancient Egyptian Portrayals

Scene and context	*Tomb owner*	*Tomb location and date*	*Disability type*
A scene of a farmer cutting grain and the cutting tool seems like an extension of the arm, in a harvesting context (Smith 1949).	Khafraankh	Giza, 4th Dynasty	Round spinal impairment
A scene of a disabled farmer catching a hanging animal from a tree, in a harvesting context (Mahran and Kamal 2016).	Akhmerutnisu, G.2184	Meidum, 5th – 6th Dynasties	Pointed spinal impairment
A male figure following the previous farmer as his work partner, while leaning against a long cane as a walking aid, in a harvesting context (Smith 1949).	Akhmerutnisu, G.2184	Meidum, 5th – 6th Dynasties	Leg impairment
A bald elderly man leaning against a long sceptre, while resting a hand on the head of a young boy in an agricultural context (McDowell 2002).	Ipuy (TT217)	Deir el-Medina, Thebes, 19th Dynasty	Leg impairment, possibly a result of old age
A farmer with a spinal impairment irrigating a garden with a "shadouf" (Wilkinson and Marsha 1983).	Ipuy (TT217)	Deir el-Medina, Thebes, 19th Dynasty	Spinal impairment

Table 8.9 Disabled Bakers in Ancient Egyptian Portrayals

Scene and context/Artefact	*Tomb owner*	*Tomb location and date*	*Disability type*
A limestone statuette of a dwarf person grinding grain, now in the British Museum, London (Karim and Amin 2018).	Not known	The precise provenance of excavation is unknown, 6th Dynasty	Dwarfism

Table 8.10 Disabled Serving Staff in Ancient Egyptian Portrayals

Scene and context	*Tomb owner*	*Tomb location and date*	*Disability type*
A scene of a dwarf man working as a sandal bearer, in a funeral procession (Figure 7) (Mahran and Kamal 2016).	Nykahem and Sekhemen-Hathor	Saqqara, 5th Dynasty	Dwarfism
A female offering bearer depicted with an angular spinal curvature, in a funeral procession (Kanawati 2001).	Seshemnefer I, (G 4940)	Giza, 6th Dynasty	Angular spinal impairment
A dwarf woman carrying an offering box over her head, in a funeral procession (Kanawati 2001).	Seshemnefer I, (G 4940)	Giza, 6th Dynasty	Dwarfism
A painted scene of **three** dwarf people following the tomb owner, on the south wall (Baramilis 2021).	Baquet III, BH No. 15	Beni Hassan, 11th Dynasty, Middle Kingdom	Dwarfism
A painted scene of **two** dwarf people following the tomb owner, on the South wall (Kanawati and Evans 2020).	Khety, BH No. 17	Beni Hassan, 11th Dynasty, Middle Kingdom	Dwarfism

Table 8.11 Disabled Elite in Ancient Egyptian Portrayals

Scene and context/ Artefact	*Tomb owner*	*Tomb location and date*	*Disability type*	*Position*
A bald man leaning against a long sceptre as a walking aid because he apparently had a leg impairment, in a marshland context (Evans 2015).	Kawab	Giza, 4th Dynasty	Leg impairment (polio)	Not clear whether he is the tomb owner or one of his supervisors
A basalt seated statue of dwarf person Pereniankh or Per-ni-ankh-w, now in the Egyptian Museum in Cairo (JE 98944) (Hawass 2004).	Pereniankh	Giza, 4th Dynasty	Dwarfism	A dancer in the great palace
The painted limestone group statue of the dwarf person Seneb and his family, now in the Egyptian Museum at Cairo, JE 51280 (Saleh and Sourouzian 1987).	Seneb	Giza (G 1036), the end of the 4th Dynasty and beginning of the 5th Dynasty	Dwarfism	Overseer of dwarf people and head of the royal treasury during the reign of Khufu and Djedefre

(*Continued*)

Table 8.11 (Continued)

Scene and context/ Artefact	*Tomb owner*	*Tomb location and date*	*Disability type*	*Position*
A bald supervisor leaning against a walking sceptre and watching male figures while crossing in two papyrus boats in marshland context (René 2005).	Ty	Saqqara, 5th Dynasty	Backwards knee impairment	Supervisor
A bald supervisor leaning against a walking sceptre while watching the animal husbandry activities (René 2005).	Ty	Saqqara, 5th Dynasty	Leg impairment (polio)	Supervisor
A partly damaged scene of a bald man, who leans forwards on to a staff which is invisible now, in a bread making workshop (Walsem 2005)	Ty	Saqqara, 5th Dynasty	Leg impairment (probably polio)	Supervisor of bread manufacture workshop, according to the text above him; "the person responsible of the workshop"
A bald man was leaning against a long sceptre as a walking aid, because he seems to have a leg impairment, in a market perspective (Daumas 1964).	Ḥetep-ḥerakheti	Saqqara, date is not confirmed but may be 5th Dynasty	Leg impairment (polio)	Supervisor
A scene of a young man leaning against a long sceptre as a walking aid, while supervising in an agricultural context, (Moussa and Altenmüller 1971).	Nefer and Ka-hay	Saqqara, 5th Dynasty	Leg impairment (probably polio)	Supervisor of herdsmen and farmers
Nikausesi leaning against a long sceptre as a walking aid (Mahran and Kamal 2016).	Nikausesi	Saqqara, 6th Dynasty	Polio	Tomb owner

(*Continued*)

Table 8.11 (Continued)

Scene and context/ Artefact	*Tomb owner*	*Tomb location and date*	*Disability type*	*Position*
A limestone statue of dwarf person Khnumḥotep, now in the Egyptian Museum in Cairo (CG 144) (El-Aguizy 1987).	Khnumḥotep	Saqqara, 6th Dynasty	Dwarfism	Overseer of clothing and Overseer of ka-priests
A scene of Mekhu leaning against a long sceptre as a walking aid while supervising agricultural activities (Moussa and Altenmüller 1971).	Mehkeu and Sabni	The rock-cut tombs of the nobles at Qubbet el-Hawa, West Aswan, 6th Dynasty	Leg impairment	Local governor in the reign of King Pepi II
A wall relief depicting Ḥerkhuf, leaning against a walking aid (long sceptre) (Bommas 2016).	Ḥerkhuf	The rock cut tombs of the nobles at Qubbet el-Hawa, West Aswan, 6th Dynasty	Leg impairment	Local governor and overseer of foreign troops in the reign of King Pepi II and Merenre
Depiction of the tomb owner Ankhwedjes, whose left arm attached backward with a small hump under the upper part of the arm (Mahran and Kamal 2016).	Ankhwedjes	Giza, late 6th Dynasty	Spinal impairment	Tomb owner (may have had a priestly position)
A scene of Pepy-ankh leaning against a long cane, while supervising different activities in his province (Kanawati and Evans 2013).	Pepy-ankh the black	Meir at Asiut, 6th Dynasty	Leg impairment	Local governor and tomb owner
A scene of Ankhtifi, whose head is damaged, leaning against a long sceptre, in a ritualistic navigation context (Vandier 1950).	Ankhtifi	Moalla at Thebes, 9th Dynasty (1st Intermediate period)	Leg impairment (possibly a result of getting old)	Local governor and military leader
A bald elderly man, leaning against a sceptre as a walking aid, in a marshland context (Kanawati and Evans 2013).	Ukhḥot-ep, son of Senbi (B2)	Meir at Asiut, 12th Dynasty	Leg impairment due to old age	Supervisor

(*Continued*)

Table 8.11 (Continued)

Scene and context/ Artefact	*Tomb owner*	*Tomb location and date*	*Disability type*	*Position*
The mummified remains of Khnum-Nakht, now in Manchester Museum, (Inv. No. 21471). Examination reveals he had a leg impairment (Galassi, Habicht, and Rühli 2017).	Tomb of the two brothers Nakht-Ankh and Khnum-Nakht	Deir Rifeh at Asiut, 12th Dynasty	Leg impairment (most probably polio)	Local governor
Ptaḥmay standing, leaning on a long staff by curving his right hand over the top while he firmly grasps the staff with his left hand. He leans slightly forward (Staring 2021).	Ptaḥmay	Provenance is not confirmed (it could be Giza or Saqqara), 18th Dynasty	Leg impairment, possibly a result of old age	Supervisor of gold workshops at the Aten temple
An elderly man leaning against a long sceptre as a walking aid in an agricultural context (Porter and Moss 1994).	Menna, (TT69)	Sheikh Abd el-Qurna, Thebes, 18th Dynasty	Polio	Supervisor
Painted limestone Stela of Roma, the door-keeper and priest now in Carlsberg Museum, Copenhagen ÆIN 0134, (Loeb and Nunn 1997).	Not confirmed	Provenance is not known, 18th and 19th Dynasties (1300 BC)	Polio	The door-keeper and priest
The mummified remains of Pharaoh Siptah, (now in the National Museum of Egyptian Civilization at Cairo CG 61080) (Galassi, Habicht, and Rühli 2017).	Valley of the Kings, Thebes KV47	Valley of the Kings, Thebes, 19th Dynasty	Polio, but alternately diagnosed as spastic cerebral palsy (CP)	Pharaoh
Granite sarcophagus of dwarf person Gjeḥu, now in the Egyptian Museum in Cairo (Kozma 2006).	Tjaiharp-ta and Gjeḥu	Saqqara, 30th Dynasty	Dwarfism	Priest and dancer of ritualistic ceremonies of the Apis bull at Saqqara

Notes

1 Mahran and Kamal (2016, 169).
2 Nyord (2013, 161).
3 Baramilis (2021, 41–44).
4 Baines (1994, 67–94) and Leary (2021, 1–18).
5 Sullivan (2001, 262–66).
6 Dasen (1988, 253–76).
7 Kozma et al. (2011, 1817).
8 Kozma (2006, 303–11).
9 Loeb and Nunn (1997, 450–54).
10 Galassi, Habicht, and Rühl (2017, 375).
11 Panteliadis, Panteliadis, and Vassilyadi (2012, 285–92).
12 Hart and Macnicol (2010, 495–515).
13 Ebbell (1937, 91).
14 Erman and Grapow (1926–1961, 22).
15 Mahran and Kamal (2016, 177–78).
16 Zaied (2020, 1–9).
17 El Shafey (1998, 38–39).
18 Nunn (1996, 57–68).
19 Morris (2022, 133–35) and Manniche (1978, 13–21).
20 Lichtheim (1945, 178–212).
21 Blackman (1915, XXI).
22 Manniche (1991, 97–107).
23 Shafik (2020, 207–26).
24 Shehab (2022, 84–107).
25 Kamal (2019, 127–79).
26 Mahran and Kamal (2016, figure 8).
27 Mahran and Kamal (2016, figure 8).
28 Kozma (2006, figure 11).
29 Al-Aboudy (2021, 69).
30 Zakrzewski (2014, 57–68).
31 Kamal (2019, 164).
32 Teeter (1987, 71–77).
33 Diab (2018, 112–23).
34 Harpur and Scremin (2008, 306, pl. 167).
35 Diab (2018, 112–23).
36 Elaboudy (2021, 231–33).
37 Elaboudy (2021, 231–33).
38 Elaboudy (2021, figures 2–5).
39 Mahran and Kamal (2016, figure 6).
40 Baramilis (2021, 43–45).
41 Gessler-Lohr (2007, 65–108).
42 Daoud (2004, 231–33).

Bibliography

Al-Aboudy, O. "Representation Modes of Dwarf Animal-Keeper." *Journal of the General Union of Arab Archaeologists* 6, no. 3 (2021): 67–82. https://doi.org/10.21608/jguaa2.2021.69919.1053.

Arnold, D. *When the Pyramids Were Built.* New York: Metropolitan Museum of Art, 1999.

Baines, J. "Merit by Proxy: The Biographies of the Dwarf Djeho and His Patron Tjaiharpta." *The Journal of Egyptian Archaeology* 78 (1992): 241–57.

Baines, J. "On the Status and Purposes of Ancient Egyptian Art." *Cambridge Archaeological Journal* 4 (1994): 67–94.
Baramilis, N. N. "Individuality in Tomb Scenes from the Old and Middle Kingdom." Thesis, Macquarie University, 2021. https://doi.org/10.25949/19430735.v1.
Barta, M. "The Sixth Dynasty Tombs in Abusir. Tomb Complex of the Vizier Qar and His Family." The Old Kingdom Art and Archaeology. Proceeding of the Conference Held in Prague, May 31–June 4, 2004. Czech Institute of Egyptology Faculty of Arts, Charles University in Prague Academia Publishing House of the Academy of Sciences of the Czech Republic Prague, 2006, 45–62.
Blackman, A. M. *The Rock Tombs of Meir: Part II: The Tomb-Chapel of Senbi's Son Ukh-Hotp: (B, no. 2).* London: Egypt Exploration Society, 1915.
Bommas, M. "Qubbet El-Hawa." The *Journal of Egyptian Archaeology* 102 (2016): 23–40. https://www.jstor.org/stable/26379070.
Daoud, K. A. "Review of the Teti Cemetery at Saqqara, II. The Tomb of Ankhmahor, by N. Kanawati & A. Hassan." *The Journal of Egyptian Archaeology* 90 (2004): 231–33. http://www.jstor.org/stable/3822258.
Dasen, V. "Dwarfism in Egypt and Classical Antiquity: Iconography and Medical History." *Medical History* 32 (1988): 253–76.
Dasen, V. *Dwarfs in ancient Egypt and Greece, Oxford Monographs on Classical Archaeology*. Oxford: Clarendon Press, 1993.
Daumas, F. "Quelques Remarques sur les Representations de pêche ă la ligne sous le'ancien empire." *BIFAO* 62 (1964): 67–85.
Diab, A. M. "Images of Leather-Workers as Sandal-Maker from the Old Kingdom to the New Kingdom." *International Journal of Heritage, Tourism and Hospitality* 12, no. 1–2 (2018): 112–23.
Ebbell, B. *The Papyrus Ebres: The Greatest Egyptian Medical Document.* Copenhagen: Levin & Munksgaard, 1937.
El Shafey, M. "Congenital Anomalies of Individuals in Ancient Egyptian Art till the End of the New Kingdom." Master's thesis, Tanta University, 1998.
El-Aboudy, O. "Representation Modes of Dwarf Animal-Keeper." *Journal of the General Union of Arab Archaeologists* 6, no. 3 (2021): Article 5. https://digitalcommons.aaru.edu.jo/jguaa/vol6/iss3/5.
El-Aguizy, O. "Dwarfs and Pygmies in Ancient Egypt." *ASAE* 71 (1987): 53–60.
El-Kilany, E., and M. Rady. "Classification of Monkey's Roles Relating to the Daily Life Scenes in Ancient Egypt." *The Journal of the Faculty of Tourism and Hotels, Mansoura University* 10, no. 10 (December 2021): 1–51. https://doi.org/10.21608/mkaf.2021.213930.
Erman, A., and H. Grapow. *Wörterbuch der Aegyptischen Sprache. Wb III* (Dictionary of Egyptian Language). Vol. III. Berlin: Akademie-Verlag, 1926–1961.
Evans, L. *Bird Behavior in Ancient Egyptian Art: Between Heaven and Earth: Birds in Ancient Egypt*, 91–98. Edited by Rozenn Bailleul-LeSuer. Chicago: The Oriental Institute for the University of Chicago, 2015.
Evans, L., and A. Woods. "Further Evidence that Niankhnum and Khnumhotep were Twins." *JEA* 102 (2016): 55–72.
Filer, J. *Disease, Egyptian Bookshelf.* London: The British Museum Press, 1995.
Galassi, F. M., M. E. Habicht, and F. J. Rühli. "Poliomyelitis in Ancient Egypt?" *Neurological Sciences* 38 (2017): 375. https://doi.org/10.1007/s10072-016-2720-9.
Gessler-Lohr, B."Pre -Amarna Tomb Chapels in the Teti Cemetery North at Saqqara." *BACE* 18 (2007): 65–108.
Harpur, Y., and P. J. Scremin. *Chapel of Ptahhotep: Scenes Details*, 306, pl. 167. Reading: Oxford Expedition to Egypt, 2008.
Hart, D. M., and M. F. Macnicol. "The Knee" *in Children's Orthopedics and Fractures*, 495–515. Edited by M. Benson, J. Fixsen, and M. Macnico. London: Churchill Livingstone, 2010.

Hawass, Z. "The Dancing Dwarf. The Ambassadors Online Magazine." *The Forum for Culture and Civilization* 7, no. 2 (2004). Accessed April 30, 2023. http://ambassadors.net./selected. study.htm.

Kamal, H. *Dictionary of Pharaonic Medicine*. Cairo: National Publication House, 1967.

Kamal, S. M. "Baldness Scenes in Ancient Egyptian Private Tombs; as an Indicator of Social Class, Activity and Physical Ability." *International Journal of Tourism and Hospitality Management* 2, no. 2 (2019): 127–79. https://doi.org/10.21608/ijthm.2019.77625.

Kanawati, N. *Tombs at Giza, Kaiemankh (G 4561) and Seshemnefer I (G 4940), Volume I. Australian Centre for Egyptology Report 16*. Warminster: Aris and Phillips, 2001.

Kanawati, N. *Deir el-Gebrawi 1*. Oxford: Aris and Phillips, 2005.

Kanawati, N., A. El-Khouli, and S. El Khouli. "The Old Kingdom Tombs at Hammaniya." Australian Centre for Egyptology Reports, Report 2, 1990.

Kanawati, N., and L. Evans. *The Cemetery of Meir. Vol. II: The Tomb of Pepyankh the Black*. Oxford: The Australian Centre for Egyptology, 2013.

Kanawati, N., and L. Evans. "Beni Hassan. Vol. VI: The Tomb of Khety." The Australian Centre for Egyptology: Reports, No. 44, 2020.

Kanawati, N., and A. Mcfarlane. "Deshasha: The Tombs of Inti, Shedu and Others." Vol. 5. Australian Centre for Egyptology Reports, Report 5, 1993.

Kanawati, N., and A. Woods. *Artists in the Old Kingdom. Techniques and Achievements*. Cairo: Supreme Council of Antiquities, 2009.

Kanawati, N., A. Woods, S. Shafik, and E. Alexakis. *Mereruka and His Family: The Tomb of Mereruka*. Oxford, England: Aris and Phillips, 2010.

Karim, S. K., and O. S. M. Amin. "Stroke in Ancient Mesopotamia." *Medical Archives* 72, no. 6 (December 2018): 449–52. https://doi.org/10.5455/medarh.2018.72.449-452; PMID: 30814779; PMCID: PMC6340609.

Kemp, B. J. *Ancient Egypt: Anatomy of a Civilization*. New York: Routledge, 1989.

Kozma, C. "Dwarfs in Ancient Egypt." *American Journal of Medical Genetics Part A* 140A (2006): 303–11. https://doi.org/10.1002/ajmg.a.31068.

Kozma, C., A. M. Sarry El Din, R. A. El Shafy El Banna, W. A. El Samie Kandeel, and R. Lachman. "The Ancient Egyptian Dwarfs of the Pyramids: The High Official and the Female Worker." *American Journal of Medical Genetics* 155 (2011): 817–1824.

Leary, N. "Fit for the Job: Proportion and the Portrayal of Cattle in Egyptian Old and Middle Kingdom Elite Tomb Imagery." *Arts* 10, no. 1 (2021): 13. https://doi.org/10.3390/arts10010013.

Lichtheim, M. "The Songs of the Harpers." *Journal of Near Eastern Studies* 4, no. 3 (1945): 178–212. http://www.jstor.org/stable/542776.

Loeb, W. Y., and J. F. Nunn. "Staffs as Walking Aids in Ancient Egypt and Palestine." *Journal of the Royal Society of Medicine,* no. 90 (1997): 450–54.

Lorenzi, R. "King Tut Re-Creation Presents a Shocking Image." *Discovery News*, 2014.

Mahran, H., and S. M. Kamal. "Physical Disability in Old Kingdom Tomb Scenes." *Athens Journal of History* 2, no. 3 (2016): 169–92.

Manniche, L. "Symbolic Blindness." *CdÉ* 53 (1978): 13–21, 105.

Manniche, L. *The Blind Harpist and His Songs*, 97–107. Londres: Music and Musicians in Ancient Egypt, 1991.

Martin, G. T., H. D. Schneider, M. J. Raven, J. Bourriau, J. Van Duk, and D. A. Aston. *The Tomb-Chapels of Paser and Ra'ia at Saqqara. ExeMem 52*. London: Egypt Exploration Society, 1985.

McDowell, A. G. *Village Life in Ancient Egypt: Laundry Lists and Love Songs*. Oxford: Oxford University Press, 2002.

Menéndez, G. "Figurines and Statuettes from the Area of TT 11–12 in Dra Abu el-Naga." *Studien Zur Altägyptischen Kultur* 40 (2011): 301–14. http://www.jstor.org/stable/41812321.

Middleton, A. "Polychromy of Some Fragments of Painted Relief from El-Bersheh." In *Studies in Egyptian Antiquities: A Tribute to T.G.H. James, Occasional Paper 123,* edited by W. V. Davies, 37–44. London: British Museum Press, 1999.

Morris, A. F. "Let the Artifacts Speak: A Look at the Physically Disabled of Ancient Egypt." MA diss., University of Pennsylvania, June 2014.

Morris, A. F. "Let that Be Your Last Battlefield: Tutankhamun and Disability." *Athens Journal of History* 6, no. 1 (January 2020): 53–72.

Morris, A. F. *Plato's Stepchildren: Disability in Ptolemaic Egypt and the Hellenistic World (332–30 BCE)*, 1–593. Middlesbrough: Teesside University, 2022.

Mourad, A. "Siege Scenes of the Old Kingdom." *The Bulletin of the Australian Centre for Egyptology* 32 (2011): 135–58.

Moussa, A. M., and H. Altenmüller. *Das Grab des Nianchchnum und Chnumhotep.* Mainz am Rhein: Philipp von Zabern, 1971.

Nunn, J. F. "Ancient Egyptian Medicine." *Transactions of the Medical Society of London* 113 (1996): 57–68.

Nyord, R. *Vision and Conceptualization in Ancient Egyptian Art.* Cambridge: Cambridge University Publication, 2013.

Panteliadis, C., P. Panteliadis, and F. Vassilyadi. "Hallmarks in the History of Cerebral Palsy: From Antiquity to Mid-20th Century." *Brain and Development* 35, no. 4 (2013, April): 285–92. https://doi.org/10.1016/j.braindev.2012.05.003; Epub: June 2, 2012; PMID: 22658818.

Porter, B., and R. Moss. *Topographical Bibliography of Ancient Egyptian Hieroglyphic Texts, Reliefs, and Paintings 3: Memphis (Abû Rawâsh to Dahshûr).* 2nd ed. Oxford: The Clarendon Press, 1931. *Memphis, Part 1 (Abû Rawâsh to Abûsîr).* Revised and Augmented by Jaromír Málek. 3rd ed. Oxford: The Clarendon Press, 1974.

Porter, B., and R. Moss. *Topographical Bibliography of Ancient Egyptian Hieroglyphic Texts, Reliefs and Paintings.* 2nd ed., Vol. III, 641–44. Oxford: Griffith Institute, Ashmolean Museum, 1994.

René, V. W. *Iconography of Old Kingdom Elite Tombs. Analysis and Interpretation, Theoretical and Methodological Aspects.* Leiden: Peeters/Ex oriente lux, 2005.

Saleh, M., and H. Sourouzian. *Matḥaf al-Miṣrī. The Egyptian Museum, Cairo: Official Catalogue.* Part 2, 40. Mainz: Organisation of Egyptian Antiquities, 1987. ISBN 978-3-8053-0942-4.

Science Museum Group. *Copy of a Statue of a Man with Kyphosis.* Cairo, Egypt: Science Museum Group Collection Online, 1920–1933. Accessed May 13, 2023. https://collection.sciencemuseumgroup.org.uk/objects/co84638/copy-of-a-statue-of-a-man-with-kyphosis-cairo-egypt-1920–1933-statue.

Shafik, S. "Representations of Distinct Physical Features in Wall Scenes of the Old and Middle Kingdoms." *International Journal of Tourism and Hospitality Management* 3, no. 2 (December 2020): 207–26.

Shehab, N. "The Identity of the Cattle Herdsman a Study in the Scenes of Ancient Egyptian Private Tombs." *Journal of the General Union of Arab Archaeologists* 7, no. 1 (2022): 84–107. https://doi.org/10.21608/JGUAA2.2021.95557.1078.

Smith, W. S. *A History of Egyptian Sculpture and Painting in the Old Kingdom.* 2nd ed. Boston: Oxford University Press, 1949.

Staring, N. "The Memphite Necropolis through the Amarna Period: A Study of Private Patronage, Transmission of Iconographic Motifs, and Scene Details." In *Continuity, Discontinuity and Change: Perspectives from the New Kingdom to the Roman Era,* edited by F. Coppens, 13–73. Prague: Charles University, 2021.

Stedman, L. *Medical Dictionary.* 24th ed., 582. London: William & Wilkins, 1982.

Sullivan, R. "Deformity-A Modern Western Prejudice with Ancient Origins." *Proceedings-Royal College of Physicians of Edinburgh* 31, no. 3 (2001): 262–66.

Teeter, E. "Techniques and Terminology of Rope-Making in Ancient Egypt." *The Journal of Egyptian Archaeology* 73, no. 1 (1987): 71–77. https://doi.org/10.1177/030751338707300107.

Vandier, J. "Mo'alla, La tombe d'Ankhtifi et la tombe de Sébekhotep." *IFAO, Bibliothèque d'étude* XVIII (1950): 1–367.

Walsem, V. *Iconography of Old Kingdom Elite Tombs: Analysis and Interpretation, Theoretical and Methodological Aspects (Mémoire de la Société d'Études Orientales 35).* Leiden: Peeters Publishers, 2005.

Wilkinson, C. K., and H. Marsha. *Egyptian Wall Paintings: The Metropolitan Museum of Art's Collection of Facsimiles.* New York: The Metropolitan Museum of Art, 1983.

Woods, A., A. McFarlane, and S. Binder, eds. *Egyptian Culture and Society: Studies in Honour of Naguib Kanawati.* 2 Vols. Cairo: SCA, 2010.

Zaied. *Copy of a Statue of a Man with Kyphosis, 1920–1933.* Cairo, Egypt: A634917 Science Museum Group Collection Online. Accessed May 13, 2023. https://collection.sciencemuseumgroup.org.uk/objects/co84638/copy-of-a-statue-of-a-man-with-kyphosis-cairo-egypt-1920-1933-statue.

Zakrzewski, S. R. "Palaeopathology, Disability and Bodily Impairments." In *Palaeopathology in Egypt and Nubia: A Century in Review. Archaeopress Egyptology.* Vol. 6, edited by Ryan Metcalfe, Jenefer Cockitt, and Rosalie David, 57–68. Oxford, GB: Archaeopress, 2014.

9 People with Spinal Curvatures of the Nile Valley

Presence, Perception and Solidarity from Naqada to the Middle Kingdom

Bénédicte Lhoyer

Among the figures presenting pathologies in Egyptian art, people with spinal disabilities are one of the most common representations, along with those of dwarf people and those with leg impairments. Contrary to what is sometimes stated, Egyptian art never concealed disability or illness. Indeed, a close observation of monuments reveals the presence of people with an atypical physique.[1] Some of those persons were named and sometimes had an administrative title, although the majority remain anonymous. The questions this chapter will address consider why the ancient Egyptians represented disabilities, what could be their significance in Egyptian art and how those persons were perceived, depending on the context.

Some Medical Considerations

A "hunchback" is an individual with kyphosis (κυφος "curved" in ancient Greek) whose characteristic is the presence of a protuberance, a bump produced by a deformity of the spine. In profile, the person has a back that follows a convex curve (round back). Conversely, someone with lordosis has a back with concave curve, with an anterior tilt of the pelvis, arched kidneys and a "hollow" back. In profile, this curve brings out both the shoulders and the lower abdomen. Modern medicine has described eight types of kyphosis, distinguished according to the location of the curves from the neck to the hips.[2] Scoliosis corresponds to a sinuous deviation of the vertebral column in three dimensions (inclination of the frontal plane, rotation of the vertebrae on the horizontal plane and inversion of curvatures in the sagittal plane). Various causes are at the origin of this impairment.[3] Kyphosis (or kypho-scoliosis) can be due to poor posture and can also be the result of a problem with the growth of the dorsal vertebrae during childhood, called "Scheuermann's disease," which affects the seventh, eighth and ninth vertebrae. In addition, several pathogenic elements can cause kyphosis. The most common is spinal bone tuberculosis (a microbial agent located in the bone tissue of the vertebra and the intervertebral disc) known as "Pott's disease." Only biological diagnosis can identify the germ associated with a radiological reading of the destructive lesions. The analyses, by sequencing of DNA fragments undertaken by É. Crubézy on a 5,400-year-old Egyptian skeleton, have detected the presence of *Mycobacterium bacilli*[4] that can be a

DOI: 10.4324/9781003440369-12

risk to humans since they can be pathogenic as agents of tuberculosis (Kock's bacillus)[5] or leprosy.

Skeletal remains of people who had Pott's disease were found during the first excavations of the nineteenth century. In Naqada, F. Petrie and J. E. Quibell excavated at least seven tombs containing vertebrae deformed either by Pott's disease or by osteoarthritis, such as the skeleton of a Predynastic woman who had an osteoarthritis dorsal with a lipping of the lumbar vertebrae as well as discarthrosis, also known as degenerative disc disease (overuse of the discs of the spine).[6] Nevertheless, since many of the skeletons discovered were not studied extensively, it is difficult to quantify the number of people affected by kyphosis at the entire site. Other cases were exhumed at Thebes (excavations by Grébaut 1891)[7] and in Giza (by Abu-Bakr in 1949–1950)[8] or in Nubia (by Derry in 1908).[9]

Senescence is also a possible cause since, with age, the bone tissue changes and can cause osteoporosis, i.e. weakening and compaction of the vertebrae. In the most serious cases, we speak of camptocormia or "curved back syndrome" for the oldest subjects, with a flattened lordosis which raises the hips. However, osteoporosis can also affect younger people. The bone remains of an individual named Nikauisesi, found in his burial chamber in Saqqara, revealed that he died between 35 and 45 years old, and that the first lumbar vertebra had been fractured by compression. The hypothesis of osteoporosis is possible, which implies that Nikauisesi experienced a chronic pathology.[10]

In addition to the discomfort caused by the curvature of the spine, it most likely reduced the quality of life of the person because of the pain associated with movement. In some cases, kyphosis can also hinder the respiratory capacities, creating serious pulmonary arterial hypertension and chronic pain.

Two Specific Cases at Adaïma

In the 2000s, the French team led by B. Midant-Reynes excavated the site of Adaïma[11] and unearthed two Naqada II period graves, S15 and S35. Two individuals with Pott's disease symptoms were buried there.

Grave S15 belonged to a woman around 30 years old. The fusion of some vertebrae demonstrates a healed tuberculosis lesion during her childhood. But the disappearance of the twelfth thoracic body and the collapse of the eleventh thoracic and first and second lumbar bodies led to a kyphosis greater than 90°. Her paraplegia could have been incomplete, and she survived with the support of her community who took care of her food and hygiene. Indeed, because of the nerve compression due to illness, she would likely have experienced sensory and sphincter disorders.

Grave S35 belonged to a child, aged between 10 and 12 years old, severely affected by bone tuberculosis. After death, an individual grave was made and the body was placed there in a contracted position, next to a funerary assemblage made up of ceramics. Nothing in the orientation nor the organization of the objects testifies to any exclusion or marginalization with regard to the whole of the cemetery concerned. But one thing is interesting: the presence of malachite on the child's back, on the affected zone. É. Crubézy explains: "On the child's skeleton, a few grains of green color, probably malachite (the basis of the traditional manufacture of make-up) were found 2 cm behind the injured vertebrae in an area where the fistulization orifice of an abscess could be located. If it is not possible to specify the exact meaning of this deposit, however because of the location, it evokes more of a magico-religious or medicinal practice rather than an element related to the adornment, with which it is usually associated."[12]

Throughout Antiquity, malachite was extracted from the eastern desert (Abu Zawal) and in the Sinai; it was the first ingredient for eye makeup until its replacement by black galena during the 4th Dynasty. The green color refers to the idea of vegetation, freshness and rebirth, and no doubt to a prophylactic concept since this make-up was applied under the eyes of certain statues, including Sepa and his wife Nesa (Musée du Louvre, A 36 – A 37 and A 38) who were from the highest nobility during the 3rd Dynasty.[13] If the "mental universe" of the ancient Egyptians during Naqada was already based on this principle of relationship between a color, a material and "magical" virtues, it is very likely that the malachite thus placed on the area of the worst pain on the back of the young disabled child served to aid him post mortem. The price of malachite was undoubtedly high, given the remoteness of the sources and the difficulties of extraction; few graves contain it. The fact that malachite was specifically used for this funeral shows that either our young child was part of a certain elite within the village, or that the community agreed to release a portion of this resource in recognition of a case requiring a particular ritual intervention. Clearly, the woman in grave S15 was not entitled to the same treatment although she likely had the same condition: her grave contained fewer ceramics and objects, suggesting that she was from a lower social level.

Apparently, there was the idea of gathering deceased persons with the same pathologies. In tomb S45, the two subjects buried side by side had scoliosis with body asymmetry (and osteoarthritis of stage 2 for one). In Nubia, D. Derry reported that in a Predynastic necropolis, four individuals (two men, a woman and a child) likely living with Pott's disease were buried in two tombs close to each other. Could it be possible that the locations of those graves responded to a "post-mortem topography" in which everyone had a place defined according to their rank and possibly to their health or appearance? In the absence of DNA studies on these human remains, it is difficult to know whether these people were part of the same family. Nevertheless, this idea of bringing together people with the same pathologies suggests a strategy for organizing the necropolis, with probable reserved "squares" – as was undoubtedly the case with the dwarf people of the Old Kingdom (like Seneb and Nyankhperu) discovered in Giza in the necropolis of Khufu's pyramid.

Appearance of the Image of the "Hunchback" and Its Development

The oldest representations of kyphosis are not, strictly speaking, images, but rather "evocations" and relate to the two skeletons of Adaïma seen previously. That of S15 is a closed pottery vessel 18.5 cm high dated from Naqada IC-IIB. If one of the profiles has a classic curve, the other side is deformed just above the center line.

The result is a protruding bump, repeating the profile of the subject who presented a 90° kyphosis and a right hump of approximately 30°. Since the pot was deformed before firing, it is likely that the potter created the bump by exerting pressure with his fist inside the vase while smoothing the outside. The state of preservation suggests little use.[14]

The pot of the S35 (Naqada IID2) is an open ceramic with an incised mark (a potter's mark or a graffito?) and streaks of use. The wall of the pottery appears to have been sunken to protrude a curve, giving the rim a straighter line than the rest of the lip. The link between the unusual shaping of the ceramics and the dorsal deformation of the subjects is notable. Indeed, for B. Midant-Reynes, "The only two pots voluntarily deformed before [firing] (S15, S35) are associated with Pott's disease (vertebral tuberculosis) at the origin, during the subjects' lifetime, of a bump in their back. These distorted vases were probably not made for the occasion since at least one of them shows obvious signs of use, but they were probably chosen because they represented the deceased, namely his physical specificity."[15]

The three examples that truly represent people with spinal disabilities are dated cautiously between "Naqada and the Predynastic." None were discovered in the context of excavations and their authenticity could be questioned. These are small statuettes between 10 and 20 cm tall, made of clay or wood. The first belongs to a private French collection, having been the property of Doctor Innès, a former professor at the Cairo School of Medicine in the first half of the twentieth century. In red clay, it features a small male figure in a little jar.[16] It might have been discovered in the Aswan desert by Bedouins. The vase and the figure are part of the same set since the rounded base of the statuette, from the ankles, perfectly fits the bottom of the container. Once inside, only the head and the shoulders of the statuette protrude from the rim. The man is seated, legs together and hands on his knees, in a curled-up position. The upper part of the thoracic spine presents a significant angular kyphosis. In the absence of context, it is easy to imagine that it was the image of a deceased, placed near him in his tomb, a more elaborate effigy than the deformed pots. One hypothesis by P. Schrumpf-Pierron in 1933 is quite different. To him, it was proof of the antiquity of heliotherapy for bone tuberculosis, or how the sun made it possible to cure the disease.[17] In reality, some deceased from the Naqada period (especially children) could be buried in jars in the same contracted position. In addition, there are other examples of statuettes placed in jars, in various positions, including one in a private collection in Boston.[18] A small male figure is seated inside a jar, curled up with his hands pressed against his face. In clay, 30.5 cm tall, W. R. Dawson interpreted it as a representation of a body in a natron bath during the mummification process, but it should rather be seen as the image of a deceased.

Moreover, section 294 § 437 of the Pyramid Texts[19] seems to refer to this remote practice. We would therefore have here an image of the resurrection of the king, emerging from the sleep of death and leaving his jar (in any case the idea of a container like a sarcophagus) to be reborn with the morning, which would reinforce the idea of a funerary practice of burial. Could these small statuettes be the first versions of the "substitutes of the dead," placed in the tomb to serve as security for the preservation of the remains?

The Royal Museums of Art and History in Brussels have a wooden statuette (E 5850), approximately 10 cm tall, of unknown origin and probably dating from the Predynastic period.[20] It is a man with a pointed beard, whose arms and the lower part of his body are missing. He must have had short hair, the nose is aquiline and protruding, the mouth is a simple incised line. A rectangular orifice at the place of the genital apparatus suggests an added part like a loincloth, a belt or a penis sheath. His body has a double protuberance: at the back and at the front like a hull. It seems that this statuette represents a man who had Pott's disease, a hypothesis refuted by A.-P. Leca who leans more for an "essential kypho-scoliosis."[21]

The Rijksmuseum van Oudehen in Leiden has a wooden statuette 17 cm tall (BA. 97), also dated from the Predynastic period. Unlike the others, the man stands with his legs slightly bent. The arms are missing, but the presence of a wooden peg shows that they must have been articulated. The upper part of the thoracic spine is misshapen by a hump, accentuated by the rounded belly which projects. The curved back responds to those of the skull, flattened at its top except towards the parietal bone where two bumps seem to protrude. As E. Warmenbol points out, who also referred to the Brussels statuette, "Now, if one has a head of the Asian 'type', the other has one of the Nubian 'type', the traditional 'enemies' of Egypt, whom Pharaoh gladly tramples under foot. It could be possible that those two statuettes represent prisoners, with their arms bound behind their bodies, or even of two fallen enemies, disarticulated like those presented on the 'battlefield' palette (London, British Museum, EA 20791), their deformity meaning disorder, order and life giving way to chaos and death."[22] The lack of context and the absence of the arms make it difficult to interpret this type of statuette. If it is indeed foreigners, we could already be in the same case as the one illustrated in the tomb of Khentika (called Ikhekhy) at Saqqara (5th Dynasty): a foreigner with a particular physique hampered, exhibited then neutralized (also ritually) in Egypt. In addition, the position of the arms behind the back, a rope tied at the elbows, projects the torso forward, as in lordosis or Pott's disease. Either we are faced with a case of statuettes of execration whereby pathology helps to neutralize the threat, or these could be funeral statuettes representing real disabled people.

The example from the Thinite period found in the publications of the Helwan excavations (1946–1947) by Z. Saad tends to prove the integration of those with spinal disabilities as servants quite early in Egyptian history.[23] The object is a small ivory vase, 8 cm tall, discovered in burial chamber 1 of tomb 1 H5, behind the pelvis of a child. The small cup with a rounded edge is attached to a representation of a man kneeling with outstretched arms. The features of his pointed face are simple, just a few incisions. A bump is on the upper part of his back. The smallness of this object, in addition to its material, suggests a prestigious article deposited in honor of the child near whom it was found.

Apart from the small wooden statuettes in the museums of Brussels and Leiden, all these examples are linked to a container. Could it be that the Egyptians were able to symbolically connect the spine bump to a container? In this case, the kyphosis-vase association would be plausible.

People who had spinal curvatures therefore already acquired a special status in statuary. Subsequently, they obtained a place in the iconographic programs of mastabas, most occupying the place of a servant, in the same way as dwarf people to whom they are sometimes linked. Between the Old and the Middle Kingdoms, I have counted five statues and fifteen bas-relief images, spanning between the 4th Dynasty and the 12th Dynasty. The only attested example from the 4th Dynasty was found in the tomb of the priestess Hetpet, opened in February 2018. Few pictures published in the press revealed the presence of a female servant with a spinal disability on the left wall of the chapel. The image seems to multiply in the 5th Dynasty, with no fewer than eleven figures listed in eight tombs: Nikauhor (Saqqara), Seshemnefer I (Giza), Ty (Saqqara), Khafreankh (Giza), Ankhudjes (unknown localization), Niânkhkhnum and Khnumhotep (Saqqara), Akhethetepher (Saqqara) and Ptahhotep II (Saqqara). In statuary, two figures present a spinal disability, a statuette is a founder-metallurgist in the tomb of Nykauinpu (Giza) and one is an anonymous wooden statuette from the tomb of Mitry (Saqqara). Two images belong to the 6th Dynasty, a servant with a dog in the tomb of Nikauisesi (Saqqara) and a prisoner in Khentika (called Ikhekhi)'s tomb. Finally, our last example is in the tomb of Baqet I, at Beni Hassan, and dates from the 11th Dynasty. The figure here is very small and belongs to the "cortege of curiosities" made up of a dwarf person and a person with double clubfoot.

Unlike the figure of the dwarf person, which enjoyed great notoriety, people with spinal disabilities do not seem to have acquired a similar status in iconography. However, they often accompany dwarf people and other physically disabled characters.

We will classify these figures into five categories:

- High-rank personalities
- Servants, companions and pet handlers
- Dancers
- Workers: herdsmen, fishmongers, harvesters, rope weavers
- Goldsmith-metallurgists

Functions and Attitudes

High-rank Personalities

The Ny Carlsberg Glyptothek in Copenhagen since 1902 has a famous image of a person with a spinal impairment on a false door (AI.E.N 942). Many Egyptologists and doctors have focused on the front of the door. Facing symmetrically on either side of it, the royal sculptor Ankhudjes is represented with a physically impaired back that the sculptor obviously did not seek to attenuate.

This impairment has been recognized as a hump, except by H. Madsen[24] and A.-P. Leca. Regarding the first, F. Jonckheere points out, "[Madsen] only wants to see in it an 'artistic essay', an attempt by the sculptor to reproduce, in a more realistic way, the shoulder turned towards the spectator in a character supposed to be in profile. Unfortunate innovation if ever there was one, with a deplorable aesthetic effect, judging by the result which, in this case, would result in considering that the root of the arm, the closest to us, is implanted in the full torso, almost halfway between the two shoulders seen from the front."

Ankhudjes is presented as a high-ranking deceased individual: standing, left leg forward, he holds in his hands the attributes of the dignitary, the *medu* cane and the *sekhem* scepter. On one figure, he wears panther skin over his short half-pleated loincloth. A small trapezoidal goatee adorns his chin only on the left pillar, and he wears a long braided and graduated wig covering his ears. This one stops at the shoulders, emphasizing the bump that stands out a little more from the back.

The case conforms to the defined canon, with a detachment of the arm which is bent at 90° in the upper part, with particular attention to the rendering of the muscles and bones. In the end, we do have an S-shaped back silhouette with a large top curve. According to H. C. Slomann: "It is the image of a deformed individual, [with] spondylitis of the upper dorsal region."[25]

I do not believe in the idea of clumsiness on the part of the sculptor(s). For me, it is the representation of a person with a physically disabled back. Although it is difficult to determine the cause of this impairment, I believe that there may be another explanation. Knowing that Ankhudjes was a royal sculptor, was this hump not the result of thousands of hours of work, bent over the blocks of stone, a sign of a common "work pathology" for this type of profession? The hump would be proof of a professional impairment acquired by accomplishment. We would then find this idea of "paradoxically qualifying" pathology which would underline his zeal.

Servants, Companions and Animal Handlers

It is in this category that the images are the most numerous since we count six two-dimensional figures: one from the 4th Dynasty, three from the 5th and one from the 6th Dynasty. Only one image dates from the Middle Kingdom, from the 11th Dynasty. Concerning the sculpture, we count two examples: one from the 5th Dynasty and the other from the Middle Kingdom. Of the entirety of this corpus, only two images are those of women with disabled backs since the rest of the representations concern only men.

The Maid with a Spinal Disability

The first image is that from the tomb of Hetpet, priestess of Hathor, discovered at Giza and dated from the 4th Dynasty. The woman is standing in the attitude of walking, her arms bent and holding in front of her two long pieces of linen. She has short black hair and seems completely naked except for jewelry: perhaps a *usekh* necklace and a gold choker necklace, as well as bracelets and anklets. Her hump is in the upper part of her back, with the head of the right shoulder raised. She is part of a procession of six female servants, next to a female dwarf person who walks in front of her.

This image is related to that of the female servant with a spinal disability from the tomb of Seshemnefer I (G 4940).[26] The woman is present in the chapel, in the fourth register of the right upright, the false door of the west wall (right side). She also stands upright and wears short hair, and the few traces of colour attest to the existence of jewellery. On the other hand, she wears a long sheath dress and holds in front of her a box with a rounded top.

There is no doubt that the bump protruding from their backs is a deliberate gesture by the sculptor. Indeed, just like Ankhudjes, the junction point of the arm, which forms a 90° elbow, is pushed forward. The profile of the left arm is also visible, accentuating an impression of a "folded figure."

The Dog Handler with a Spinal Disability

A large number of men with spinal disabilities can also be in charge of pets. Contrary to the dwarf people who were depicted taking care of both dogs and monkeys, the people with spinal disabilities only keep leashed dogs. In the 5th Dynasty, they can be found in the tombs of Nikauhor, Ty and Nikauisesi, and this only in Saqqara. So far, I have not found the equivalent in the tombs of Giza.

These men appear standing and walking, holding on a leash one or two dogs. In Nikauhor's,[27] the man with a spinal disability is the first in a line of servants (while a sandal-bearing dwarf person closes the procession). Holding a long staff with a curved top in his right hand, followed by a dog, he walks to the left in an outdoor scene.

In Ty's, the disabled man is at the end of a procession of servants carrying furniture for the deceased, in relation to a dwarf person who is in the upper register.[28] Naked, with short hair and the tendons of his legs underlined, the curve of his back and the position of his right arm take up exactly the same features as the disabled servant of Hetpet. On the other hand, his left arm is outstretched, barely far from his body, hence this impression of discomfort emerges, the arms being exactly parallel to each other. F. Jonckheere proposed to see a dwarf person[29] but, in this perspective, I think that the sculptor would not have hesitated to make his legs much stockier and more arched. In my opinion, the small size is due to the organization of the composition of this part of the relief, which associates the servant with the animal on two distinct registers. A taller character would have made this division of space impossible and would have thus relegated the dwarf person to the last position with too much space around him, which would have undoubtedly destabilized the balance of the scene.

In Nikauisesi's of the 6th Dynasty, the dog-master merges with the servant since the character, under the seat of his master, holds in his hands both a small, closed chest and a dog on a leash which sits in front of him **(Figure 9.1)**. This is one of the rare cases in which the identity of the man is indicated: "The bearer of the seal, Itchi." This mention could tell us that it is a servant who really existed. The rib cage of this disabled man is imposing, with a carina thorax where four ribs have been highlighted. The large curve that forms the upper part of his back has caused the sculptor to implant the left arm very far back, with this characteristic slight drop.

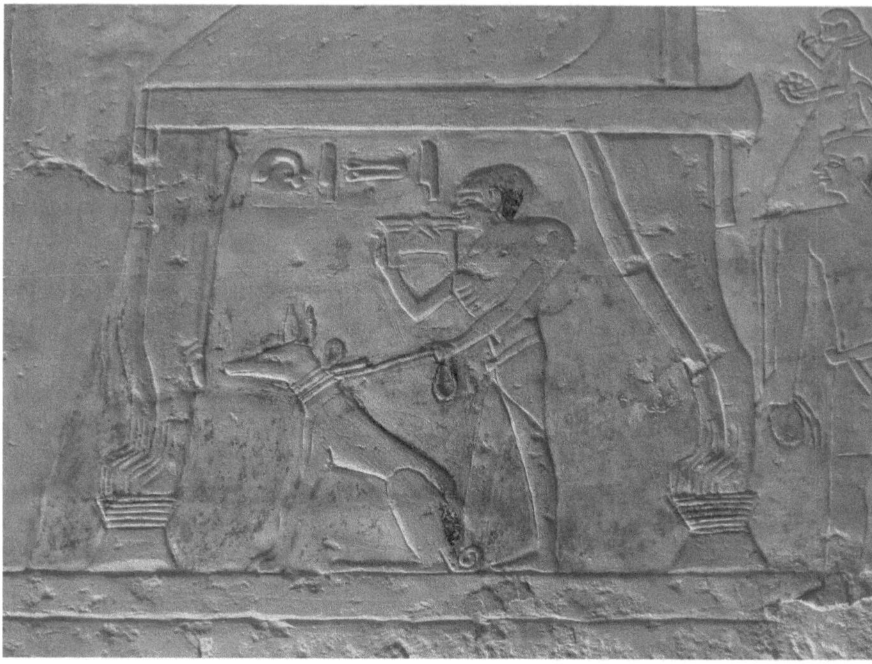

Figure 9.1 A servant of the tomb of Nikauisesi (Saqqara), on the west wall of room I, above the door. © Dominique Farout

The Companion or Servant of Prestige

In the mastaba of Niankhkhnum and Khnumhotep at Saqqara, a small figure in the fifth register of the north wall of room II seems to be waiting to receive treatment.[30] The general scene depicted is that of a massage/pedicure and manicure "cabinet." The figure of this disabled man stands out among the others due to its large size. In comparison with the character on the left, his waist is thinner, his buttocks are higher and his thighs longer. A crack erased the part located at the top of the thorax, preventing us from understanding how the sculptor managed to connect the right shoulder to the right arm, which seems to take along the body. The hieroglyphs in front of him seem to indicate his title: "companion." The curvature of his back lets us think first of spinal problem, but the odd position of the arm, with the elbow almost turned, makes us lean more towards a person who has a dislocation. In this case, the representation of this bump would be more the representation of the head of the humerus sticking out towards the back, which would correspond to a posterior dislocation of the shoulder. Thus, this character would be waiting to be treated by the massage specialists.

Finally, the last two-dimensional image is from the tomb of Baqet I (tomb No. 29)[31] at Beni Hassan **(Figure 9.2)**. Unlike the two servants in the upper register who

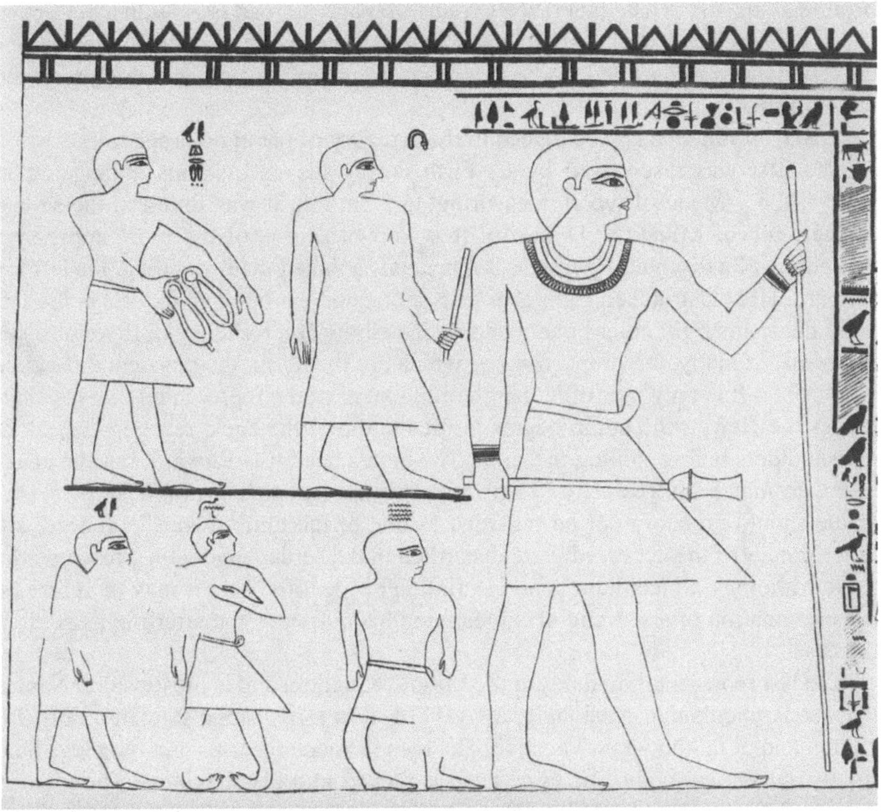

Figure 9.2 The dwarf person, the man with clubbed feet, and the person with a spinal disability from the tomb of Baqet I, in the first register of the south wall of the chapel. From Newberry, Percy Edward. *Beni Hasan*. Part II. London: Kegan Paul, Trench, Trübner & Co., 1893, pl. XXXII.

carry the master's sandals or staff, the three small figures in the lower register do not seem to have any particular service function. The person with a spinal disability is the very last in line but damage has erased the central part of the paint. Few anatomical details have been rendered on the representation, but we can still see that the bump was rendered by an elevation of the right arm as well as a lower-than-average head. Each character has an inscription above him: "dwarf person," "disabled" [i.e. lower limb impairment] and the word *jw* above the person with a spinal disability, which is a hapax. P. E. Newberry[32] considered that it could be the name of the character, while for A. Erman and H. Grapow, the word designates infirmity: "a physically disabled man."[33] I think that this word is to be compared to the homophone *jw* "dog." Since the dwarf person is related to the monkey in the Egyptian mentality, could the person with spinal disability possibly be related to the dog by task and posture association? The fact that a kyphosis creates a broad back with a hump that sits behind the head, causing the back and head to be on the same line with the face curved towards the ground – like a dog – is arguably the element which resolved to amalgam.[34]

In 3D, two figures can be placed in the category of prestigious servants.

The first was discovered by C. Firth during his excavations at Saqqara in 1925–1926.[35] Made of wood, measuring 45.5 cm tall, it was found in the serdab of the tomb of Mitry (5th Dynasty). It is known as one of the most impressive depictions of a disabled Egyptian. It represents a naked man, standing, his left leg forward. His outstretched right arm rests alongside his body as he brings his left hand flat to his right collarbone, bending his elbow at a right angle. If we observe this work frontally, the proportions of which are the norm, the physical difference is invisible. It is only in profile that the full extent of the represented disease challenges the viewer: the bump begins in the middle of the back, reaches its peak at the shoulders before joining the neck. The man's head tilts forward, but the effect seems to match his gesture of respectful attitude. According to J. Harvey, "This statue should probably not be regarded as one of the tomb owner."[36] Indeed, six other statues of the deceased were unearthed in the serdab, and none presented the same pathology. Since there is no inscription or identification, it may therefore be a representation of a servant, accompanying his master in the afterlife, as is often the case.

The last representation dates to the Middle Kingdom and is preserved in Naples (Museo Archeologico Nazionale, inv. 417).[37] It is a limestone statuette, only 3.8 cm tall and of unknown provenance. The man is kneeling, arms and long legs held tightly against his body. His large head is tucked into his shoulders. The torso is projected forward in "keel," while the back has a bump in its upper part, making him raise his head. Again, in the absence of context and inscription, it is difficult to determine the function of this object.

Dancers

The Louvre Museum has a tamarisk statuette 13.80 cm tall, of unknown provenance and dated from the Middle Kingdom (probably 12th Dynasty), E 11562.[38] The arms were held by a wooden peg while the legs were inserted using a mortise-and-tenon system, allowing them to be articulated; perhaps it is a child's toy. The good state of preservation shows an elongated skull surmounted by small buns, three tighter on the top of the forehead and three more spaced out at the back. He wears a green choker necklace, as well as a white cross-belt across his chest. A belt, also white, surrounds the loins and is tied just above the genitals, the two sides falling diagonally on the upper thighs. In profile, the statuette presents a characteristic curve of lordosis, a pathology that dancers know well. Indeed, this and lumbar hyper-lordosis are often observed in dancers and acrobats because of jumps, arabesques and lifts that solicit the lumbar region. The Egyptians had therefore noted this bodily characteristic in their performers and translated it into statuary by exaggerating the hollow of the spine.

The Workers: Herdsmen, Fishmongers, Rope Weavers, Harvesters

The Herdsman

The tomb of Ptahhotep II at Saqqara (5th Dynasty) contains two images of disabled herdsmen.[39] The first is located at the entrance to room II of the chapel, on the left wall. The highest register is occupied by a herdsman whose upper part is very damaged. He holds the reins of the five oxen that follow him, the first of which has a twisted horn that descends towards its muzzle. Only wearing a belt, the man advances to offer the animals to the deceased, although the curve of his legs shows difficulty in moving. Similarly, the curvature of his back, with the belly which seems to project forward, may possibly suggest a back impairment. In this case, this image would be linked to that of its counterpart a little further on (east wall of the chapel, right part, fourth register), seated near the master in front of a tethered ox whose left horn is itself also distorted.

The general composition of the scene is as follows: the deceased, very tall, stands on the far right, his head turned to the left, towards seven registers, some of which are divided in two. The seated herdsman is turned to the left, and one of his raised knees can still be seen with the hem of his short loincloth. His skull is particularly elongated (hydrocephalus?). The left hand was probably holding the reins, but a crack has damaged the scene, while his right hand is plunged into the mouth of the lying ox, to feed it.

Y. Harpur devoted an extensive commentary to it:

> Evidently the ageing man is a hunchback, and his cranium is far too distorted to be anything but a natural deformity at the back of the head. . . . Perhaps the unfortunate condition of the man . . . prompted the designer to associate him with a particular type of ox, because the animal has a deformed left horn, deliberately made to curve downwards over its face in the opposite direction to the other normal-looking horn. . . . The intact backline of the lower ox-feeding man reveals that he is not a hunchback but simply a thin individual. Moreover, no horn-tip is visible level with the ox's eye, therefore the lower group was probably free from deformities and served as a visual contrast to the atypical group above.[40]

Indeed, in the lower register, another herdsman presents a different dorsal curve, with a hump towards the middle of the back, which would correspond to the idea of arduous work. In any case, the Egyptians, being fond of associations, did not hesitate to bring together two figures which seemed to them to share common characteristics, such as the dwarf person with the monkey, the person with a spinal disability with the dog, and the crooked herdsman with an animal with a twisted horn.

The Fishmonger and the Rope Weaver

In the tomb of this same Ptahhotep at Saqqara, still on the east wall but on the left side, two figures on the fourth register have a rounded back.[41] Their humps are not as obvious as the previous cases, but the suspicious curvature prompts us to point them out, especially since the work carried out by these two men – clearly related to fishing – requires them to bend in their work, which can have consequences if performed extensively over time.

The first character on the left is an old man. Seated and turned to the right, legs against his chest, the man guts fish with a knife on a diagonal board. The back is shaped like a "C," giving the impression of a shrunken man, executing gestures in a tight space. The second character, whose features and attitude are close to his companion above, seems to respond to him since he is turned in the direction of the left. He too is bald and, sitting on a mat, he makes ropes with the help of a young boy. The back – or even the entire body – is more "D" shaped than "C" shaped. First, we have a straight oblique line starting from the neck which rounds towards the middle of the thoracic column and then becomes a slightly concave curve up to the waist. It was undoubtedly a way for the sculptor to suggest the effort deployed to stretch the rope.

Surprisingly, the four images of people with spinal curvatures in the tomb of Ptahhotep II are all located in the fourth register of the east wall (entrance wall and hall wall). The alterations would serve here as an "iconographic border" (with the workers affected by bilharzia) thus separating the world of domesticated animals (lower registers) and the world of wild animals or disorder to be mastered (upper registers).

The Goldsmith-metallurgist

The serdab of the tomb of Nikauinpu (late 5th Dynasty) contained limestone statuettes. Twenty-six of them were sold in 1920, and most of them are now at the Oriental Museum in Chicago, except for one which is in the MET in New York. The statuette OIC E10631[42] represents a kneeling man, carrying a long pipe to his mouth to feed the fire at the base of a crucible. Wearing short hair and a short loincloth, his spine appears to protrude from the middle of his back, forming a bump that gradually tapers down to his nape. In profile but also from the front, the impression is that of an abrupt deformation, due to the arduousness of the work more than to an illness like Pott's disease. It is, to date, the only copy known.

Conclusions

Thus, even if the characters who had spinal disabilities did not experience the same iconographic presence as the dwarf people, they indicate a particular interest for this type of alteration. Their attestations are found above all in the 5th Dynasty, whereas the images of people with a different physique often tended to multiply in the 6th Dynasty. Moreover, the association made between those with spinal curvatures and other bodily differences (dwarf people, those with clubfoot, oxen with twisted horns or workers affected by bilharzia) testifies once again of the strong associations between the atypical bodies.

It seems that the motif of people with spinal disability have continued in wooden statuary, such as this impressive statuette from the Brooklyn Museum (37.1595E) representing a seated man with the upper part of the back facing horizontally. Likewise, a few people with spinal disabilities may appear in some scenes realized in limestone reliefs, like these dockworkers on relief 48.112 in the Brooklyn Museum of Art, one with lordosis and his compere with kyphosis.

The presence of people with disabilities responds to multiple issues. They are images of people who really existed, possibly symbol figures of a threat, but above all the expression of the multiplicity of bodies and of creation as a whole. By showing the difference, Egyptian art and texts wish above all to illustrate the plurality of the living.

Thus, they allow us to understand ancient Egyptian mentality and, in addition to all the other representations, remind us that some domains in ancient Egypt were sometimes more inclusive than those in our modern society.

Notes

1 Lhoyer (2018), Jeffreys and Tait (2002, 87–95).
2 Dimeglio, Hérisson, and Simon (1995).
3 Bourke (1971, 363–75), Roberts and Buikstra (2019, 321–439).
4 Crubézy et al. (1998, 941–51).
5 Nerlich et al. (1997, 1404).
6 Moodie (1931, pl. II).
7 Smith and Ruffer (1910, 9–16).
8 Abu-Bakr (1953, 85, pl. XLII).
9 Derry (1938, 196–99).
10 Kanawati and Abder-Raziq (2000, 68–72).
11 Crubézy, Duchesne, and Midant-Reynes (2008, 289–310).
12 Duchesne et al. (2010, 47).
13 Ziegler (1997, 112–15, 141–47).
14 Crubézy, Janin, and Midant-Reynes (2002, 525).
15 Ibid., 472.
16 Leca (1971, 241).
17 Schrumpf-Pierron (1933, 299).
18 Dawson (1928, 126–27, pl. XV).
19 Piankoff (1968, 51).
20 Jonckheere (1948, 24–35).
21 Leca, *Médecine*, 235.
22 Warembol (2002, 142).
23 Saad (1969, pl. 46 et 47).
24 Madsen (1905, 65–69), Leca (1971, 241).
25 Slomann (1927, 62–86).
26 Kanawati (2001, 63, pl. 42).
27 Quibell (1909, 115, pl. LXII).
28 Murray and Sethe (1937, pl. IV).
29 Jonckheere (1948, 28).
30 Harpur and Scremin (2010, 144).
31 Aufrère (1999, 11–17).
32 Newberry (1893, 36).
33 *Wb* I, 43, 11.

34 Lhoyer (2018, 177).
35 Firth (1926, 101).
36 Harvey (2001, 171).
37 Cantilena and Rubino (1989, 42–43).
38 Vandier (1958, 478, 675).
39 Harpur and Scremin (2008, 5, 188).
40 Harpur and Scremin (2008, 323).
41 Harpur and Scremin (2008, 117, 123).
42 Breasted (1948, 50, pl. 45a).

Bibliography

Abu-Bakr, Abdel-Moneim. *Excavations at Giza 1949–1950.* Cairo: Government Press, 1953.

Aufderheide, Arthur C. and Conrado Rodríguez-Martín, "Ankylosing Spondylitis (AS)" In *The Cambridge Encyclopedia of Human Paleopathology, UK: Cambridge University Press*, 2011: 102–104.

Aufrère, Sydney. "L'énigme du nain, du pied-bot et du bossu dans les tombes de Baqet I et de Khety à Béni-Hassan." *BSEG* 23 (1999): 11–17.

Bourke, J. B. "A Review of the Palaeopathology of the Arthritic Diseases." In *Diseases in Antiquity. A Survey of the Disease, Injuries and Surgery of Early Populations*, edited by Don Brothwell and A. T. Sandison, 358–59. Springfield: Charles C. Thomas, 1967.

Bourke, J. B. "The Palaeopathology of the Vertebral Column in Ancient Egypt and Nubia." *Medical History* 15 (1971): 363–75.

Bourke, J. B. "Trauma and Degenerative Diseases in Ancient Egypt and Nubia." *Journal of Human Evolution* 1, no. 2 (1972): 225–32.

Breasted, James Henry. *Egyptian Servant Statues, The Bollingen Series XIII.* Washington: Pantheon Books, 1948.

Cantilena, Renata, and Paola Rubino. *La Collezione egiziana del Museo Archeologico Nazionale di Napoli.* Naples: Arte tipografica, 1989.

Crubézy, Éric, Sylvie Duchesne, and Béatrix Midant-Reynes. "The Predynastic Cemetery at Adaïma (Upper Egypt). General Presentation and Implications for the Populations of Predynastic Egypt." In *Egypt at Its Origins 2*, edited by Béatrix Midant-Reynes and Yann Tristant, 289–310. Leuven: Peeters Press, 2008.

Crubézy, Éric, Thierry Janin, and Béatrix Midant-Reynes. "Adaïma 2. La nécropole prédynastique." In *FIFAO*. Vol. 47, 511–23. Cairo: IFAO, 2002.

Crubézy, Éric, Bertrand Ludes, Jean-Dominique Poveda, John Clayton, Brigitte Crouau-Roy, and Daniel Montagnon. "Identification d'ADN de *Mycobacterium* dans un mal de Pott égyptien de 5400 ans." *Comptes rendus de l'Académie des Sciences, series III* 321, no. 11 (1998): 941–51.

Dawson, Warren R. "Note on an Ancient Egyptian Figure." *JEA* 14, no. 1–2 (1928): 126–27.

Derry, Douglas E. "Pott's Disease in Ancient Egypt." *The Medical Press and Circular* 197, no. 1 (1938): 196–99.

Dimeglio, Alain, Christian Hérisson, and Lucien Simon. *Les cyphoses: de l'enfant à l'adulte, Collection de pathologie locomotrice 30.* Paris: Masson, 1995.

Duchesne, Sylvie, Henri Dabernat, Béatrix Midant-Reynes, and Éric Crubézy. "Handicap, tuberculose et représentation symbolique dans l'Égypte prédynastique." In *Décrypter la différence: Lecture archéologique et historique de la place des personnes handicapées dans les communautés du passé*, edited by Valérie Delattre and Ryadh Sallem, 45–48. Paris: CQFD, 2010.

Firth, Cecil M. "Preliminary Report on the Excavations at Saqqara (1925–1926)." *ASAE* XXVI (1926): 101.

Fischer-Elfert, Hans-Werner. *Abseits von Ma'at. Fallstudien zu Außenseitern im Alten Ägypten, Wahrnehmungen und Spuren Altägyptens 1.* Würzburg: Ergon Verlag, 2005.
Harpur, Yvonne, and Paolo Scremin. *The Chapel of Ptahhotep: Scene Details, Min.* 2. Oxford: Oxford Expedition to Egypt, 2008.
Harpur, Yvonne, and Paolo Scremin. *The Chapel of Niankhkhnum & Khnumhotep: Scene Details.* Min. 3. Oxford: Oxford Expedition to Egypt, 2010.
Harvey, Julia. *Wooden Statues of the Old Kingdom, a Typological Study, EM 2.* Leiden: Brill, 2001.
James, Thomas Garnet Henry. *The Mastaba of Khentika, called Ikhekhi, ASE 30.* Oxford: University Press, 1953.
Jeffreys, David, and John Tait. "Disability, Madness, and Social Exclusion in Dynastic Egypt." In *Madness, Disability and Social Exclusion. The Archaeology and Anthropology of "Difference"*, edited by Jane Hubert, 87–95. London: Routledge, 2002.
Jonckheere, Frans. "Le bossu des Musées Royaux d'Art et d'Histoire de Bruxelles." *Chronique d'Égypte* 45–46 (1948): 24–35.
Kanawati, Naguib. *Tombs at Giza I: Kaiemankh (G4561) and Seshemnefer I (G4940), ACE Reports 16.* Warminster: The Australian Centre for Egyptology, 2001.
Kanawati, Naguib, and Mahmud Abder-Raziq. *The Teti Cemetery at Saqqara. Vol. VI: The Tomb of Nikauisesi, ACE Reports 14.* Warminster: The Australian Centre for Egyptology, 2000.
Leca, Ange-Pierre. *La médecine égyptienne au temps des pharaons.* Paris: R. Dacosta, 1971.
Lhoyer, Bénédicte. "Les altérations corporelles dans l'image à l'Ancien Empire." PhD diss., Université Paul-Valéry Montpellier 3, École du Louvre, 2018.
Madsen, Henry. "Ein künstlerisches Experiment im alten Reiche." *ZÄS* 42 (1905): 65–69.
Ménard, Victor. *Étude pratique sur le mal de Pott.* Paris: Masson et Cie, 1900.
Moodie, Roy Lee. *Roentgenological Studies of Egyptian and Peruvian Mummies.* Chicago: Field Museum of Natural History, 1931.
Murray, Margaret A., and Karl Sethe. *Saqqara Mastabas.* Part II. London: British School of Archaeology, 1937.
Nerlich, Andreas G., Christian J. Haas, Albert Zink, Ulrike Szeimies, and Hjalmar G. Hagedorn. "Molecular Evidence for Tuberculosis in an Ancient Egyptian Mummy." *The Lancet* 350, no. 9088 (1997): 1404.
Newberry, Percy Edward. *Beni Hasan.* Part II. London: Kegan Paul and Trench, Trübner & Co., 1893.
Petrie, William Matthew Flinders. *Diospolis Parva. The Cemeteries of Abadiyeh and Hu.* London: The Egypt Exploration Fund, 1901.
Piankoff, Alexandre. *The Pyramid of Unas, Egyptian Religious Texts and Representations.* Vol. V. New York: Pantheon Books, 1968.
Quibell, James Edward. *Excavations at Saqqara 1907–1908.* Cairo: IFAO, 1909.
Roberts, Charlotte A., and Jane E. Buikstra. "Bacterial Infections." In *Ortner's Identification of Pathological Conditions in Human Skeletal Remains,* edited by Jane E. Buikstra, 321–439. Harvard: Elsevier Science & Technology, 2019.
Ruffer, Marc Armand. "Arthritis Deformans and Spondylitis in Ancient Egypt." *The Journal of Pathology* 22, no. 2 (1918): 152–96.
Saad, Zaki Yusef. *The Excavations at Helwan: Art and Civilization in the First and Second Egyptian Dynasties.* Norman: University of Oklahoma Press, 1969.
Schrumpf-Pierron, Pierre. "Le mal de Pott en Égypte 4000 ans avant notre ère." *Æsculape* 12 (1933): 299.
Slomann, Herman Christian. "Contribution à la paléo-pathologie égyptienne." *Bulletins et Mémoires de la Société d'anthropologie de Paris, VII series* 8, no. 1–3 (1927): 62–86.
Smith, Grafton Elliot, and Marc Armand Ruffer. "Pott'sche Krankheit an einer ägyptischen Mumie aus der Zeit der 21 Dynastie (um 1000 V. Chr.)." In *Zur historischen Biologie der Krankheitserreger,* edited by Karl Sudhoff, 9–16. Leipzig: Druck von C. G. Röder GmbH, 1910.

Stevenson Smith, William. *A History of Egyptian Sculpture and Painting in the Old Kingdom.* Boston: Hacker Art Books, 1978.
Vandier, Jacques. *Manuel d'archéologie égyptienne, 3, Les grandes époques. La statuaire.* Paris: A. et J. Picard, 1958.
Warembol, Eugène. *Beautés d'Égypte.* Bruges: Cedarc, 2002.
Ziegler, Christiane. *Les statues égyptiennes de l'Ancien Empire.* Paris: Musée du Louvre, 1997.

10 Defining the Idealized Body

A Reexamination of Depictions of Dwarfism in the Old Kingdom

Emily Smith-Sangster

Introduction

Historical analyses of the body in Egyptian art often defaulted, and still default, to a discussion of the *ideal* – a term with differing definitions based on a milieu of factors; many of which have only tangential relation, if any, to the culture being discussed. The antithesis to this bodily representation of the ideal has always been 'the other,' often used to describe bodies that do not fit the expected 'idyllic' form many familiarize themselves with in the study of Egyptian artistic representation.[1] This has been particularly impactful in prior studies of depictions of dwarf individuals[2] – depictions that have typically been assigned a semiotic role, or used to discuss the 'assigned roles' of disabled people in the past;[3] a discussion that usually relies on a modern, ableist perspective,[4] or singular datapoints drawn through time and space to make generalizations. Although many scholars may disagree with the conclusions drawn in these past studies, the continued use of these methods of analysis in the literature, and their colloquial use within the field, continues to other these individuals, and hinders any true discussion about the actual significance behind the depiction of this multivalent group in the artistic corpus.

This paper works to address these issues through the reexamination of depictions of dwarf individuals, using the Old Kingdom material as a case study. The analysis demonstrates that, in contrast to prior conclusions on this topic, depictions of dwarf individuals in this period serve no iconographical role. Further, there is no artistic evidence to suggest that dwarf individuals were pigeonholed into specific social roles, such as dancer, due to their bodies. Instead, this paper proposes that depictions of this body type are as equally idealized as any other in the artistic corpus of the Old Kingdom. In doing so, this reanalysis will help the field to move closer to understanding the way dwarf individuals were perceived and represented in Old Kingdom society.

Methodology

The present study collated depictions of dwarf individuals from Old Kingdom tomb decorative programs and private statuary, then analysed for method of depiction,

DOI: 10.4324/9781003440369-13

indicators of status of the individual, and depicted societal role. The data is separated into 'known' individuals, which encompass the named individuals for whom we have multiple depictions, statuary, and often a tomb; and individuals who are depicted in the tombs of others, henceforth referred to as 'unknown' individuals.[5] Depictions are identified based on the representation of individuals with specific bodily proportions, primarily shortened limbs. While scholars like Dasen have suggested that the primary attribute in the depiction of dwarf individuals was small body size, this is an oversimplification, likely based on assumptions of size-based hierarchy being the paramount indicator of status, and cannot be relied on to properly identify these individuals.[6]

Although viewed as a continuum at many times in the past, no attempt is made in this paper to discuss the depictions of dwarf individuals in prior or later periods. The constant fluctuation of Egyptian ideology and imagery throughout the culture's history necessitates a more period-specific study of depictions of topics, like disability, to add depth to our understanding of the subject. The significance of this data for understanding the meaning behind the formalized depiction of dwarfism and its implication for further study is discussed further in the following.

The Old Kingdom Data

Representations of Known Individuals

Looking to the artistic representation of dwarf individuals in the Old Kingdom, we can begin with an overview of depictions of known individuals, a category in which we find three persons – Seneb, Perniankhu, and Khnumhotep – each for whom we have differing levels of artistic evidence.[7] The most commonly cited in prior studies of dwarfism and disability is Seneb,[8] a high-status individual who, based on the dating of his Giza tomb, likely lived around the late 4th to early 5th Dynasty.[9] Depictions of Seneb were found by Junker on his large false door, offering slab, and as part of the now famous statue of Seneb, his wife Senetites, and their two children, Ankhmaredjedef and Auibenkhufu (JE 51280).

Across all of the pieces, the depictions of Seneb's body are notably consistent, depicting the deceased as possessing the shortened proportions of an individual with achondroplasia dwarfism. The proportions of his body, however, do not interfere with his depiction as the primary focus of the tomb decoration, nor with conventions of size-based hierarchy. In the scenes in which he is depicted in front of individuals without dwarfism, Seneb is proportionally larger than the secondary figures, or is positioned so that his head is above those in his presence, leaving no doubt regarding his position in the hierarchy. In fact, his representation as a tomb owner can be classified as remarkably conventional. In no scene is he shown with a different body, nor is there 'hinting' at or suggested desirability of a differently proportioned body as has been suggested in the past.[10] In fact, this evidence seems to suggest that there was no difficulty in representing Seneb's body as fulfilling the ideal for the body of a male tomb owner at all.

A similar conclusion can be drawn regarding the statue of Seneb and his family. While Seneb is cross-legged, there is no aspect of the depiction that seems to suggest an undesirability of his body type. Indeed, his pose can be regarded as scribal in nature, not only allowing the artist to adapt the statue type to Seneb's proportions, but also to allow for the maintenance of a high-status representation. When taken together with the decorative program of his tomb, it seems clear that Seneb was a high-status individual of great wealth and importance – conclusions also well supported by his titles as well as the architecture and placement of his tomb.[11] It is also notable that there is nothing about Seneb's representation that is suggestive of his form serving an iconographical purpose, nor do the depictions insinuate a social identity dictated by his body, as has been suggested for others with dwarfism.

For some, however, Seneb represented the 'exception' the individual who was able to exceed expectations or was 'allowed' to rise to such a status in society. However, while the other two individuals, Perniankhu and Khnumhotep, are only depicted artistically in their statues, similar conclusions can be drawn about their representations and social roles in Old Kingdom society, demonstrating that Seneb was by no means an exception to the rule.

The tomb of Perniankhu was rediscovered by Hawass and his team in 1990.[12] It appears, based on the material remains discovered in the remains of his mastaba, that Perniankhu was, like Seneb, a high-ranking individual of the 4th or 5th Dynasty. In fact, their tombs were found quite close to one another in the Western Giza Necropolis. While the body of Perniankhu was discovered and found to possess evidence of dwarfism,[13] of interest to this analysis is the basalt statue also discovered in the tomb. The statue, which depicts Perniankhu as a seated man in a short wig holding a staff between his right and left hands, and a scepter in his right, was noted for its delicate and accurate carving and "perfectly formed face."[14] The proportions of Perniankhu's body appear to emphasize his shortened proportions significantly less than Seneb's statue; however, it is unclear how much of this is based on the fact that this is a solo statue. The negotiation of the size of his body and even the base on which he sits, suggests the ease through which, again, the body of an individual with dwarfism could still fit within the ideal representation of a male at this period in time. Further, neither evidence from his statue nor from his titles suggest Perniankhu held a position associated with entertainment, again negating the conclusions of former studies.[15]

The final individual, Khnumhotep, is known via a limestone statue (CG 144) which was rediscovered by Mariette in 1888 in the badly destroyed remains of a mastaba at Saqqara.[16] The statue depicts an adult male with dwarfism, with closely cropped hair and a white kilt. Although composed like a striding statue, Khnumhotep is shown stationary, with both feet next to one another. While his proportions differ from statues of individuals without dwarfism, he is suitably depicted with the fit and youthful body of a male in the Old Kingdom. Overall, the quality of the piece, the find spot, and the high-ranking titles inscribed on the base[17] suggest that Khnumhotep was an elite individual who, like the others, was easily represented as such in his statuary.

Representations of Unknown Individuals

Even more convincing than the analysis of known individuals, however, is the analysis of the depictions of dwarf individuals in the tombs of others. Surely, if the physical differences of dwarf people were used iconographically, or if individuals with this body type were primarily slotted into social roles such as dancer or entertainer, it would be seen in these depictions. This turns out not to be the case. Utilizing the *Porter and Moss Topographical Bibliography*,[18] Dasen's catalogue of depictions of dwarfism,[19] and field visits to Old Kingdom necropolises and museum collections, 115 carved relief and painted depictions of dwarf individuals across 71 scenes in 56 tombs are identified.[20] These depictions show individuals possessing one of ten social roles, with the role of dancer second lowest. Instead, the resulting statistical demonstrates an arguably high rate of variation in the social positions held by these individuals.[21] Furthermore, these depictions also utilized an

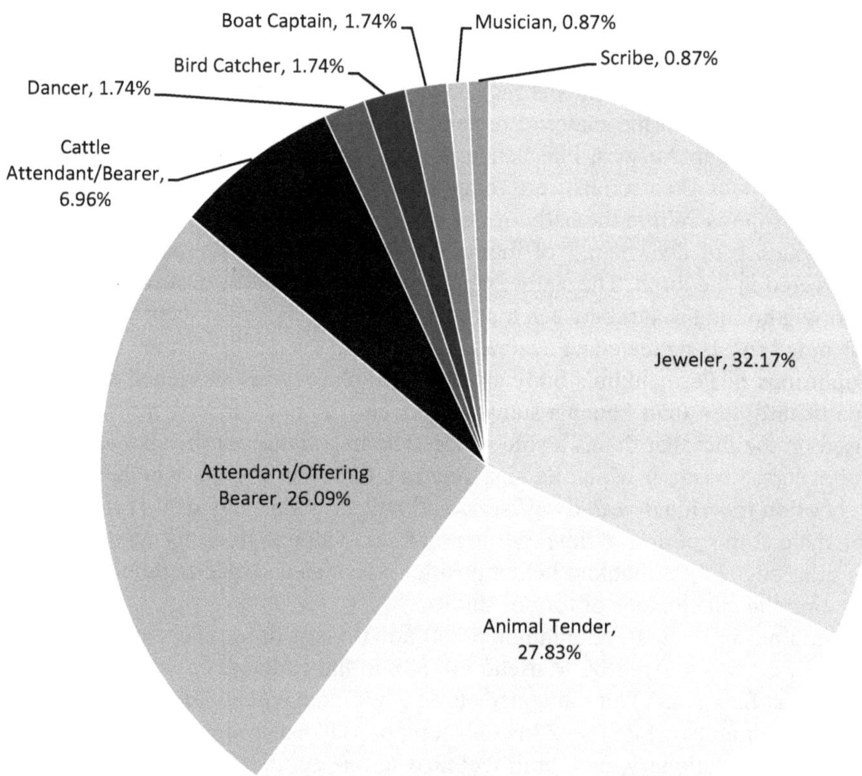

Figure 10.1 Distribution of positions held by dwarf individuals in Old Kingdom tomb decoration.

extremely idealized and formalized approach to the representation of dwarf bodies, as was seen in the depictions of known individuals.

The breakdown of the data across the ten roles includes an emphasis on dwarf individuals fulfilling the role of jeweler (32.17%), animal tender (27.83%),[22] and attendant (26.09%)[23] most often. There is no evidence to suggest that these individuals possessed these roles due to their body structure. Instead, in each of the depicted roles, dwarf individuals can be found depicted side by side with individuals without dwarfism.[24] There is nothing within these depictions to suggest a different status between these individuals either, instead with the emphasis seemingly on the varying population fulfilling these roles.

Women with dwarfism are depicted only holding two of these positions, dancer or attendant, while men with dwarfism are present in the depiction of every role type. It is likely that this has more to do with traditional gender representations rather than the bodies of these individuals.[25] Men, however, are intermittently shown as naked when possessing the role of attendant; however, it is unclear what this depiction meant. While previous scholarship assumed that nudity in adults marked a lower status individual, most of the nude men are the only named attendant in the scene, inversely suggesting higher status or favor from the tomb owner. It is possible that this was meant as a status indicator referential to other individuals in the scene with dwarfism, such as is seen on the false door of the tomb of Nisut-nefer (G4970).[26]

As for the bodily representation of these individuals, the bodies are depicted as fitting an idealized and formalized artistic canon, which only differs in the representation of differing limb proportions. At times, such as in the depiction of dancers in tomb of Nunetjer at Giza (E45), the individual is depicted as smaller, likely because the artist was attempting to add an aspect of realism.[27] In other tombs, however, such as that of Watetkhethor at Saqqara,[28] individuals with and without dwarfism are shown as the same hierarchical size, possibly in an attempt to depict status based on the social position these women held as attendants. As such, as a basic bodily form, it seems that the depiction of an individual with dwarfism was treated almost as a secondary bodily ideal included in whatever manner deemed necessary for the execution of the scene, and usable by individuals of varying social status.

Notably, when viewed overall, there is no evidence to suggest that these individuals were being used in an iconographical manner. There is also no emphasis on including these individuals in scenes of entertainment or scenes associated with comedy. In fact, only 1.74% of individuals were found to serve a role associated with dancing, making it the second least common social role depicted (on par with boat captain and bird catcher), and only 0.87% found to serve a role associated with music (on par with scribe). Further, many of these individuals in the tombs of others are named, suggesting they represent actual individuals as opposed to ideas. Thus, it seems clear that there is no emphasis on dwarf individuals serving specific roles, or an iconographical purpose in the art of the Old Kingdom. Instead, it appears that the statistical breakdown is one of a cross-section of roles across Egyptian society.

Data Analysis

What is apparent from this collection of evidence is that dwarf individuals were depicted throughout the Old Kingdom in a strikingly conventional manner, which followed all necessary artistic decorum for the depiction of any other tomb owner, attendant, or generic individual in a decorative program. Individuals, like Seneb, are presented with smaller proportions, but in a completely idealized manner, comparable in clothing, hair, status, and pose to any other contemporary elite. Likewise, depictions of named and unnamed individuals in tombs differ only from their peers in the proportions of their bodies, with no evidence that they were utilized in a comedic or symbolic manner. Instead, it seems that these individuals possessed a body type that was easily included in the depiction of an idealized body. While appearing physically different, it suggests that scholars' 'othering' of this body type is less based on the evidence at hand, and more on the modern conceptualization of how society views these individuals.

It should be noted that there is also no reason to believe that Seneb or any dwarf person *had to* be shown as possessing such a body due to their highly visible 'condition,' as Bolshakov concluded.[29] Instead it should be suggested that this body type was seen as *equally as valid* of an artistic option as a differently proportioned one. The possible manipulation of the proportions of individuals like Perniankhu in his statue also suggests that, while valid, choosing to be depicted with such body may not have been required at all, further separating the depiction of the body in art from the physical body of the deceased, and placing the agency back in the hands of the patron and artist.

Regarding the secondary suggestion that dwarf people were dancers or entertainers, only three tombs depict dwarfs in such a role out of 115 depictions. In fact, looking at the data, it seems that there is no specific connection between dwarf individuals and a specific social position. These former conclusions were likely based on later evidence, as well as the letter of Pepi II to Harkuf. While the concentration of depictions identified as animal tenders, jewelers, and attendants was noted earlier, there is nothing that identifies these as the *only* positions held by dwarf individuals, nor are these dwarf people the *only* individuals depicted in such roles. In sum, the distribution of representations seems to epitomize a rather generic spread of possible roles that could be held by a group of people, regardless of their physical appearance. If anything, the data seems indicative of the well-integrated nature of the dwarf people population into Old Kingdom society.

The treatment of the bodies of dwarf people as an 'ideal' body type raises questions about the historical grouping of all disability in the study of Egyptian art; a practice that presents the depicted as fitting into a binary category – disabled or not disabled – and then assigning characteristics associated with membership in one of those groups. By complicating this approach and, instead, utilizing specific case studies as has been demonstrated here and across the chapters of this book, we can begin to understand more closely the integration of these previously 'othered' populations into society. In addition, we can begin to challenge the role that modern thought has played in this othering.[30] Thus, instead of associating dwarf individuals together with individuals with curved spines, and then drawing widespread conclusions regarding the categorization and representation of these people[31] as has been done in the past, we can begin to understand that these groupings are often based on modern perceptions and each bodily experience, or disability, should be studied on its own before such conclusions are made.[32] By doing this, preconceptions about the representation of disability in Egyptian artwork can be broken down and corrected, hopefully stopping their transmission as popular knowledge.

Conclusions

It seems clear that dwarfism and the representation of the body of dwarf individuals in the Old Kingdom cannot be essentialized to a symbolic explanation, nor are the overly simplistic suggestions by earlier scholars of individuals serving in roles such as dancers or 'pets' supported by the evidence at hand. Instead, the complex representations of these people speak to a subsect of the general population, who had many roles, existed in multiple socio-economic classes, and were represented in art in a clearly conventional, idealized, and formalized manner. This highlights a twofold issue, the first being the essentializing of the entirety of the disability community in ancient Egypt into a typified form and attempting to understand the treatment of these individuals from a single example. Not only was the disability community not a monolith, but, as exemplified here in reference to dwarf people, treatment does not seem to have been based on an individual's body type or perceived difference.

Secondly, this highlights the way that modern historians have often removed disabled individuals from the canon of Egyptian art history. When recontextualized in the periods from which these examples of dwarf individuals come, the depictions fit well with the artistic patterns of experimentation and use of realism seen in areas like Giza during the Old Kingdom. Thus the portrayal of dwarf individuals should not be considered as odd or to have been othered by the artists who depicted them in such a manner. The integration of depictions of dwarf individuals into the canonical representation of bodies and thematic artistic shifts of the time period seems to be the perfect reflection of the way that these individuals, othered by modern scholarship, were perceived by the Egyptian population: a typical subset of the societal whole.

Appendix I: Depictions Utilized in This Analysis[33]

Depicted social role	*Tomb*	*Location*	*Date*
Pet Attendant	LG 90 Debhen	Giza	4th Dynasty
	Neferma'et	Maidum (relief now in Ny Carlsberg Glyptotek, AEIN 1133)	4th Dynasty
	G7530 Meresankh III	Giza	4th Dynasty
	Kaemnefert	Saqqara (relief now in Boston, MFA, 04.1761)	5th Dynasty
	D 55 Neferirtenef	Saqqara (relief now in Brussels, Musées Royaux, E 2465)	5th Dynasty
	Itisen	Giza	5th Dynasty
	G2150 Kanufer	Giza	5th Dynasty
	G7837/7843 (2)	Giza	5th Dynasty
	N 60 Ty (2)	Saqqara	5th Dynasty
	Ka'aper	Saqqara	5th Dynasty
	Seshemnūfer-Theti	Giza	6th Dynasty
	Neferseshemre Sheshi	Saqqara	6th Dynasty
	Kagemni Memi	Saqqara	6th Dynasty
	Mereruka	Saqqara	6th Dynasty
	Serfka (2)	El-Sheik Sa'id	6th Dynasty
	Nekhebu (2)	Giza	6th Dynasty
	Nyankhnefertem	Saqqara	6th Dynasty
	G2430 Hetepniptah	Giza	6th Dynasty
	G5550	Giza	6th Dynasty
	Nufer (2)	Giza	6th Dynasty
	Ankhmahor	Saqqara	6th Dynasty
	Hesy, Hapi	Saqqara	6th Dynasty
	Niankhnesut (2)	Saqqara	6th Dynasty
	Nikauisesi (2)	Saqqara	6th Dynasty
	No. 481 Ipi	Beni Hasan	6th Dynasty
Jeweler	LG 86 Nebemakhet	Giza	4th Dynasty
	Wepemnefert (4)	Giza	5th Dynasty
	N. 79 Kaemrehu (2)	Giza (relief now in Cairo Museum, CG 1534)	5th Dynasty
	Ptahhotep (4)	Saqqara	5th Dynasty
	Nufer (4)	Saqqara	5th Dynasty

Depicted social role	*Tomb*	*Location*	*Date*
	G2378 Senedjemib (4)	Giza	5th Dynasty
	Neferseshemre Sheshi	Saqqara	6th Dynasty
	Mereruka (4)	Saqqara	6th Dynasty
	Ibi (2)	Deir el-Gabrâwi	6th Dynasty
	Inti (2)	Dishasha	6th Dynasty
	Ankhmahor (6)	Saqqara	6th Dynasty
	Kairer (2)	Saqqara	6th Dynasty
	Serfka	El-Sheikh Sa'id	6th Dynasty
Cattle Bearer/ Attendant	Nikauhathor	Giza	4th Dynasty
	Ireru	Giza	5th/6th Dynasty
	Kakhent	Hammamiya	5th Dynasty
	Tjenti	Saqqara	5th Dynasty
	Inti	Dishasha	6th Dynasty
	Inpuhotep (2)	Giza	6th Dynasty
	Niankhkhnum	Giza	6th Dynasty
Attendants/Offering Bearers	G7540	Giza	4th Dynasty
	G7530 Meresankh III	Giza	4th Dynasty
	G4970 Nisutnefer (2)	Giza	5th Dynasty
	Nebt	Saqqara	5th Dynasty
	D117 Wehemka	Giza	5th Dynasty
	Niankhkhnum and Khnumhotep	Saqqara	5th Dynasty
	S915 Nikauhor	Saqqara	5th Dynasty
	Kaemnefert	El-Hagarsa	5th Dynasty
	G4940 Seshemnefer	Giza	5th Dynasty
	Mereruka	Saqqara	6th Dynasty
	Khentka	Saqqara	6th Dynasty
	Whatetkhethor (8)	Saqqara	6th Dynasty
	Sebknufer	El-Hagàrsa	6th Dynasty
	Mereri	Saqqara	6th Dynasty
	Inti	Dishasha	6th Dynasty
	Nenankhpepy	Hierakonpolis	6th Dynasty
	Khentika	Saqqara	6th Dynasty
	Mereri	Saqqara	6th Dynasty
	Nikauisesi	Saqqara	6th Dynasty
	Ibi	Deir el-Gabrâwi	6th Dynasty
	Khentkaus	Giza	6th Dynasty
	Meryteti	Saqqara	6th Dynasty
Dancer	LG 90 Debhen	Giza	4th Dynasty
	Nunuter	Giza	6th Dynasty
Overseer of Linen	Seshemnufer Tjeti (title given to one of the animal tenders)	Giza	6th Dynasty
	Khentika (title given to one of the attendants)	Saqqara	6th Dynasty
	Mereri (title given to one of the attendants)	Saqqara	6th Dynasty

(*Continued*)

Depicted social role	*Tomb*	*Location*	*Date*
	Nikauisesi (title given to one of the attendants)	Saqqara	6th Dynasty
Bird Catchers	Hesy, Hapi	Saqqara	6th Dynasty
	Akhtihotep	Saqqara	6th Dynasty
Scribe	Nufer	Saqqara	5th Dynasty
Boat Captain	Kakhent	Hammamiya	5th Dynasty
	Inti	Dishasha	6th Dynasty
Musician/Singer	Ka'aper	Saqqara	5th Dynasty
Treasurer	Nikauisesi (title given to one of the animal tenders)	Saqqara	6th Dynasty
	Niankhnesut (title given to one of the animal tenders)	Saqqara	6th Dynasty

Notes

1 For examples of associations of dwarfism with negative characteristics such as the 'monstrous' or 'grotesque' and of the assigning of an 'othered' body see Fischer (1987, 22–23), David (2016, 82–83), Fischer-Elfert (1996, 101, 103), and Jeffreys and Tate (2010, 89).

2 The author has decided to primarily use identity-first terminology, since it is noted as being the preferred language for many disabled people (see Morris and Sneed 2021).

3 See for example Buszek (2008, 43), Sampsell (2001, 63), Dasen (1993, 126, 156), and David (2016, 83).

4 See for example Fischer-Elfert finding comedy in the depiction of a dancer with dwarfism due to her size (Fischer-Elfert 1996, 101–2), or the suggestion by Dasen that some individuals served as "human pets" (Dasen 1993, 126), an idea that is never suggested for individuals tending animals who are not dwarf people.

5 It should, however, be noted that some of the individuals depicted in the tombs of others are named and likely referential to actual individuals. They have been included in this category because we do not possess data from their tombs to draw additional conclusions regarding self-representation and social role, as we do in the cases of known individuals.

6 Dasen (1993, 35, 44). Further, the suggestion that small size of these individuals was referential to a lower status does not seem to be supported by the data. Instead, the bodies of these individuals are manipulated to either represent a more realistic image in reference to the bodies of others, or, to properly participate in the hierarchy of size in tomb vignettes, as is seen in the tomb of Seneb. This conclusion seems to ignore the fact that a large majority of depictions show dwarf people and their counterparts as the *same* size (see for example the bottom register of the carrying chair scene from chamber B3 in the tomb of Watekhethor), but with differing proportions. It seems instead that the size of dwarf individuals, like other figures, was adjusted depending on the scene and the role the individual was filling.

7 While it has been suggested that the statue of Petpennisut (JE 37719) schematically portrays a dwarf person from the 5th Dynasty through the depiction of a large head, there is not enough data to securely confirm that this is a dwarf individual. As such, this statue was left out of this analysis.

8 See for example Fischer-Elfert (1996, 97), Dasen (1993, 104–6), Buszek (2008, 43), Sampsell (2001, 65). This popularity also extends beyond the direct field of Egyptology as well – see for example Tassinari and Sisti (2016, 489).

9 The date of Seneb's tomb is often debated. For a good overview of past arguments and the reason for this date see Woods (2010, 301–31).
10 See Bolshakov (1994, 29) and Fischer-Elfert (1996, 94).
11 Seneb's titles included Companion, Friend of the Palace, Beloved of his Lord, Overseer of Weaving in the Palace, Overseer of the Dwarfs in Charge of Linen, Overseer of the Administration of *mw,* Overseer of *jwHw,* Great One of the Litter, Overseer of the Crew of *kz* Ships, Keeper of the God's Seal of the wn-H-bAw Boat, Priest of Wadjet, *ka* Priest of Khufu and Radjedef, Priest of the Large Bull Which is at the Head of Stpt, and Priest of the Bull mrHw, among others. Translations of Seneb's titles can be found in Junker (1941, 6–8), and Dasen (1993, 127–28). Discussion of the tomb's location can be found in Junker (1941, 3–4).
12 Hawass (1991, 157).
13 See Kozma et al. (*2011*, 1818).
14 Hawass (1991, 158).
15 The title present on Perniankhu's serdab was that of Royal Acquaintance, while his statue included an inscription which Hawass translated as "The one who delights his lord every day, the king's dwarf, Pr-nj-anx-w of the great palace" (Hawass 1991, 157, 160). Fischer, however, argued in 2002, that the term Hawass translated as dwarf was actually *jwHw* disrupting the proposed translation (Fischer 2002, 35–36). Fischer suggests it may be referential to a title held by dwarf individuals; however, it is present in the titles of individuals without dwarfism as well and the translation is debated.
16 See Sampsell (2001, 64) and Mariette (1889).
17 Additional titles include Overseer of Linen, *ka*-Priest, and Overseer of *sem*-Priests. Maspero (1913, 85), Thompson (1991, 92). As El-Aguizy points out, it appears that while Khnumhotep was of high status, his titles suggest a lower status than that held by Seneb (El-Aguizy 1987, 56).
18 Porter and Moss (1962), Porter, Moss, and Burney (1968), Porter, Moss, and Burney (1972), and Porter, Moss, and Burney (1981).
19 See Dasen (1993, 253–66).
20 These are all listed in Appendix I. It should be noted that none of the known individuals discussed in the previous section have been identified in any of these tombs, and that the depictions of Seneb found within his tomb are not included in the statistical analysis performed in this section.
21 The author recognizes that there is a margin of error present in this data, due to our inability to know whether or not the scenes depict the same dwarf people across multiple tombs. That said, the conclusions are the same, even if the analysis is done by scene rather than by individual depiction.
22 It should be noted that three of these depicted individuals are given titles in addition to their depicted role as animal tender. This includes two with the title of Treasurer, and one with the title Overseer of Linen. These are recorded in the Appendix. Since an analysis of titles is outside the scope of this paper, these roles were not included in the data distribution.
23 It should be noted that three of these depicted individuals are given the title of Overseer of Linen in addition to their depicted role as Attendant.
24 See for example the depiction of goldsmiths in the tomb of Mereruka (Duell 1938, pl. 32).
25 For an overview of gendered social roles see Roth (2020, 91–94). It should be noted, however, that it is possible that the scope of female social roles was larger than previously believed and not as based on heteronormative beliefs as earlier scholarship has led some scholars to conclude. The suggestion of gendered representation by the author of this paper here is based solely on what is represented in these specific tombs, rather than an overall conclusion of gender representations in the Old Kingdom.
26 Kanawati (2002, pl 18).
27 Interestingly, in some depictions, such as the depiction of the boat captain in the tomb of Inti at Dishasha (E59a) (see Petrie 1898, pl. XIII), the heads of the individuals without dwarfism are shrunk or lowered allowing the individual with dwarfism, the head of the

ship, to maintain the highest headline. Thus, this practice was not only executed in the case of a tomb owner, like Seneb, but in the depiction of all individuals.

28 Kanawati and Abder-Raziq (2008, pl. 69).

29 Bolshakov (1994, 29).

30 For an additional example of how we can challenge the role of modern thought in othering disability in the ancient world see Vogel and Power (2023).

31 Although a single individual with a curved spine does appear in a banquet scene in the mastaba of Ty holding a dog, while a dwarf person stands in the register above holding a monkey, there is no additional evidence to group representations of dwarfism and other disabilities together in a way that convincingly proves that the Egyptians saw them as part of the same group. While it could be argued that the statistical likelihood of dwarfism could have been higher than that of a curved spine in Egypt, the large percentage of dwarf individuals who are clearly depicted as members of the elite class, and the complete absence of representations of individuals with curved spines in the same positions, suggest that there was another factor at play.

32 For example, claims that disability is only shown in Old Kingdom artwork in the lower, working classes cannot be mapped onto the representation of dwarf individuals, and instead can only be used in the discussion of individuals with hyper-extension of the knees (see Mahran and Kamal 2016, 16–17).

33 For a complete list of known depictions of dwarf people throughout Egyptian history as of 1993, see Dasen (1993, Catalogue E).

Bibliography

Bolshakov, Andrey. "Hinting as a Method of Old Kingdom Tomb Decoration. I: The Offering-Stone and the False Door or the Dwarf Snb." *Göttinger Miszellen* 139 (1994): 9–33.

Buszek, Artur. "Dwarf Figurines from Tell El-Farkha." *Studies in Ancient Art and Civilization* 12 (2008): 35–56.

Dasen, Véronique. *Dwarfs in Ancient Egypt and Greece. Oxford Monographs on Classical Archaeology*. Oxford: Clarendon Press, 1993.

David, Rosalie. "Egyptian Medicine and Disabilities: From Pharaonic to Greco-Roman Egypt." In *Disability in Antiquity*, edited by Christian Laes, 75–89. New York and London: Routledge, 2016.

Duell, Prentice. *The Mastaba of Mereruka: Part I: Chambers A 1–10*. Chicago: University of Chicago Press 1938.

El-Aguizy, Ola. "Dwarfs and Pygmies in Ancient Egypt." *Annales du Service des antiquités de l'Egypte* LXXI (1987): 53–60.

Fischer, Henry G. "The Ancient Egyptian Attitude Towards the Monstrous." In *Monsters and Demons in the Ancient and Medieval World: Papers Presented in Honor of Edith Porada,* edited by Ann Farkas, Prudence Harper, and Evelyn Harrison, 13–26. Mainz on Rhine: P. von Zabern, 1987.

Fischer, Henry G. "Some Titles Associated with Dwarfs and Midgets." *Göttinger Miszellen* 187 (2002): 35–40.

Fischer-Elfert, Hans-Werner. "'Lache nichet über einen Blinden und verspotte nicht einen Zwerg!' Über den Umgang mit Behinderten im Alten Ägypten." In *Behinderung als Pädagogische und Politische Herausforderung: Historische und systematische Aspekte*, edited by Max Liedtke, 93–116. Bad Heilbrunn: Klinkhardt, 1996.

Hawass, Zahi. "The Statue of the Dwarf Pr-n(j)-anx(w) Recently Discovered at Giza." *Mitteilungen des Deutschen Archäologischen Instituts, Abteilung Kairo* 47 (1991): 157–62.

Jeffreys, David, and John Tait. "Disability, Madness, and Social Exclusion in Dynastic Egypt." In *Madness, Disability and Social Exclusion: The Archaeology and Anthropology of Difference*, edited by Jane Hubert, 87–95. London and New York: Routledge, 2010.

Junker, Hermann. *Giza V: Die Mastaba des Snb (Seneb) und die umliegenden Gräber*. Wien and Leipzig: Hölder-Pichler-Tempsky, 1941.

Kanawati, Naguib. *Tombs at Giza. Vol. II: Seshathetep/Heti (G5150), Nesutnefer (G4970), and Seshemnefer II (G5080).* Warminster: Aris and Phillips Ltd., 2002.

Kanawati, Naguib, and M. Abder-Raziq. *Mereruka and His Family, Part II, The Tomb of Waatetkhethor*. Oxford: Aris and Phillips, 2008.

Kozma, C., A. M. Sarry El Din, R. Abd El Shafy El Banna, W. Abd El Samie Kandeel, and R. Lachman. "The Ancient Egyptian Dwarfs of the Pyramids: The High Official and the Female Worker." American Journal of Medical Genetics *Part A* (2011): 1817–24.

Mahran, Heba, and Samar Mostafa Kamal. "Physical Disability in Old Kingdom Tomb Scenes." *Athens Journal of History* 2, no. 3 (2016): 169–92.

Mariette, Auguste. *Les Mastabas de l'ancien empire*. Paris: Vieweg, 1889.

Maspero, Gaston. "The Dwarf Khnoumhotpou (Vth or VIth Dynasty)." In Egyptian Art: Studies, translated by Elizabeth Lee, 85–89. London: T. Fisher Unwin, 1913.

Morris, Alexandra, and Debby Sneed. "A Brief Guide to Disability Terminology and Theory in Ancient World Studies." *Society for Classical Studies*, August 30, 2021. Accessed May 25, 2023. https://classicalstudies.org/scs-blog/alexandra-morris/blog-brief-guide-disability-terminology-and-theory-ancient-world-studies.

Petrie, William Flinders. *Deshasheh*. London: Egyptian Exploration Fund, 1898.

Porter, Bertha, and Rosalind Moss. *Topographical Bibliography of Ancient Egyptian Hieroglyphic Texts, Reliefs, and Paintings. V. Upper Egypt: Sites (Deir Rîfa to Aswân, Exclusing Thebes and the Temples of Abydos, Dendera, Esna, Edfu, Kôm Ombo, and Philae).* Oxford: Oxford University Press, 1962.

Porter, Bertha, Rosalind Moss, and Ethel Burney. *Topographical Bibliography of Ancient Egyptian Hieroglyphic Texts, Reliefs, and Paintings. IV. Lower and Middle Egypt (Delta and Cairo to Asyût).* Oxford: Oxford Clarendon Press, 1968.

Porter, Bertha, Rosalind Moss, and Ethel Burney. *Topographical Bibliography of Ancient Egyptian Hieroglyphic Texts, Reliefs, and Paintings. III. Memphis, Part I. Abû Rawâsh to Abûsir*. Oxford: Oxford University Press, 1972.

Porter, Bertha, Rosalind Moss, and Ethel Burney. *Topographical Bibliography of Ancient Egyptian Hieroglyphic Texts, Reliefs, and Paintings. III. Memphis, Part II. Saqqâra to Dahshûr*. Oxford: Oxford Clarendon Press, 1981.

Roth, Ann Macy. "Gender Roles in Ancient Egypt." In *A Companion to the Ancient Near East*. 2nd ed., edited by Daniel C. Snell, 87–96. Hoboken: Wiley Blackwell, 2020.

Sampsell, Bonnie. "Ancient Egyptian Dwarfs." *KMT: A Modern Journal of Ancient Egypt* 12, no. 3 (2001): 60–73.

Tassinari, J., and A. Sisti. "First Dwarf Represented: Ancient Egypt 2520 B.C." *Journal of Endocrinological Investigation* 39 (2016): 489.

Thompson, Elizabeth. "Dwarfs in the Old Kingdom in Egypt." *The Bulletin of the Australian Centre for Egyptology* 2 (1991): 91–98.

Vogel, Hannah, and Ronika K. Power. "Recognising Inequality: Abelism in Egyptological Approaches to Disability and Bodily Differences." *World Archaeology* (2023). https://doi.org/10.1080/00438243.2023.2170911.

Woods, Alexandra. "A Date for the Tomb of Seneb at Giza: Revisited." In *Egyptian Culture and Society: Studies in Honour of Naguib Kanawati*. Vol. 2, edited by Alexandra Woods, Ann McFarlane, and Susanne Binder, 301–31. Cairo: SCA, 2010.

11 Bes or the Offense of Physiognomy in Egyptology

Livia Bergerot

The god Bes, the object of many studies since the nineteenth century, has often been subjected to prejudices and biases from Egyptologists. As early as the end of the eighteenth century, Bes was misunderstood by several interpretative errors. This is primarily due to the fact that his physical appearance was judged to be out of step with that of the other major deities. Bes is the only Egyptian god to be the subject of a human-animal hybridization, unlike the other gods who have clearly defined physical parts, represented either entirely as humans, entirely as animals, or as zoomorphic.[1]

This misinterpretation on the part of Egyptologists in the nineteenth and part of the twentieth century is also because there is no apparent evidence of Bes in the classical literature (Greco-Roman) that early Egyptology typically used. Furthermore, once they were able to translate the Egyptian texts, early scholars realized that the few representations of Bes that were not anonymous, particularly in the Greco-Roman mammisi, could also bear the name Hyt. For nearly a century, Bes was therefore named Typhon, referring to the Typhon of Greek mythology who was a fearsome being, a primitive and malevolent deity. It seems that it was Sir Gardner Wilkinson who first proposed the name Bes (Besa) in the second edition of *Manners and Customs* in 1841: "The name of this Deity is as yet doubtful. . . . May this Deity have been Besa, whose oracle is placed by ancient writers in the vicinity of Abydus or of Antinoë? His name in some of the hieroglyphic legends resembles that of the unkhnow Besa; and if his character appears little likely to justify the notion of his possessing an oracle, it will cease to present an objection, when we recollect that, in Greece, even the monster Geryon, slain by Hercules, was deemed worthy of a similar honour".[2]

It is because of these few characteristics that make him a unique deity in history and pharaonic art that Bes has been the subject of certain bitterness from several authors who have considered him a somewhat contemptible minor entity. Thus, the figure of Bes was a victim of censorship as soon as it was rediscovered. Indeed, when the scholars accompanying Bonaparte on his famous Egyptian expedition passed through the temple of Ermant between 1798 and 1801, the artist who reproduced a bas-relief from the mammisi of Cleopatra VII on plate 97, vignette 3 of the *Description de l'Égypte* literally erased the highly characteristic features of Bes to give a more 'classical' appearance to the great figure carrying a tambourine and

DOI: 10.4324/9781003440369-14

following the procession (Figure 11.1). Represented only by a circle, his head was not reproduced; his belly was reshaped to appear slimmer, and a skirt covered the nudity of a more elongated body. Although this relief from the temple of Ermant has since disappeared under the construction of a sugar refinery in 1861, we can have a more realistic glimpse of it under the pen of Dominique Vivant Denon in his book *Voyage dans la Basse et la Haute Égypte* (Figure 11.2). Bes – then called Typhon – holds a large tambourine near his head. While he has his typical stocky limbs and a large beard, the person is immense. Indeed, Bes is twice as tall as the priests carrying the statue of Min in front of him.

"No Egyptian deity is as little known so far as the monstrous god ⟨Bes⟩".[3] This sentence written by Viscount Emmanuel de Rougé in 1865, then curator of the Egyptian Department at the Louvre Museum, is representative of the comments that followed for nearly a century.

In his *Histoire de la Caricature Antique* published the same year, Champfleury led the way with a chapter devoted to Bes:

> In these sun-drenched lands, no trace of comedy appears on Pharaonic sculptures. However, there is a short, stout, pot-bellied and thick-lipped god, an

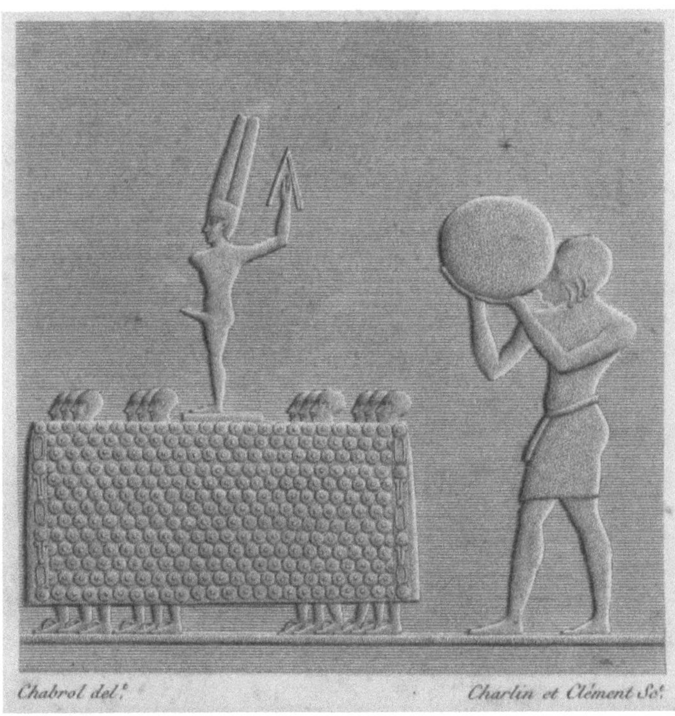

Figure 11.1 Engraving depicting a procession scene from a now-lost bas-relief of the mammisi of Ermant. From *Description de l'Égypte*, Vol. 1: Antiquités, 1809, pl. 97, 3.

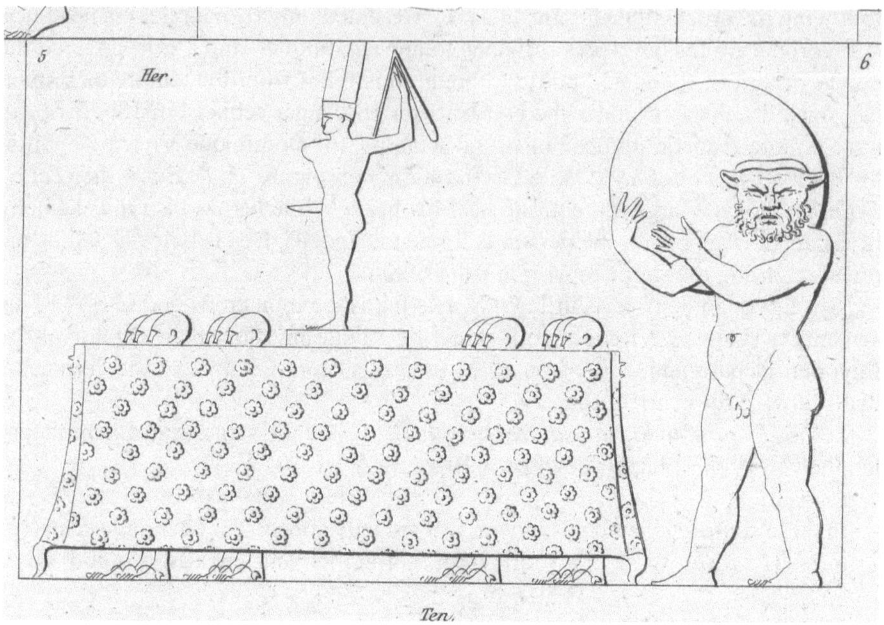

Figure 11.2 Drawing depicting a procession scene from a now-lost bas-relief of the mammisi of Ermant. From Dominique Vivant Denon, *Voyage dans la Basse et la Haute Égypte*, 1802, pl. 121.

> apoplectic dwarf, grotesque and puppet-like, whose pretentious seriousness provokes laughter; it is an Egyptian god, the god Bes . . . Amidst the silent granites that disturb with their serious gravity, a gouty old man raises his leg with difficulty, and if his joyful mouth and thick lips did not indicate one of those good-natured beings who join in the amusements of youth, one would fear the consequences of these follies for the stiffened limbs of the god Bes, who can be compared, despite the respect due to any god, to an old frog threatened with ankylosis.[4]

Champfleury illustrated his remarks with a drawing reproducing a fragmentary Bes from the Louvre[5] (Figure 11.3). His friend Victor Hugo was inspired by his drawing (and probably the text) for his passage on the king of the Auxcriniers in his novel *Toilers of the Sea* published the following year. Here is an excerpt that rivals Champfleury's "old frog threatened with ankylosis": "Only the ignorant are unaware that the greatest danger in the English Channel is the king of the Auxcriniers. There is no more formidable sea character. Those who have seen him shipwreck between Saint-Michel and the other. He is small, being a dwarf, and he is deaf, being a king. . . . A massive head at the bottom and narrow at the top, a stocky body, a slimy and deformed belly, nodules on the skull, short legs, long arms, fins for feet, claws for hands, a broad green face – such is this king".[6]

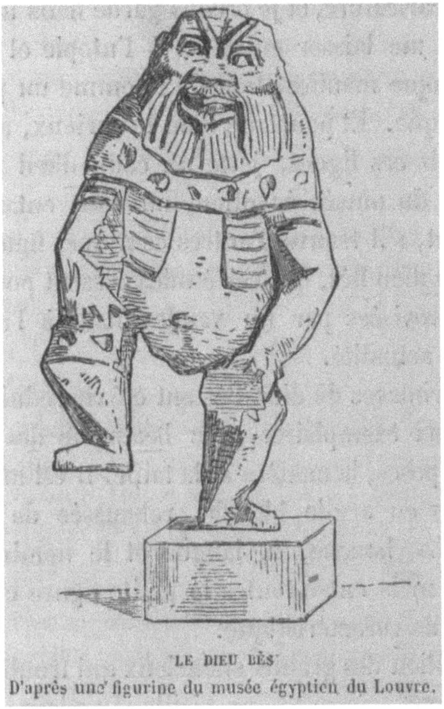

Figure 11.3 Drawing of a fragmented statue of Bes. From Champfleury, *Histoire de la Caricature Antique*, p. 16.

Another object from the Louvre also has been at the center of attention.[7] Between January 1 and March 15, 1851, while Auguste Mariette thought he was excavating the Serapeum of Saqqara, he discovered a statue of Bes in the courtyard of the temple of Nectanebo II dedicated to Apis. In his notes published posthumously by Gaston Maspero, Mariette recounted a scene that occurred after he had the statue put back upright on its pedestal:

> It's lunchtime, and the sun is beating down directly on the statue, emphasizing its powerful reliefs. Women from Abusir and Saqqara have joined our workers. A sort of procession forms. Of course, Bes is mistaken for the devil. The parade begins. Each person acts according to their temperament. The women stand in front of the statue and insult it, making frantic gestures. Generally, the men spit on it. Among my workers, there are two or three Africans. They look directly at the impassive deity, and suddenly burst into loud laughter as they run away.[8]

This statue has been held since 1952 at the Louvre Museum under inventory number N 437. In 1897, in an article by the physician and anthropologist Félix Regnault titled "Le dieu égyptien Bès était myxœdémateux" the same statue was described as follows: "The ears are broad, not bordered, set apart from the head, a sign of degeneration but not of myxedema. Remove the flesh from this skull in your mind, and it will resemble that of the cretin from Batignolles that I studied".[9] And the author adds further on:

> The Egyptian god Bes was, therefore, myxedematous[10] or cretinous. Why did the Egyptians raise a cretin to such a role? It should be noted that in countries that have cretins, these individuals are respected and revered. The families who have them consider them to bring good luck. Therefore, it is indeed a symbol of life, and it is understandable that the Egyptians perceived a monster as such.[11]

The author concludes his remarks as follows: "It is useful to demonstrate the support that certain sciences, such as history, can find in medicine".[12] It is important to note that while the term "cretin" became an insult in the twentieth century, in the nineteenth century it was a medical term. Cretinism referred to a set of physical and intellectual disabilities related to thyroid deficiency due to environmental iodine deficiency.

In disagreement with Félix Regnault, Dr. Pierre Vassal noted that Bes' developed body hair and the disharmony between his torso and limbs were not indicative of myxedema, and preferred to see in him a psychiatric disorder characterized by an expansive mood: "Bes behaves mostly like a hypomanic,[13] which aligns perfectly with his short, stocky build".[14]

In 1894, the Egyptologist Ollivier-Beauregard was not gentle when describing the physical appearance of Bes:

> From head to toe, the figure of Bes is hideous and deformed; everything about it is coarse, bloated, and repulsive; it is a big inflated dwarf. . . . Bes's figures have absolutely nothing of the biases, qualities, and flaws of Egyptian statuary. Everything about them is strange and, above all, foreign to Egypt. . . . Bes, with the singular embellishments adorning his face and the brutal whimsy of his posture, is a monster whose origin seems unable to be explained. . . . In these conditions of grotesque activity or subordinate employment, Bes, among the divine figures of Egypt, appears to have been a jack-of-all-trades character.[15]

The Egyptologist, like many others still today, assumed that with such a 'monstrous' physique, Bes could only occupy subordinate, minor, and 'grotesque' functions in the Egyptian cult landscape.

The transition to the twentieth century was not easy for Bes. In 1933, Marcelle Werbrouck had some harsh words when she said that "in Pharaonic civilization, he became the god of the common people, pitiful in his reception, so close to mortals that he is invoked with naive trust and faith". The author comments on the bas-relief EA 994 from the British Museum that notably depicts juvenile individuals from the

5th Dynasty dancing and playing, among whom a boy wears a lion mask and holds a "scepter terminated by a hand". About this attribute, Marcelle Werbrouck writes: "[T]his object, depicted in a few other mastabas, is between the fingers of deformed dwarfs, true jesters of the great of the Old Kingdom, and servants taking care of the master's familiar monkeys".[16] As we can see, the biased view that the author has of Bes is sadly equal to the one she seems to have of people with dwarfism.

In 1938, Jeanne Vandier d'Abbadie also taints her words with a certain disgust towards a "different" physical aspect, which is therefore foreign to Egypt since it is not "majestic":

> Who was this god, always depicted as deformed, grotesque, familiar, and often joyful? His face, almost always depicted facing forward, affirms his foreign origin: he had come from the land of Punt. He is not encountered in Egyptian art before the New Kingdom. Clearly, he does not belong to the lineage of the grand Egyptian gods, so majestic and distant.[17]

It is Bernard Bruyère who, in 1939, has the harshest words describing dwarfism as a "pathological monstrosity" while considering the small stature of Pygmies a "racial deformity":

> Summing up in himself so many characters and attributes, Bes is a somewhat obscure upstart whom luck has elevated to the rank of supreme god, a Pantheon with a thousand aspects. One can conceive the ardor of the struggle that Christianity had to undertake against this malicious spirit that, hunted in one form, was reborn in another before admitting defeat. . . . Is the small, stocky body that of a pygmy or that of an Egyptian dwarf? Sometimes one hesitates between a pathological monstrosity and a racial deformity.[18]

All these remarks, while they may seem extremely shocking to us today, must be put into their historical and social context. Note, however, that they are mostly the work of French-speaking authors. The main Anglophone or Germanophone authors who wrote about Bes were not so insistent in their remarks. Only a few comments on his physique are noteworthy: thus, Sir Gardner Wilkinson described Bes as a "short deformed man",[19] while Eduard Meyer spoke of a "ghastly deformity in the form of a dwarf".[20]

If negative comments on the physical appearance of Bes have reduced over time, it is still regularly argued that he is a grotesque or coarse genius, a monstrous and whimsical character, that he is ugly, hideous. Associating his "horrible silhouette" with his actions, some comments even go so far as to speak of "noise" when Bes plays a musical instrument, regardless of whether it is to calm down after returning from the Distant Goddess.[21]

Despite the attempts of physicians Félix Régnault and Pierre A. Vassal to diagnose Bes as myxedematous or hypomanic,[22] he has always been associated with achondroplastic dwarfism in recent literature. However, a new association has recently been proposed. In "La perception des handicapés mentaux dans le

Proche-Orient ancien" and more specifically in a paragraph titled "Un dieu handicapé",[23] the theologian Edgar Kellenberger addresses the figure of Bes as a caricatured god whose ugliness, which opposes the custom of representing an ideal form of gods, is intended to drive away evil spirits. The author suggests that his protruding tongue is a characteristic feature of Down syndrome, while also linking individuals with Down syndrome to Bes through their flat nose as well as their certain joviality, strong affinity for music and dance, and attachment to family. Despite an additional proposal to link the name Bes with the word *pèti*, which relates to mild mental disability in late Jewish texts, Edgar Kellenberger's hypothesis is not convincing. Indeed, the author fails to mention that a lion primarily characterizes Bes' face. Furthermore, some characteristics oppose Bes to a person with Down syndrome, such as his large, round eyes that contrast with almond-shaped eyes, a muscular and powerful body against muscular hypotonia, and above all, a very imposing head and large, lion-like ears. In contrast, individuals with Down syndrome have a relatively small head and ears proportional to their body.

Indeed, Bes is a composite image from the Egyptian imagination (Figure 11.4). His primary components, even before dwarfism, are frontality and animal like. The

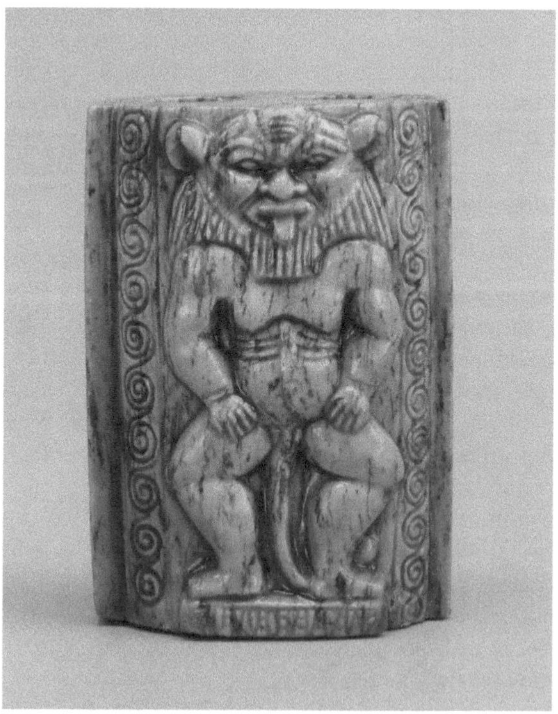

Figure 11.4 Kohl container decorated with Bes-image, Metropolitan Museum of Art, 26.7.1277, 18th Dynasty. H.: 6 cm, Credit Line: Purchase, Edward S. Harkness Gift, 1926.

latter corresponds to his leonine nature and recalls the formidable fauna in which he operates and controls. His leonine mask is more or less pronounced depending on the era, but his ears are always round and hairy, while his eyes are invariably wide open and piercing. The protruding tongue is an animal characteristic not attested in representations of humans. Bes is constantly in motion, with bent or thrown legs and a muscular body, and his particular bodily attitude certainly breaks with the hieratic stance of most other deities.

Additionally, his hybrid appearance is a significant marker, often revealing protective entities. In fact, Bes is one of the few expressive deities. He grimaces, bares his teeth, sticks out his tongue, furrows his brow and nose – sometimes to display genuine joviality, sometimes terrible anger. Frontality highlights his facial expressions, which testify to his apotropaic nature. Indeed, in two-dimensional Egyptian representations, a front-facing face is unusual, designed to evoke fear: either the fear that the subject must inspire or the fear that he/she experiences. This frontality allows the eyes to scan danger and the mouth to recite some imprecation in its direction. In this characteristic attitude, protective deities, with their tongues sticking out to frighten, also have two ears facing forward (i.e., folded forward), wide open to listen attentively. This is what Dominique Farout calls 'facial' or 'absolute' frontality.[24]

In 1963, H. Wild stated, "These bearded dwarf gods originally played a very insignificant and subordinate role. After serving the great gods to entertain them through music and dance, and to watch over their children and the children of humans, they saw their favor grow to the point that in the Late Period they became their equals or even surpassed them".[25] Even today, for the majority of Egyptologists, Bes remains confined to a subordinate role in an intimate and family domain, especially with mothers in childbirth and their infants. However, his attributes are not limited to the strictly domestic sphere.

The assumed form of dwarfism that Bes appears to have, which he shares with the deity Ptah-Pataikos, is called achondroplasia. It is a genetic disease that disrupts the cartilage growth in all limbs – only the trunk grows normally while the limbs remain short with retraction of the elbows and bowed legs. The belly is prominent and the rounded buttocks are due to a strong back arching. The skull can also be brachycephalic, meaning wider than it is long, and sometimes hydrocephalic due to increased cerebrospinal fluid volume as seen in depictions of Ptah-Pataikos. This is not the case with Bes: he is a hybrid deity, part-human and part-lion, so we should not try to categorize him precisely. What is interesting to understand, however, is the symbolism of this dwarfism.

In ancient Egyptian, there are mainly two terms related to the figure of the dwarf person: *dng* (*d3ng*, *d3g*, or *dlg*) 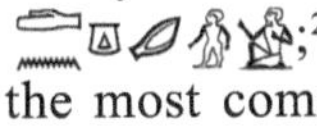;[26] and *nmw* (*nmi*) 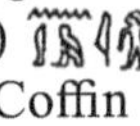 and variants, ;[27] 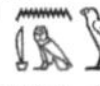, 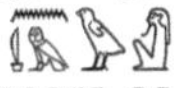 [28] are the most common. From the Coffin Texts, the dwarf person appears as belonging to the divine world; *spell* 132 states: "I am Atum, who created the great ones. I am the one who begot Shu and gave birth to Tefnut. It is I who broke my passivity at the time of Nun. These lands of the dwarf people belong to me";[29] *spell* 136 takes up the same theme, and the divine determinative appears in *spell* 1442: "Ra, Atum, Nun, the Ancient, Shu, Iky, Nemu and Hetep."

According to Bénédicte Lhoyer, "[T]he dwarfs would here be the first manifestations of the creative power of the divine, linked to the earth and to light, since the pair Geb and Nut succeeded Shu and Tefnut in the divine genealogy".[30]

Dimitri Meeks identified a connection with the term *bs* found in a passage in the *Pyramid Texts*: "[Y]ou are a *bs* who does not know his father and does not know his mother" (Pyr. § 1186 a), and later in the *Ritual of the Four Balls*: "the little one, the *bs*, the short one, the dwarf person (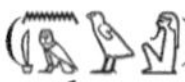)".[31] The author indicates that the generic term *bs* is equivalent to the other three, designating a being whose gestation is not complete, an "apotropaic transposition of the premature", and reminds us that the dwarf person (*nmi*) is itself associated with childhood, the fetus, and miscarriages.[32]

The oldest case of dwarfism discovered in Egypt dates back to the fifth millennium BCE (around 4,500 years before our era),[33] and already during the Old Kingdom, representations of so-called everyday life show that the Egyptians integrated them into their universe, both earthly and divine. They were already associated with childhood, joy, and fertility, but also with dance and music. According to Bénédicte Lhoyer, for the Egyptians, they were "perceived as the result of a divine action, making them irrefutable physical proof of a supernatural will".[34]

And for good reason: being children in size and adults in age, the stout appearance of short, twisted limbs attached to a long trunk has linked dwarf people to the iconography of the scarab as well as to the different aspects of the sun, young at the beginning of its course and old at the end of the day. The figure of the dwarf person thus embodies both the notion of growth and also that of regeneration. This solar aspect of the dwarf in religious thought is particularly well illustrated in papyrus 37 of the Meermanno-Westreenianum museum dating from the 21st Dynasty: in the solar disk where the ram, the evening star, takes place, a dwarf person replaces the usual representation of the scarab, the morning star. Regarding this play of imagery, Véronique Dasen explains that "unfinished, the dwarf symbolizes that which takes shape, that which constantly grows and regenerates, much like the ever-renewing sun, which at its rise presents the same ambiguity as the dwarf, as it is both eternally young and old".[35]

As Ptah-Pataikos regularly carries a scarab on his cranial cap, Bes is also closely linked to the beetle, as evidenced by his many representations on the flat side of scarab amulets. One object is particularly remarkable in this regard: a Greco-Roman period faience scarab preserved in the August Kestner Museum. Instead of the usual head, it features a Bes head with a beard replacing the beetle's serrated visor, while the god's headdress fans out on the pronotum (Figure 11.5). The object is as valuable for its rarity as it is for perfectly illustrating the symbiosis between Bes, dwarfism, the scarab, and the solar disk.

In the Chapel of the Throne of Ra at the Temple of Edfu, a text concerning the birth of the divine child from a lotus compares the young sun to a bud in which a dwarf person (*nmw*) was located: "A lotus emerged in which there was a beautiful child who illuminated the earth with his rays . . . a bud in which there was a dwarf person whom Shu loved to see".[36] Due to its yellow heart surrounded by blue petals, the *Nymphaea caerulea*, which blooms at sunrise and withdraws into the water at dusk, was associated with the solar orb appearing each morning in the sky

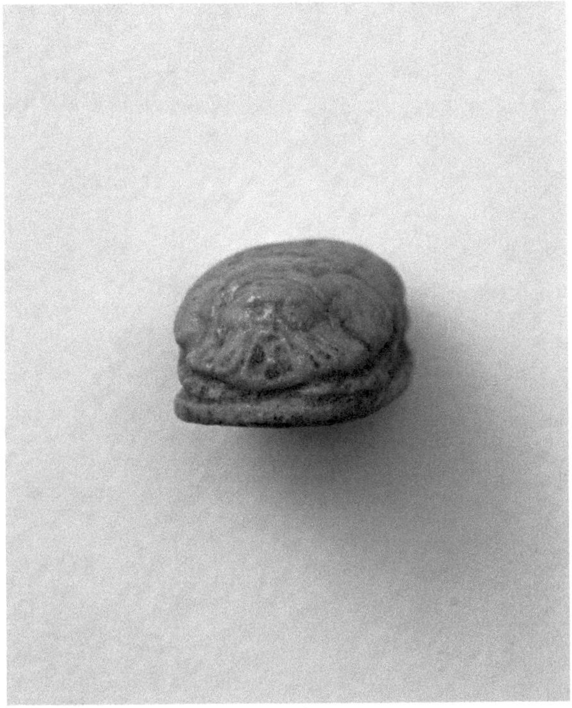

Figure 11.5 Scarab with Bes' head, Museum August Kestner L17.2019. Kunst- und Kulturstiftung Hannover collection. Permanent lending © Museum August Kestner

and disappearing on the horizon at the end of the day. This, of course, echoes the numerous representations of Bes emerging from a lotus flower – representations that make this deity 'a form of solar creator god' as proposed by Michel Malaise.[37]

A bronze statuette of the pan-iconic deity, placed on a rectangular base that was originally meant to fit onto a stick to serve as a sign. The body is human and male, muscular and covered with eyes, with an erect phallus, two pairs of clenched fists, and two pairs of wings. The main head is that of Bes, topped with two pairs of broken horizontal ram horns. The rest of the headdress is missing. On either side of Bes' head, four animal heads are presented in profile, one above the other. The entity is standing and in a walking position, with the left leg in front of the other and the left arm folded forward, which once held a now lost was scepter. Its feet end in the shape of raised cobra heads. A snake climbs up each leg to the knee while an Ouroboros, a serpent biting its own tail, occupies the space around the entity's feet on the base. The object still bears traces of gold inlays, especially in the eyes, beard, and animal skin placed on the entity's shoulders.

Bes' involvement in solar beliefs is extensive.[38] In addition to his role as protector of the child gods Horus, Harpocrates, and Shed, to whom he lends his strength, from the Late Period onward, Bes with his dwarfism and mask has widely lent his image to the powerful pan-iconic figure improperly called "Bes Pantheos" in the form of statuettes, amulets, stelae, etc. (Figure 11.6). In the Harris Magical Papyrus

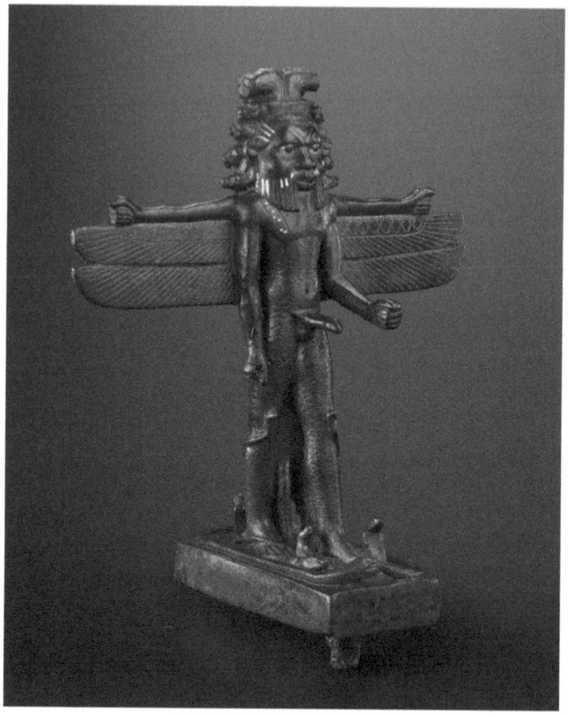

Figure 11.6 Pan-iconic statuette with head of Bes, bronze with gold inlay, FGA-ARCH-EG-0170. © Photographic credit: Fondation Gandur pour l'Art, Geneva. Photographer: André Longchamp

(VIII, 9–10), Michel Malaise rightly proposed to recognize Bes through the invocation addressed to an anonymous deity qualified as the "dwarf person of the sky", "dwarf person with a large face, high-backed and short-legged, the great support that extends from the sky to the underworld", described in the Harris Papyrus (VIII, 9–10).[39] This same entity is also described in the Brooklyn Magical Papyrus as "he whose name (itself) is hidden from the gods, the g[iant] of a million cubits, the [god with] the powerful arm who supports the sky above him, whose feathers are high; [the wind] comes forth from his mouth to give life to every nostril; he rises in the form of the light-god (Shu) [to] illuminate the two lands . . . the man of a million [cubits who] has seven faces on a single [neck]; one with a face of Bes".[40] The two vignettes of the papyrus show the entity with the face of Bes as the main one of the nine heads that compose it. In this regard, two other representations associating Bes with this giant of a million cubits who supports the sky are remarkable for their iconographic composition. One is a register of the sarcophagus of Ankhrui where a Bes takes the place of Shu and holds up Nut with both arms (Figure. 11.7), and the other is a register of the sarcophagus 6270 of the Kunsthistorisches Museum in Vienna where, once again, Bes lifts up the sky goddess while holding a pillar-*djed*, a symbol of stability[41] (Figure 11.8). On the sarcophagus of Ankhrui, it can be seen

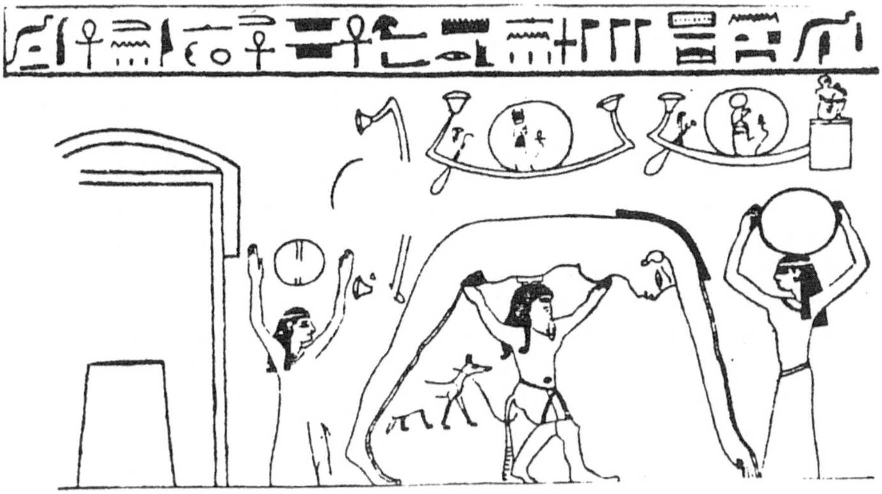

Figure 11.7 Bes in the role of Shu. Lid of the sarcophagus of Ankhrui, fourth register. From William Matthew Flinders Petrie, Hawara, Biahmu and Arsinoe, London, 1889, pl. II.

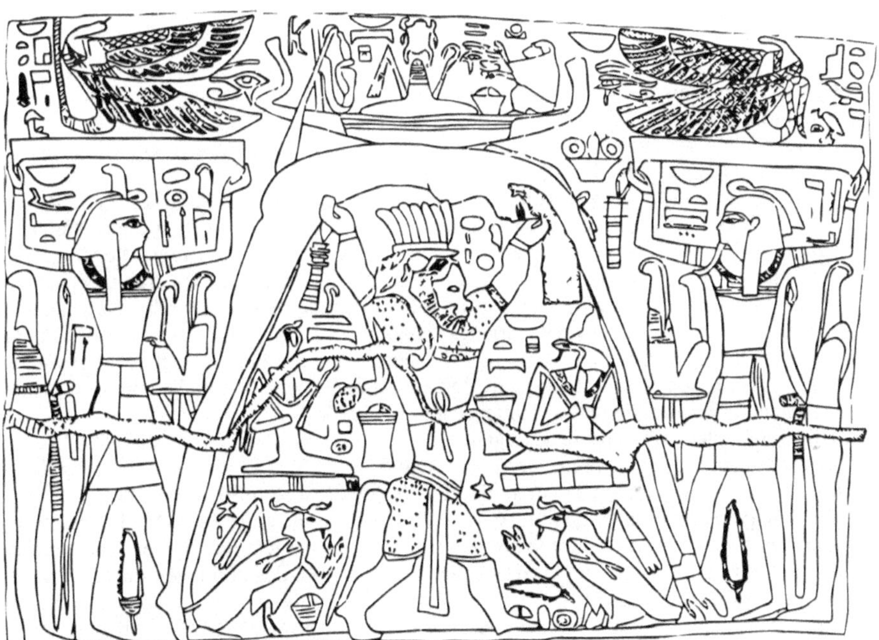

Figure 11.8 Bes supporting Nut in the place of the god Shu. Vienna, Kunsthistorisches Museum, sarcophagus 6270. From Dasen, Veronique. *Dwarfs in Ancient Egypt and Greece*, 52. Oxford, 2004, fig. 5.4.

that Nut's belly rests directly on Bes' modius. His head, therefore, as well as his arms, serves as a support for the sky.

Finally, Bes' dwarfism turns out to be much more positive than many comments throughout history have shown. Dwarf people were not rejected but, on the contrary, were considered in ancient Egypt. Dwarfism, particularly that of Bes, is indicative of divine and solar power. His face, still considered "ugly" today to the point of being ridiculous, is bearer of powers so powerful that they were as useful to other deities as to the Egyptian population. Enjoying constant popularity, with hands resting on his thighs and feet firmly planted in the ground, Bes was in an ideal position to become a solid and unshakable support for worship.[42] Obviously, the abundance of his representations attests to the attachment that Egyptians had for him, but also to his formidable effectiveness, day and night. The deity revealed himself in an Atlantean role, both physically and figuratively, as an architectural support, a pillar of worship, a protector of the divine space, and a mediator for all Egyptians.

Georges Michailidis wrote, "Bes in his various forms would therefore be the divine soul of the Cosmos, as gradually conceived by the Egyptian people throughout the centuries".[43] So, if we consider the significance of these words, rather than viewing Bes as a secondary, subordinate deity, it would be more accurate to say that he is an essential deity in the history of ancient Egypt.

Notes

1 Hathor also stands out when depicted frontally, with a human face and cow ears.
2 Wilkinson (1841, 431–35).
3 De Rougé (1865, 143). [Aucune divinité égyptienne n'est aussi peu connue jusqu'ici que le dieu monstrueux ⟨Bès⟩.]
4 Champfleury (1865, 30). [Dans ces pays d'ardent soleil, nulle trace de comique n'apparaît sur les sculptures pharaoniques. Cependant il est un dieu court, ramassé, ventru et lippu, nain apoplectique, grotesque et fantoche, dont la prétentieuse gravité provoque le rire; c'est un dieu égyptien, le dieu Bès . . . Au milieu des granits silencieux qui troublent par leur gravité sérieuse, un vieillard podagre lève la jambe avec peine, et si sa bouche joyeuse et ses lèvres lippues n'indiquaient un de ces êtres de bonne humeur qui se mêlent aux divertissements de la jeunesse, on craindrait les suites de ces folies pour les membres engourdis du dieu Bès, qu'on peut comparer, malgré le respect dû à tout dieu, à une vieille grenouille menacée d'ankylose.]
5 This fragmented Bes is preserved under the inventory numbers E 320 and N 4236.
6 Victor Hugo, *Les Travailleurs de la mer* (1866, I.I–IV). [Les ignorants seuls ignorent que le plus grand danger des mers de la Manche, c'est le roi des Auxcriniers. Pas de personnage marin plus redoutable. Qui l'a vu fait naufrage entre Saint-Michel et l'autre. Il est petit, étant nain, et il est sourd, étant roi (. . .). Une tête massive en bas et étroite en haut, un corps trapu, un ventre visqueux et difforme, des nodosités sur le crâne, de courtes jambes, de longs bras, pour pieds des nageoires, pour mains des griffes, un large visage vert, tel est ce roi.] This text was written in the spring of 1865. See also the drawing made by the author.
7 In addition to the following lines, also see the depiction of this Bes N 437 in *The Triumph of Alexander* painted by Gustave Moreau in: Bergerot (2021, 59–66).
8 Mariette (1882, 17). [C'est l'heure du repas de midi, et le soleil tombe d'aplomb sur la statue dont il fait saillir puissamment les reliefs. Il est venu des femmes d'Abousyr et

de Saqqarah se joindre à nos ouvriers. Une sorte de procession se forme. Évidemment on prend Bès pour le diable. Le défilé commence. Chacun agit alors selon son tempérament. Les femmes se posent devant la statue et l'injurient, avec des gestes de forcenées. En général, les hommes crachent dessus. J'ai parmi mes ouvriers deux ou trois nègres. Ils regardent en face l'impassible divinité, et subitement se sauvent en riant aux éclats.]

9 Regnault (1897, 436). [Les oreilles sont larges, non ourlées, écartées de la tête, signe de dégénérescence, mais non de myxœdème. Décharnez ce crâne par la pensée, et il rappellera celui du crétin des Batignolles que j'ai étudié.]

10 Myxedema is a term used synonymously with severe hypothyroidism. It is a condition caused by the insufficiency or atrophy of the thyroid gland, characterized by edema and a whitish discoloration of the skin, a slowing down of physiological functions, genital and psychological disorders, or a decrease in basal metabolism.

11 Regnault (1897, 438). [Le Dieu Égyptien Bès était donc myxœdémateux ou crétin. Pourquoi les Égyptiens ont-ils élevé un crétin à ce rôle? Notons que dans les pays qui possèdent des crétins, ces idiots sont respectés, révérés. Les familles qui les possèdent les regardent comme devant leur porter bonheur. C'est donc bien là le symbole de la vie, et on s'explique ainsi que les Égyptiens aient pris pour tel un monstre.]

12 Regnault (1897, 439). [Il est utile de montrer l'appui que certaines sciences, comme l'historique, peuvent trouver dans la médecine.]

13 Hypomania is a psychiatric mood disorder characterized by a euphoric and excited mood, sometimes irritable, accompanied by disturbances in thinking and behavior with abnormally high levels of energy.

14 Vassal (1956, 173). [Bès se comporte d'ailleurs surtout comme un hypomane, ce qui s'accorde tout à fait avec sa constitution bréviligne]

15 Ollivier-Beauregard (1894, 107, 108, 111). [De la tête aux pieds, la figure de Bès est hideuse et difforme; tout est en elle grossier, empâté et repoussant; c'est un gros nain en baudruche. . . . Des partis-pris, qualités et défauts, de la statuaire égyptienne, les figures de Bès n'ont absolument rien. Chez elles tout est étrange et surtout étranger à l'Égypte. . . . Bès, par la singularité des agréments qui décorent sa face, par la brutale fantaisie de son attitude, est un monstre dont la provenance semble de pas pouvoir être expliquée. Dans ces conditions de grotesque activité ou d'emploi subalterne, Bès, au cénacle des divines figures de l'Égypte, nous semble avoir été un personnage à tout faire.]

16 Werbrouck (1933, 28–29). [⟨Bès⟩ est devenu, dans la civilisation pharaonique, le dieu des petites gens, pitoyable d'accueil, si proche des mortels qu'on l'invoque avec une confiance et une foi naïves. . . . cet objet, représenté sur quelques autres mastabas, est entre les doigts de nains difformes, véritables bouffons des grands d'Ancien Empire, et de serviteurs s'occupant des singes familiers du maître.]

17 Vandier d'Abbadie (1938, 34–35). [Qui était ce dieu représenté toujours difforme, grotesque, familier et souvent joyeux? Son visage presque toujours dessiné de face affirme son origine étrangère: il était venu du pays de Pount. On ne le rencontre pas dans l'art égyptien avant le Nouvel Empire. De toute évidence, il n'appartient pas à la lignée des grands dieux égyptiens si majestueux et lointains.]

18 Bruyère (1939, 94–102). [Résumant en lui tant de personnages et d'attributions, Bès est un parvenu un peu obscur que la chance a conduit au rang de dieu suprême, de Panthée aux mille aspects. On conçoit l'âpreté de la lutte que le christianisme eut à entreprendre contre cet esprit malin qui traqué sous une forme, renaissait sous une autre avant de s'avouer vaincu. . . . Le corps petit et trapu est-il celui d'un pygmée ou celui d'un nain égyptien? On hésite quelquefois entre une monstruosité pathologique et une difformité raciale.]

19 Wilkinson (1841, 431).

20 Ballod (1913, 23). [Schauerlichen Missbildung in Gestalt eines Zwerges]. The author does not specify where he found these statements by Meyer, and we have not found them in *Geschichte des Altertums*, the only bibliographic element mentioned by Ballod.

21 Goddess-lioness, daughter and eye of Ra, whose legend is attested by various versions under different names and aspects, the Distant One is sometimes identified as

Hathor-Sekhmet, sometimes as Tefnut. She is called the Distant One because she lives in Nubia after having distanced herself from her father due to a series of events that provoked a violent and insatiable anger within her. Shu, under the name of Onuris, "The One Who Brings Back the Distant One", is sent by Ra, along with Thoth, to retrieve his sister whose fury spreads terror in the Nubian desert. To welcome her upon her return, Bes and Hity dance and sing joyfully to appease her. See Hermann Junker, *Der Auszug der Hathor-Tefnut aus Nubien, Abhandlungen der preussischen Akademie der Wissenschaften*, vol. 3 (Berlin: G. Reimer, 1911), Stephanie West, "The Greek Version of the Legend of Tefnut," *Journal of Egyptian Archeology* 55 (1969): 161–83. London: The Egypt Exploration Society; Danielle Inconnu-Bocquillon, *Le Mythe de la Déesse Lointaine à Philae, Bibliothèque d'étude 132* (Cairo: Institut Français d'Archéologie Orientale 2001).

22 See footnotes 11 and 14 for definitions.

23 Kellenberger (2019, 274–82). For Bes, "Un dieu handicapé," see 281.

24 Farout (2017, 48).

25 Wild (1963, 84–85). [Ces dieux nains barbus n'ont joué à l'origine qu'un rôle très insignifiant et subalterne. Après avoir été au service des grands dieux pour les réjouir au moyen de musique et de danse et pour veiller sur leurs enfants et sur ceux des hommes, ils ont vu leur faveur grandir au point qu'à la Basse Époque ils sont devenus leurs égaux ou même les ont supplantés.]

26 Erman, Grapow, *Wörterbuch der Aegyptischen Sprache. Die Belegstellen V*, vol. 470 (Berlin: Akademie Verlag, 1992), 5–7; "Zwerg, Faulkner", *A Concise Dictionary of Middle Egyptian* (Oxford: Griffith Institute, 1962), 314; "Pygmy, Hannig", *Ägyptisches Wörterbuch I, Hannig-Lexica 4* (Mainz: Philipp von Zabern, 2003), 1478, {39080}: "Zwerg, Pygmäe".

27 *Wb* II, 267, 4–6: "Zwerg, Faulkner", *CD*, p. 133: "Dwarf, Hannig" (2003, 630), {15721}: "Zwerg, Verwachsener".

28 Hannig (2003, 1286), {15721}: "Zwerg (a. göttlich), Verwachsener".

29 Barguet (1986, 255 et 257).

30 Lhoyer (2018, 174).

31 Meeks (1992, 423–36).

32 The topic of the name of Bes, however, is far too important to be more extensively addressed in these pages.

33 Lhoyer (2018, 203).

34 Lhoyer (2021, 20).

35 Dasen (2006, 99). See also Dasen (2004, 55–83). [Inachevé, le nain symbolise ce qui prend forme, ce qui croît et se régénère sans cesse, comme le soleil renaissant, qui présente à son lever la même ambiguïté que le nain, puisqu'il est à la fois éternellement jeune et âgé.]

36 Koenig (1981, 69), Émile Chassinat and Marquis de Rochemonteix, *Le temple d'Efou I, Mémoires publiées par les membres de la mission archéologique française au Caire X*, ed. Sylvie Cauville and Didier Devauchelle, vol. 1, 2nd ed. (Cairo: IFAO, 1984), 289.

37 Malaise (2004, 272).

38 These were skillfully analyzed in Malaise (1990, 680–729).

39 Lange (1927, 75).

40 Sauneron (1970, 23–24).

41 Architectural element, the djed is to be read as a central pillar of the universe in its form of four superimposed columns. See Livia Bergerot and Thierry-Louis Bergerot, "Ptah et l'énigmatique sceptre djed," in *Égypte Afrique & Orient*, vol. 91 (Montségur: Centre d'égyptologie, 2018), 31–40; Livia Bergerot, Thierry-Louis Bergerot, and Tristan-Louis Bergerot, "Ouvrir les vantaux du ciel," in *Égypte Afrique & Orient*, vol. 99 (Montségur: Centre d'égyptologie, 2020), 3–28.

42 This subject has been more discussed at length in Livia Bergerot, "Bès. À propos d'un pilier cultuel divin," in *Bes kleine God in het Oude Egypte. Proceedings of the*

colloquium of 6 and 7 March 2020 in Amsterdam, ed. Tina Bagh, Olaf E. Kaper, and Christian E. Loeben (Forthcoming).

43 Georges Michaïlidis, "Bès aux divers aspects," in *Bulletin de l'Institut français d'archéologie orientale*, vol. 45 (Cairo: IFAO, 1963–64), 7. [Bès multiforme serait, par conséquent, l'âme divine du Cosmos tel que l'aura progressivement conçue à travers les siècles le peuple égyptien.]

Bibliography

Ballod, Franz. *Prolegomena zur Geschichte der bärtigen Zwerghaften Götter in Ägypten*, 23. Moscow: H. Liessner & D. Sobko, 1913.

Barguet, Paul. *Les Textes des sarcophages égyptiens du Moyen Empire*. Paris: Éditions du Cerf, 1986.

Bergerot, Livia. "À propos de quelques Bès memphites." Master's degree thesis, Université PaulValéry – Montpellier 3, 2018. Unpublished.

Bergerot, Livia. "Le Bès N 437 du Louvre. Du Sérapeum au Triomphe d'Alexandre." In *Égypte Afrique & Orient*. Vol. 100, 59–66. Montségur: Centre d'égyptologie, 2021.

Bruyère, Bernard. *Fouilles de Deir el-Médineh 1934–1935, FIFAO 16*, 94–102. Cairo: Institut Français d'Archéologie Orientale, 1939.

Champfleury. *Histoire de la caricature antique*, 30. Paris: Dentu, 1865.

Dasen, Veronique. *Dwarfs in Ancient Egypt and Greece*. 2nd ed., 55–83. Oxford: Oxford University Press, 2004.

Dasen, Veronique. "Nains et pygmées. Figures de l'altérité en Égypte et Grèce anciennes." In *Penser et représenter le corps dans l'Antiquité*, edited by Francis Prost and Jérôme Wilgaux, 99. Rennes: Presses universitaires de Rennes, 2006.

Dasen, Veronique. "Des Patèques aux nains ventrus: Circulation et transformation d'une image." In *Figurines grecques en contexte. Présence muette dans le sanctuaire, la tombe et la maison*, edited by Stéphanie Huysecom-Haxhi and Arthur Muller, 39–55. Lille: Presses Universitaires du Septentrion, 2015.

De Rougé, Emmanuel. *Notice sommaire des monuments égyptiens exposés dans les galeries du Musée du Louvre*, 143. Paris: de Mourgues frères, 1865.

Farout, Dominique. "La frontalité contrariée dans l'iconographie égyptienne." *Pallas* 105 (2017): 41–66. https://doi.org/10.4000/pallas.8022.

Kellenberger, Edgar. "La perception des handicapés mentaux dans le Proche-Orient ancien." In *Archéologie de la santé, anthropologie du soin*, edited by Alain Froment and Hervé Guy, 274–82. Paris: La Découverte, 2019.

Koenig, Yvan. *Le Papyrus Boulaq 6, Bibliothèque d'Étude 87*. Cairo: IFAO, 1981.

Lange, Hans Ostenfeldt. *Der magische Papyrus Harris*. Copenhagen: Biancos Lunos Bogtrykkeri, 1927.

Lhoyer, Bénédicte. "Les Altérations corporelles dans l'image à l'Ancien Empire." PhD diss., Université Paul-Valéry – Montpellier 3, École du Louvre, 2018.

Lhoyer, Bénédicte. "Bès et les nains." In *Égypte Afrique & Orient*. Vol. 100, 15–26. Montségur: Centre d'égyptologie, 2021.

Malaise, Michel. "Bès et les croyances solaires." In *Studies in Egyptology Presented to Miriam Lichtheim*, edited by Sarah Israelit-Groll, 680–729. Jerusalem: Magnes Press, 1990.

Malaise, Michel. *Bès et la famille isiaque, Chronique d'Égypte 79*, 266–92. Bruxelles: Brepols, 2004.

Mariette, Auguste. *Le Sérapeum de Memphis 1 published by Gaston Maspero*. Paris: Gide, 1882.

Meeks, Dimitri. "Le nom du dieu Bès et ses implications mythologiques." In *The Intellectual Heritage of Egypt. Studies presented to László Kákosy by friends and colleagues on the occasion of his 60th birthday, StudAeg 14*, edited by dans U. Luft, 423–36. Budapest, 1992.

Ollivier-Beauregard, Gratien-Michel. *La caricature égyptienne. Histoire, politique et morale*, 107–39. Paris: Thorin et fils, 1894.
Regnault, Félix. "Le Dieu Égyptien Bès était myxœdémateux." *Bulletins de la Société d'anthropologie de Paris* 4, no. 8 (1897): 434–39. Paris: Masson.
Sauneron, Serge. *Le papyrus magique illustré de Brooklyn.* New York: The Brookklyn Museum, 1970.
Vandier d'Abbadie, Jeanne. "Une fresque civile de Deir el Médineh." In *Revue d'Égyptologie 3,* 27–35. Paris: Peeters, 1938.
Vassal, Pierre A. "La physio-pathologie dans le panthéon égyptien: les dieux Bès et Ptah, le nain et l'embryon." *Bulletins et Mémoires de la Société d'anthropologie de Paris* 10, no. 7 (1956): 168–81. Paris: Masson.
Werbrouck, Marcelle. "À propos du dieu Bès." In *Egyptian Religion I,* edited by Samuel Mercer, 28–32. New York: Alma Egan Hyatt Foundation, 1933.
Wild, Henri. "Les danses sacrées de l'Égypte ancienne." In *Les danses sacrées, Sources Orientales 6,* 33–118. Paris: Le Seuil, 1963.
Wilkinson, John Gardner. *Manners and Customs of the Ancient Egyptians 1.* 2nd ed., 431–35. London: John Murray, 1841.

12 Dwarfism in Ancient Egypt/Nubia

Utilising the Bioarchaeology of Care Approach to Investigate Léri-Weill Dyschondrosteosis

Katie M. Whitmore and Michele R. Buzon

Introduction

The cemetery of Tombos is located at the Third Cataract of the Nile River in modern-day Sudan and started being used in the New Kingdom. Nubians and Egyptians cohabitated at Tombos and there is evidence that over time individuals at Tombos formed an entangled community.[1] Isotopic analysis demonstrates that Egyptians came to Tombos late into the New Kingdom.[2] Egyptian mortuary practices, including monumental pyramid complexes and Egyptian-style artifacts, are prevalent in the New Kingdom structures of the cemetery. An individual (U36.Sh2.B10) with Léri-Weill dyschondrosteosis (LWD), a form of disproportionate dwarfism, was excavated from one of these Egyptian-style chapel tombs and is the focus of this investigation.

The prevalence of disability and impairment studies has increased in the bioarchaeological literature and over the last several years, increasing attention has been placed on the bioarchaeology of care methodology and associated Index of Care.[3] The case of U36.Sh2.B10 provides a compelling opportunity to utilize the bioarchaeology of care perspective to examine health-related care provisioning in New Kingdom-period Egypt/Nubia, especially within the context of numerous publications discussing dwarfism in ancient Egypt. Additionally, many case studies utilizing the bioarchaeology of care methodology focus on individuals with severely physically and potentially socially limiting conditions. U36.Sh2.B10 highlights how the bioarchaeology of care methodology can be used to examine conditions that are less severe in physical limitations in the past.

Disability and Bioarchaeology

Disability and impairment have been discussed within archaeological and bioarchaeological contexts for several decades.[4] However, consideration of disability has not entered the archaeological canon with the same attention as other aspects of identity, such as gender, ethnicity, and age. There are several contributing factors to the lack of integration of disability studies into archaeology, including undertheorization and a perceived inability to investigate disability and impairment outside the context of case studies.[5] However, recently the Bioarchaeology of Disability

DOI: 10.4324/9781003440369-15

model was proposed by Bohling and colleagues.[6] This model provides an approach for the consideration of disability, impairment, and care in archaeological contexts at a population level, moving the scale of analysis from the individual to the community. Theory and methods to investigate impairment and disability in the past have increased dramatically.[7]

Defining Impairment and Disability

Several terms are fundamentally important to disability studies; however, there is no consensus on their definitions. Impairment and disability are conceptually distinct in some models. The World Health Organization defines impairment as "any loss or abnormality of psychological, physiological, or anatomical structure or function"[8] and impairment is viewed as a biological "fact," and therefore without any social connotations, whether positive or negative. In contrast, disability is "the loss or limitation of opportunity to take part in the normal life of the community on an equal level with others, due to physical or social barriers."[9] There is a lot of room for interpretation when these definitions are used, which is reflected in their use within bioarchaeological and paleopathological literature.

While there is variability in the acceptance of these terms, unless otherwise noted, this paper uses the social model approach. Namely, when the term impairment is used here, it will refer to the loss of function or functional limitation; for example, the inability to fully extend or bend the leg. The term disability on the other hand will be used to refer to a cultural construct, in which the impairment restricts the ability to participate fully in the life of a community in the manner considered culturally appropriate. Disability and impairment should not be universalized, and cross-culturally these terms have varied definitions and experiences. However, methods for considering impairment and disability can provide outlines for the investigation of these topics. Disability studies of past populations are influenced by modern, and often Western, perspectives of disability, which often emphasize the relative degree of need, health care provisioning, and dependency.[10] The perspective of an impairment as a disability is culture-specific and can be related to the prevalence of the impairment within a community. Conversely, an impairment that is especially rare might also not be viewed as a disability, rather as an example of divine touch, or special ability. In ancient Egypt, dwarf women were associated with midwifery due to the association of fertility and pregnancy with the venerated dwarf god Bes.[11]

Bioarchaeology of Care

Since its introduction, an increasing number of publications have utilized the bioarchaeology of care approach. Tilley and Schrenk bring together a number of case studies that use the bioarchaeology of care approach and are emblematic of the diversity of cases possible in the bioarchaeological literature, including those from Precontact Southwest United States, Medieval Poland, Prehistoric Peru, and Bronze Age United Arab Emirates.[12] Additionally, a number of other publications utilize the bioarchaeology of care methodology to investigate health-related caregiving from a wide geographic and temporal range, including nineteenth-century Kentucky,[13] Late Intermediate period Peru,[14] Neolithic China,[15] and in Neanderthals[16] and focusing on a variety of topics such as traumatic injuries,[17] analysis of hair and soft tissue,[18] and pathophysiology.[19] However, the majority of publications using the bioarchaeology of care approach focus on individuals with physically severe impairments. In comparison, there are relatively few case studies of individuals with more minor functionally limiting impairments.

Limitations to Finding Disability in the Past

There are several limitations to the investigation of disability in the past, especially when considering archaeological populations. The visibility of impairment can have a profound impact on how individuals are perceived in their community, and there are many non-visible conditions that do not leave skeletal marks but can still impact daily life.[20] In addition, many diseases do not exhibit visible external manifestations and therefore may not be perceived as impairments or disabilities by a given society. Less visible conditions, or conditions that do not have skeletal manifestations, are rarely considered as an impairment or disability within paleopathology, despite the potential for these conditions to impact how individuals are perceived within their community and an individual's ability to participate in daily activities. All individuals will experience periods when health-related care might be necessary, such as during infancy, the hours/days surrounding childbirth, instances of acute illnesses or injury, and so on. Disability and ability are fluid and relate to a society's or community's ideas of "normalcy."[21] Assessing disability in the past stems from assumptions of what constitutes a disabling condition, without critical exploration of the assumptions underlying these conclusions. Minor bone damage can cause extreme pain, while other physical impairments might not impact an individual's ability to function on a day-to-day basis.

Impairment and Disability in the Ancient Nile Valley

The individual who is the focus of this study was excavated from an Egyptian cemetery in Nubia and was buried in an Egyptian-style tomb. However, given the context of the site, it is possible this individual could be a local Nubian who was buried using Egyptian traditions. Very few resources are available for documenting concepts of impairment, disability, or dwarfism in ancient Nubia. Thus, we rely on ancient Egyptian sources to contextualize this case study. There are investigations into impairment and disability in ancient Egyptian contexts on a general level, as well as more specifically within paleopathology and bioarchaeology.[22] Additionally, several case studies explore specific conditions, including dwarfism, and relate these conditions to impairment and disability in ancient Egypt.[23] There are a variety of sources from which researchers can investigate themes of impairment and disability in ancient Egypt, including skeletal remains,[24] mummified remains,[25] artistic depictions,[26] and texts.[27] Many publications considering disability in ancient Egypt include discussions of dwarfism, and if a specific type of dwarfism is discussed, it generally is attributed as achondroplasia. However, individuals with other types of disproportionate dwarfism are found in the ancient Nile Valley[28] and identification of a specific type of dwarfism from artistic depictions or texts is problematic. It is likely that some cases that have been identified solely as achondroplasia may represent different types of dwarfism or combined skeletal dysplasia, as has been identified in other revisited cases.[29]

Dwarf people are documented in all parts of Egyptian society, from personal attendants, to jewelers, to entertainers, to high-ranking officials in the Egyptian hierarchy. Three words have been identified as relating to individuals with short stature (*dng*, *nmw*, and *ḥw*ʿ) and are often associated with determinatives of dwarf people.[30] While many of the documented high-ranking dwarf people lived during the Old Kingdom (*c.* 2600–2150 BCE), evidence of the importance of dwarf people are found throughout ancient Egyptian history. Perhaps one of the most well-known examples is Seneb and his family from the 4th Dynasty.[31] Seneb and his family are depicted in a statue that was excavated in the 1920s at the Giza necropolis. The statue of Seneb shows him in the seated position of a scribe with his wife and two children (Figure 12.1). Seneb appears to have disproportionate

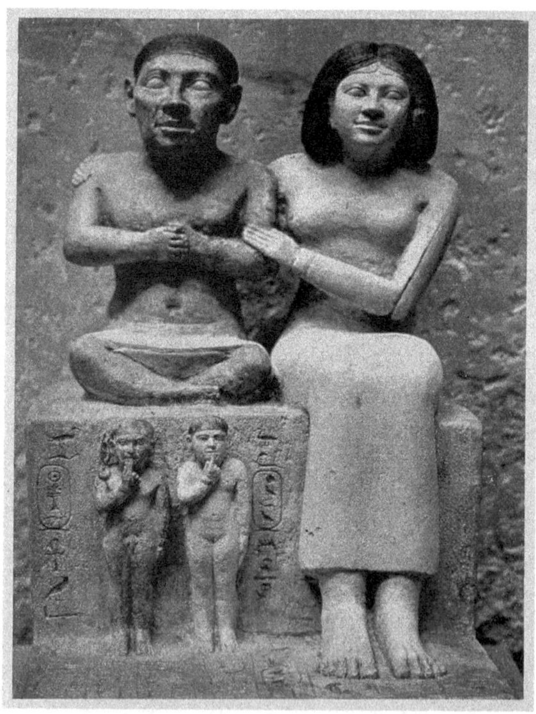

Figure 12.1 Seneb, a dwarf person with his family. Reproduction, 1934, of a photograph of a statue. © Wellcome Collection.

dwarfism. Another example is the statue of Perniankhu who was approximately 40 years old at death and had a form of disproportionate dwarfism.[32] The statue of this individual mimics the skeletal remains found in association with the statue, both in terms of proportions and measurements. Perniankhu also lived during the Old Kingdom and was a court official during the 5th or 6th Dynasty. The statue includes the inscription "the King's acquaintance, (the dwarf) of the Great Palace, *Pr-n(j)-'nḫ(w)*."[33] However, some translations of the description include references to "the dancing dwarf," which may reference Perniankhu's role in society as an entertainer with important status.[34] Djeho lived during the 30th Dynasty and his sarcophagus includes a life-sized side profile/figure of Djeho and displays the characteristics associated with disproportionate dwarfism.[35] There are several other cases of individuals who did not hold high ranking positions, such as the female worker found with fetal bones from an Old Kingdom cemetery near the pyramids at Giza[36] and an adult female with proportionate dwarfism from the Third Intermediate period cemetery in the Dakhleh Oasis, Egypt.[37] Medical papyri do not reference dwarfism specifically, perhaps because ancient Egyptians did not view it as a medical condition.[38]

In the New Kingdom, magical spells invoke the protection and assistance of both dwarf people and dwarf gods against a myriad of dangers, including snakes and fire.[39] For example, "O you dwarf of heaven! You whose face is big, whose back is long, and whose legs are short" is part of a New Kingdom magical spell beseeching the intervention of a divine dwarf.[40] New Kingdom wisdom texts also reference dwarf people and indicate a level of tolerance for impaired individuals, including dwarf people. For example, the *Instruction of Amenemope* advises its readers,

> Do not laugh at a blind man, Nor tease a dwarf, Nor cause hardship for the lame. Don't tease a man who is in the hand of the god [meaning one who is ill or insane], Nor be angry with him for his failings.[41]

The examples of New Kingdom magical spell and the passage from the *Instructions of Amenemope* suggest very different social implications for dwarf people in ancient Egypt. However, both demonstrate that dwarf people were marked as "different" in some way.

There are several ancient Egyptian gods who are depicted with dwarfism, although the best known are probably Bes and Ptah. Bes was a popular god in ancient Egypt, especially during the New Kingdom[42] as well as in Nubia during this period.[43] Bes is often depicted with a combination of animal and human features and is presented with a form of disproportionate dwarfism and is often displayed in objects including amulets and figurines, such as these examples from Tombos (Figure 12.2). Bes is also found in reliefs and paintings associated with childbirth in the New Kingdom.[44] Furthermore, papyri from the New Kingdom describe magical spells for protection during birth, appealing to dwarf people, probably Bes, for their assistance.[45] Ptah is associated with regeneration and rejuvenation and is sometimes depicted with disproportionate dwarfism, frequently so in amulets

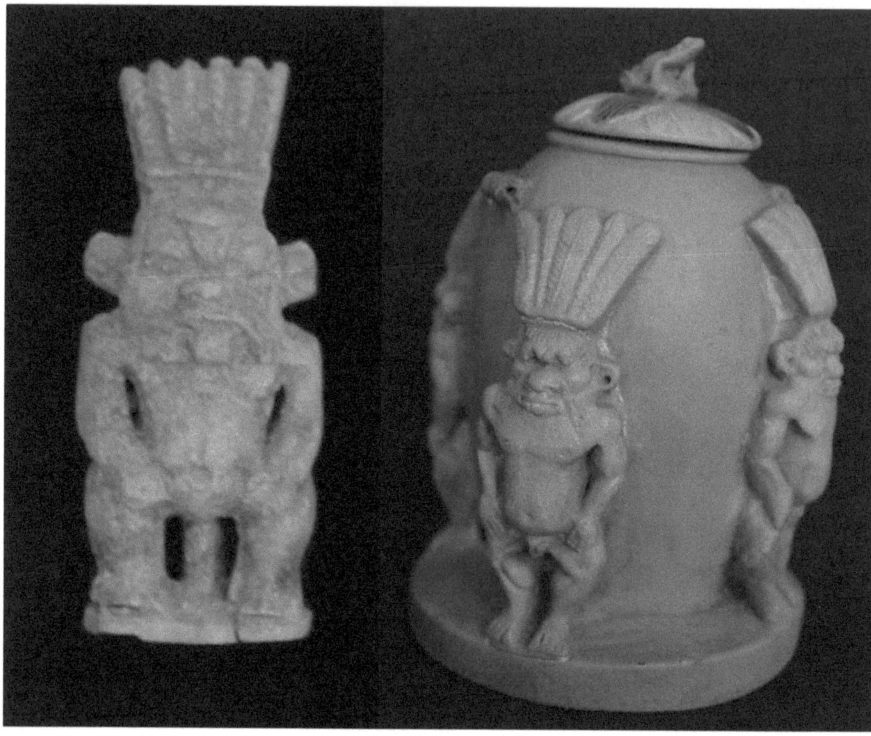

Figure 12.2 Amulet of Bes from Tombos (left); figure of Bes is shown in a crouched position with a fine detailed feathered headdress. Four figures of Bes on a faience cosmetic vessel from Tombos (right). Image by M. Buzon.

during the New Kingdom.[46] Ptah is the patron god of craftspeople and was particularly revered at Deir el-Medina, the New Kingdom village associated with the building of the tombs in the Valley of the Kings[47] and dwarf people in ancient Egypt were associated with certain crafts. Dwarf people are shown making jewelry in tomb scenes from the tomb of Mereruka (vizier to the Pharaoh Titi of the 6th Dynasty) and are also associated with nursing and midwifery, perhaps due to the close association with Bes and Ptah with these professions.[48]

Materials and Methods

The focus of this study is the individual referred to in this chapter as U36.Sh2.B10, an older adult female who exhibits a form of disproportionate dwarfism, most likely LWD. This individual was excavated during the 2017 field season of the Tombos Archaeological Project (Directors: Drs. Stuart Tyson Smith and Michele R. Buzon). The skeletal remains from this project are housed at the Purdue University Bioarchaeology Laboratory. A complete differential diagnosis and description for U36.Sh2.B10, including photographs, can be found in

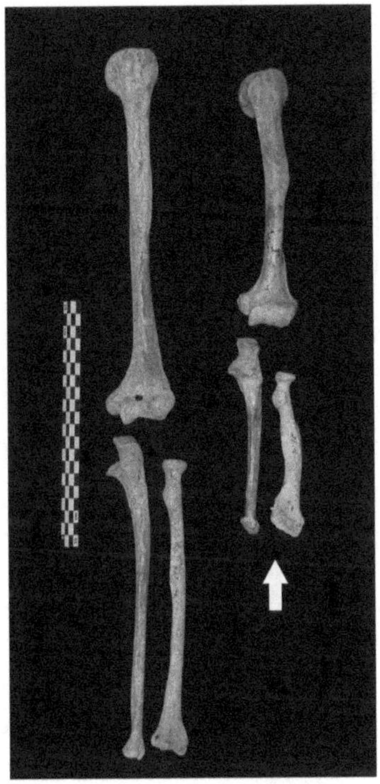

Figure 12.3 U36.Sh2.B10's upper limb (right, with arrow pointing) compared to the upper limb of a New Kingdom female of average stature (based on femur length) from Tombos (left). Image by K. M. Whitmore.

Whitmore and Buzon (2019).[49] Briefly, U36.Sh2.B10 exhibits several characteristics associated with LWD including short stature, mesomelia (relative shortening of the middle elements: radii, ulnae, tibiae, and fibulae), and characteristics of the arm and wrist known as Madelung's deformity, which result in abnormalities including the deformation of the distal radius (including angulation of the articular surface) and a shortened and thickened styloid processes of the ulnae and radii (Figure 12.3).

Bioarchaeology of Care Approach and the Index of Care

The bioarchaeology of care approach[50] and the Index of Care[51] are used here to understand the possible health-care provisioning to support U36.Sh2.B10 in the Tombos community. Tilley and colleagues use the terms "health-related care," "care," "caregiving," and "care provision" interchangeably. These terms are defined as "the delivery of assistance to an individual experiencing short, medium, or long-term disability as an outcome of pathology."[52] Health-related caregiving is loosely divided into "direct support" that relates to activities such as provisioning, hygiene maintenance, nursing, and physical therapy, and "accommodation," which is related to activities in which strategies are adopted to enable or facilitate participation in cultural, social, and/or economic activities. The bioarchaeology of care methodology comprises four distinct stages of analysis, each building on the observations and conclusions of the previous stages, with the goal of achieving the most comprehensive understanding of the individual's experience of impairment and/or disability and health-related care. Researchers can use different portions of the model depending on the types of evidence and resources available. Data gathering and interpretation protocols corresponding to each stage of the bioarchaeology of care analysis were developed into the Index of Care, with the goal of achieving consistency in data collection and analytical approach across studies into past health-related caregiving.[53]

U36.SH2.B10 and the Bioarchaeology of Care Approach

Index Step 1: Document, Describe, and Diagnose

Lifeways Context

U36.Sh2.B10 was excavated within a New Kingdom structure in the cemetery at Tombos. Tombos' location on the Nile River at the Third Cataract is important, because it lies on the border of direct and indirect Egyptian control during this period. Given recent findings within the Tombos settlement, it is likely that Tombos is the fortress of Taroy.[54] Regardless of whether Tombos is Taroy, the site's location at the Third Cataract would have been important in controlling the movement of people and goods along the Nile. Tombos was an Egyptian administrative center that facilitated the tribute to Egypt from Upper Nubia, with documented evidence of a high-level administrator, Siamun, "Scribe Reckoner of the Gold of Kush." As such, individuals at Tombos were connected to an Egyptian network to the north and a Nubian network to the south.[55] The area surrounding Tombos includes sandy terrain, with small steep areas around the Nile embankment. Next to the cemetery are rocky outcrops, which in later periods were mined and used, such as for a large statue of an unnamed ruler, perhaps Taharko (25th Dynasty).[56]

Even with differences between mortuary treatments, previous studies suggest that the individuals living in New Kingdom Tombos were relatively healthy, had low incidences of traumatic injury, and were not participating in strenuous labor.[57] Most individuals do have evidence of oral health issues, especially dental attrition, which can likely be attributed to the sand and grit from quern stones that would have been present in bread.[58]

Mortuary Treatment

There is evidence for socioeconomic differentiation in the Tombos cemetery. Some Egyptian-style structures in the cemetery are more modest underground burial chambers, while other structures in the cemetery consist of pyramid and chapel complexes that may have included elite individuals, family, and household members. In addition, the cemetery has Nubian-style tumuli, circular mounds with underground shafts and side niches. Most individuals in the cemetery in structures from the New Kingdom are buried using typical Egyptian practices, including the use of coffins, body position, orientation of the body, and inclusion of artifacts with burials. However, these standardized Egyptian mortuary practices found in most of the adult burials do not extend to the youngest members of the Tombos community, and burials of individuals under approximately four to five years of age demonstrate variability in the position and orientation of the remains. There are a few exceptions to these trends, which may be related to factors other than age. One four- to six-year-old individual (U36.Sh2.B5) was interred flexed, on the left side, inside of a basket and associated with a ceramic vessel. However, this individual was much smaller than other four- to six-year-old individuals at Tombos as a result of a type of skeletal dysplasia, possibly LWD.[59] Despite the near ubiquitous use of Egyptian mortuary traditions, there is some variability in mortuary treatment. Some individuals are buried with numerous and expensive grave goods, ceramics, and offerings, while other individuals have few or no grave goods. Many individuals are buried supine and extended with head to the west, following Egyptian standards. However, there is variability in the use of burial furniture such as reed mats, wooden coffins, and ceramic coffins. Nubian-style beds are also found in some graves, sometimes in association with Egyptian-style burial furniture; other graves have no trace of burial furniture. U36.Sh2.B10 is buried in a manner similar to other individuals from this period at Tombos. U36.Sh2.B10 is interred in a chapel tomb in an extended and supine position with the head to the east. While many adult individuals at Tombos are buried with their head oriented to the west, the majority of individuals in the same structure as U36.Sh2.B10 are buried with their head to the east. U36.Sh2.B10 was found with a green glazed steatite scarab on the right hand with an inscription of Amun Re.

U36.Sh2.B10 Description

U36.Sh2.B10 is estimated to be female and approximately 50+ years of age at death. The majority of U36.Sh2.B10's postcrania were consolidated *in situ* by an archaeological conservator and recovered; the skull, however, was extremely fragmented and could not be reconstructed.

U36.Sh2.B10 has an estimated stature of ~130 cm when the stature regression formula developed by Raxter and colleagues[60] for ancient Egyptians is used. However, given the difficulty in estimating stature in individuals with disproportionate dwarfism, U36.Sh2.B10's skeletal elements were compared to the elements of other New Kingdom-period females in Whitmore and Buzon.[61] To summarize, U36.Sh2.B10 displays a reduction in length for all recorded long bones, with standard z-scores ranging from -6.38 to -4.34 (note, measurements for the fibulae were not available from the reference population). A mesomelic pattern of dysplasia (in which the middle elements of a limb, i.e. the ulnae, radii, tibiae, and fibulae, are more shortened compared to the proximal and distal elements) is observed in U36.

Sh2.B10, with the greatest reductions in maximum length as compared to the reference population being found in the radii and ulnae.

In addition to the shortened limb bones, U36.Sh2.B10 displays additional bilateral changes to the forearm, including characteristics associated with Madelung's deformity and decreased carrying angle of the elbow. U36.Sh2.B10's forearm extension would have been limited to approximately 130 to 135 degrees and is a result of constrained humero-ulnar articulation. Specifically, the distal radius is malformed in both the coronal and sagittal planes, which increases radial inclination/volar tilt.[62] Individuals with Madelung's deformity, including U36.Sh2.B10, have shortened and thickened styloid processes of the ulna and radius and increased radial angulation of the distal radial articular surface of the ulna.[63]

U36.Sh2.B10 Diagnosis

A differential diagnosis of U36.Sh2.B10 was conducted; however, the full suite of characteristics associated with different skeletal dysplasias could not be analyzed given the extremely fragmented nature of U36.Sh2.B10's skull.[64] However, the most likely diagnosis is LWD, a form of mesomelic dwarfism associated with haploinsufficiency of the short stature homeobox-containing gene (*SHOX*).[65]

Index of Care Step 2: Determine Disability

Clinical Impacts

The symptoms, and the severity of the symptoms, of LWD can vary widely between individuals, even those within the same family. However, females tend to have more severe symptoms as compared to males.[66]

Compromised mobility: there is a potential for compromised mobility due to short stature and shortened lower limb lengths, which may impact gait. This can lead to early-onset osteoarthritis, although osteoarthritis is not apparent in U36.Sh2.B10, who has few indicators of degenerative joint disease in the spine (minimal osteophytic growth on six vertebral bodies) and few indications of osteoarthritis (minimal lipping and minimal porosity in the upper body) of the limb joints. Short stature and differences in gait may have impacted U36.Sh2.B10's ability to move throughout the landscape, especially in the rocky and sandy terrain surrounding the settlement and the steep inclines around the Nile River.

Restricted forearm and hand use (wrist): characteristics of the upper limbs include incomplete elbow extension to approximately 130–35 degrees. This is a common complication for individuals with LWD. However, the restriction of elbow extension may not fully develop until late childhood or adolescence.[67] The restricted forearm extension may have impacted U36.Sh2.B10's ability to participate fully in certain activities. Madelung's deformity was originally described in 1878 as a painful malformation of the wrist and forearm that begins in adolescence.[68] However, in modern clinical settings not all individuals with Madelung's deformity report discomfort or pain, and those that do, report variability in the severity of these symptoms.[69] Individuals with Madelung's deformity and incomplete elbow extension may also be unable to fully pronate or supinate their arms (rotate their palms face down or face up). These types of conditions are also associated with degeneration, stiffness, tenderness, and pain at the elbow joint.[70] However, as discussed earlier, U36.Sh2.B10 has limited indications of osteoarthritis throughout the body. Individuals with Madelung's deformity can display limited range of motion or pain, but more commonly exhibit a loss or decrease in wrist extension. Often pain is a result of the dorsal displacement of the ulna and radiocarpal pain often occurs when the wrist is forcibly extended, such as during upper limb weight-bearing activities.[71] Malformations of the wrist associated with Madelung's deformity generally become more apparent around puberty and in some cases can be visually observed.[72] However, in clinical settings many patients are unaware of the abnormal radius or the volar subluxation of the hand and wrist.[73] Mesomelia is often not noticed until children reach school age and may increase in severity as individuals age.[74] The spectrum of *SHOX* deficiencies is highly variable in phenotype, and because the main characteristics of mesomelia disproportions and Madelung's deformity develop over time and may not appear until the second decade of life, these characteristics may go unnoticed during early ages. In children under six, short stature might be the only visible characteristic of LWD and the limb disproportions may be less pronounced.[75]

The symptoms of LWD tend to be more severe in females as compared to males, so it is possible that U36.Sh2.B10 may have experienced some of the more significant symptoms associated with LWD. Characteristics associated with LWD, such as mesomelic shortening of the limbs and Madelung's deformity, were likely not immediately visible during the earliest years of life but would have become more apparent as U36.Sh2.B10 aged, starting around the second decade of life/puberty. Short stature would have been apparent in U36.Sh2.B10 beginning in early life.

Functional Impacts

Intellectual impairment is not associated with LWD and U36.Sh2.B10 would likely not have faced any developmental delays as a result of this condition.[76] In clinical settings, LWD is often not identified until later childhood or puberty, and it is possible that members of U36.Sh2.B10's community would have only noted U36.Sh2.B10's short stature in infancy and early childhood. However, during the second decade of life when the physical manifestations of LWD, such as Madelung's deformity and mesomelia, would have increased in observability and symptom severity, these characteristics would have become more visible to U36.Sh2.B10 and other members of the community.

It is possible that U36.Sh2.B10 experienced increased difficulty with mobility due to short stature and the sandy and rocky terrain around Tombos. However, given that Tombos was an administrative town, and possibly a fortress, day-to-day mobility within the town would have likely been easier than the surrounding countryside. U36.Sh2.B10 does not display indications of osteoarthritis except for minimal lipping and porosity in the joints of the upper limbs or indications of degenerative joint disease of the spine, except for minimal osteophytic growth on approximately 25% of the vertebrae, which is not uncommon for older adults at Tombos. In fact, U36.Sh2.B10 is similar to other older adults at Tombos in that U36.Sh2.B10 displays few indications of osteoarthritis.[77] Long-distance travel may have been more difficult for U36.Sh2.B10. However, overall U36.Sh2.B10's mobility would not have been severely limited.

Elbow and wrist limitations may have impacted U36.Sh2.B10's ability to participate fully in all activities without difficulty, discomfort, and/or pain. Using the upper arm to lift the weight of the body from a lying or standing position, pushing a heavy object using the hands/wrists, and other activities requiring full extension of the elbow, extension of the wrist, or supination or pronation of the hands would have been more difficult. While individuals with LWD may have a reduction in upper arm mobility, activities can be easily modified to remove potential discomfort. For example, if an individual is pushing a heavy object with the hand/wrist, another part of the body, such as the shoulder, could be used instead as the point of contact. Other activities, such as those associated with agriculture, may have been more difficult for U36.Sh2.B10. However, there is little evidence that the individuals buried in the Tombos cemetery were participating in physically strenuous labor during the New Kingdom.[78] Individuals with Madelung's deformity may not be able to fully supinate or pronate their hand/wrist, which may limit object manipulation. Again, activities requiring these movements can be easily adapted for individuals experiencing a decrease in movement, discomfort, or pain. Movement and dexterity of the hand are not generally impacted in individuals with Madelung's deformity and U36.Sh2.B10 could have engaged in activities requiring finger and hand dexterity such as craftwork. U36.Sh2.B10's participation in some activities at Tombos might have been hindered or required modification, but were not necessarily prevented.

Estimating the Need for Health Care Provisioning

There is no skeletal evidence that U36.Sh2.B10 required daily direct care as an adult. During early childhood, U36.Sh2.B10 might not have been perceived as being different outside her short stature, since mesomelia and Madelung's deformity are often not visibly identified until adolescence/puberty. Individuals providing care to U36.Sh2.B10 during the younger years likely would not have required additional effort, outside the limitations related to short stature. As U36.Sh2.B10 entered later adolescence and adulthood, differences would have become more noticeable. U36.Sh2.B10 would have been much shorter than peers and the mesomelic pattern of the limbs would have become more noticeable in appearance. Around the same time, characteristics of LWD in the upper limbs would have become more pronounced, including the decreased carrying angle of the elbow, visible malformation of the wrist, difficulty with wrist extension, and the inability to fully supinate or pronate the wrists and hands. These symptoms might be accompanied with other symptoms associated with LWD including joint stiffness in the wrist and elbow and pain at the radioulnarcarpal joint. However, the physical limitations associated with LWD would likely have been relatively mild. Potential physical issues could be overcome through simple modifications by U36.Sh2.B10. Wrist pain may have impacted U36.Sh2.B10's living experience. However, it is impossible to understand the degree of pain or stiffness that U36.Sh2.B10 would have experienced from skeletal remains alone; even within modern clinical settings, patients report differing pain levels.

It is likely that individuals at Tombos regarded U36.Sh2.B10 with special consideration. Dwarf people are known throughout Egypt from skeletal remains, artistic depictions, historical documentation, and religious iconographies, such as those related to the gods Ptah and Bes. If U36.Sh2.B10 were restricted from participating in certain activities with ease, like agriculture-related activities, then other professions, such as craft work or midwifery, may have been considered more appropriate due to the association of these professions with dwarf gods. There is nothing in U36.Sh2.B10's burial context that indicates that U36.Sh2.B10 was viewed differently, whether positively or negatively. In fact, U36.Sh2.B10's interment follows a similar pattern found throughout the New Kingdom-period Tombos cemetery. The only difference in U36.Sh2.B10's mortuary treatment was the direction of the body. However, the majority of the individuals buried in the same structure as U36.Sh2.B10 are buried in this orientation and variation in body orientation is observed in the Tombos cemetery. This supports other research concluding that dwarfism may have been considered a difference and possibly an impairment, but likely was not considered a disability by ancient Egyptians, according to the model used in this chapter.[79]

The bioarchaeology of care approach was previously used to examine an individual with a form of skeletal dysplasia. Romito 2 is an individual with acromesomelic dysplasia and the discussion about the case of Romito 2[80] and subsequent reevaluations of the case, including through the lens of the bioarchaeology of care approach,[81] provides a useful comparison to U36.Sh2.B10. Differences between the cases of Romito 2 and U36.Sh2.B10 highlight the importance of considering the historical, environmental, economic, and cultural contexts in conjunction with clinical information when utilizing this approach and avoiding broad interpretations related to specific conditions or specific impairments. Both individuals likely had a mesomelic condition falling on the *SHOX* spectrum, Romito 2 with acromesomelic dysplasia (possibly Maroteaux type) and U36.Sh2.B10 with LWD. Romito 2 and U36.Sh2.B10 would have shared some similar clinical characteristics including short stature, mesomelia, and possibly Madelung's deformity.[82] However, the functional impacts on daily life and potential healthcare provisioning would have likely differed. Romito 2 (estimated to be 17 to 20 years old at death) lived in a hunter-gatherer community in southern Italy. This area is mountainous, and the site is surrounded by heavily forested terrain. Archaeological evidence suggests that the economic and cultural activities of Romito 2's community were quite different from U36.Sh2.B10's community and included the reliance on medium to large herbivores. Tilley evaluated Romito 2 from a bioarchaeology of care perspective and concluded that Romito 2 would "*not* have conformed to the normative role demands of his community – demands dictated by the realities of an active, mobile, periodically-stressed, subsistence lifestyle"[83] and would have likely received care in the form of accommodation. It seems unlikely that U36.Sh2.B10 required much health care provisioning in the form of accommodation and little to none in the form of direct support, emphasizing the importance of cultural context in interpretation. Analysis of U36.Sh2.B10's skeletal remains and mortuary treatment using a bioarchaeology of care approach indicates that LWD might have constituted an impairment or have been considered a difference, but would likely have not been perceived as a disability at Tombos during the New Kingdom. In death, U36.Sh2.B10 was treated in a similar manner as other individuals who were buried at the Tombos cemetery. Additionally, U36.Sh2.B10 was perhaps not the only individual with LWD who was buried at Tombos. A juvenile individual possibly had the same condition and was interred in the same pyramid and chapel complex as U36.Sh2.B10.[84] An important aspect of considering impairment and disability in the past is the specific consideration of the participation and agency of the individual in their own health care provisioning. The bioarchaeology of care model is well suited to consider these topics when incorporating the clinical and functional impacts to estimate the need for healthcare provisioning. However, there are limitations in the skeletal and archaeological record, where observations of the manifestations of human agency may be limited or absent.

Conclusion

Many of the published cases utilizing the bioarchaeology of care methodology have focused on cases of impairment in which the condition was at times severely limiting. The case of U36.Sh2.B10 demonstrates the utility of the bioarchaeology of care methodology in contexts in which the condition is less severely physically limiting by providing a thorough model to investigate how an individual would have physically and socially engaged in the local community.

The bioarchaeology of care method and the Index of Care provide useful groundwork for investigating health care provisioning in the past. However, caution should be utilized when using this method, especially in cases in which the community environment is unsure or unknown. Additionally, the manifestations of human agency might be absent in the archaeological or skeletal record. For example, analysis of textual documentation, art, etc. indicates that generally dwarfism was not perceived with disfavor by ancient Egyptians. However, that does not necessarily suggest that the members of U36.Sh2.B10's community or immediate family held this individual in high or low regard, with compassion, with hostility, and so on. These critical aspects of an individual's life experience are unfortunately, often absent in the bioarchaeological record.

Skeletal manifestations of conditions do not always correlate directly with the experience of symptoms. However, the bioarchaeology of care approach provides a useful model for the consideration of impairments in the past, including those that were not severely physically limiting. Additionally, the approach highlights the importance of considering the historical, cultural, social, environmental, and economic contexts of cases, by emphasizing that even individuals with overlapping clinical symptoms, like Romito 2 and U36.Sh2.B10, may experience very different impacts to daily life. The paleopathological, archaeological, textual, artistic, clinical, and skeletal data provide the opportunity to integrate multiple lines of evidence, allowing for more nuanced interpretations. While U36.Sh2.B10 was likely viewed as different, the combination of archaeological, artistic, textual, clinical, and skeletal data under the bioarchaeology of care approach suggests that dwarfism, including LWD, was not perceived as a disability in ancient Egypt and Nubia.

Notes

1 Buzon, Smith, and Simonetti (2016).
2 Buzon, Smith, and Simonetti (2016).
3 Tilley (2015a), Tilley and Cameron (2014), Tilley and Schrenk (2018).
4 e.g., Dettwyler (1991), Frayer et al. (1987), Frayer, Macchiarelli, and Mussi (1988), Hawkey (1998).
5 Byrnes and Muller (2018), Tilley (2015a).
6 Bohling, Croucher, and Buckberry (2022).
7 e.g., Byrnes and Muller (2018), Powell, Southwell-Wright, and Gowland (2017), Tilley (2015a), Tilley and Schrenk (2018).
8 WHO (1980, 47).
9 Roberts (1999, 83).
10 Zakrzewski (2014).
11 Kozma (2006), Kozma (2010).
12 Tilley and Schrenk (2018).
13 Worne (2017).
14 Palma Málaga and Makowski (2019).
15 Halcrow et al. (2020).
16 Spikins et al. (2018).
17 Dittmar et al. (2023), McKenzie, Murphy, and Watt (2022).
18 Brown and Wilson (2019).
19 Beckett and Conlogue (2019).
20 Zakrzewski (2014).
21 Zakrzewski (2017).
22 e.g., Jeffreys and Tait (2013), Zakrzewski (2014), Zakrezewski (2017).
23 e.g., Kozma (2006), Kozma (2008), Kozma (2010), Kozma et al. (2011), Molto and Kirkpatrick (2018).
24 Kozma et al. (2011).
25 Nerlich et al. (2010).
26 Dasen (1993), Hawass (1991), Kozma (2008), Kozma (2010).
27 Baines (1992), Dasen (1993).
28 e.g., Whitmore and Buzon (2019).
29 Cormier, Buikstra, and Osterholtz (2017).
30 Dasen (1993).
31 Kozma (2006).
32 Kozma (2006).
33 Hawass (1991, 158).
34 Kozma (2006), Hawass (1991).
35 Baines (1992), Dasen (1993).
36 Kozma et al. (2011).
37 Molto and Kirkpatrick (2018).
38 Kozma (2006).
39 Dasen (1988).

40 Dasen (1988, 258).
41 Lichtheim (1984, 165).
42 Dasen (1993).
43 Budka (2018).
44 Dasen (1993).
45 Kozma (2008).
46 Dasen (1988), Dasen (1993).
47 Kozma (2006).
48 Kozma (2006).
49 Whitmore and Buzon (2019).
50 Tilley (2015a).
51 Tilley (2015a), Tilley and Cameron (2014).
52 Tilley (2015a, 3).
53 Tilley (2015a), Tilley and Cameron (2014).
54 Smith and Buzon (2018).
55 Smith and Buzon (2018), Smith (2003).
56 Schrader and Buzon (2017).
57 Buzon (2006), Buzon and Richman (2007), Schrader and Buzon (2017).
58 Buzon and Bombak (2009).
59 Whitmore and Buzon (2019).
60 Raxter et al. (2008).
61 Whitmore and Buzon (2019).
62 Whitmore and Buzon (2019).
63 Kozin and Zlotolow (2015).
64 Whitmore and Buzon (2019).
65 Binder (2011), Bunyan et al. (2015), Ross et al. (2005).
66 Ross et al. (2005).
67 Olney (2012).
68 Felman and Kirkpatrick (1969).
69 Al Kaissi et al. (2016).
70 Olney (2012).
71 Kozin and Zlotolow (2015).
72 Heath (2020).
73 Kozin and Zlotolow (2015).
74 Heath (2020).
75 Binder (2011).
76 Heath (2020).
77 Schrader (2012), Schrader (2013).
78 Schrader (2012), Schrader (2013).
79 Dasen (1993), Kozma et al. (2011), Sullivan (2001), Zakrzewski (2014), Zakrzewski (2017).
80 Frayer et al. (1987), Frayer, Macchiarelli, and Mussi (1988).
81 Bower (2002), Dettwyler (1991), Tilley (2015b).
82 see Cummings and Rega (2008).
83 Tilley (2015b, 70).
84 Whitmore and Buzon (2019).

Bibliography

Al Kaissi, Ali, Maher Ben Ghachem, Farid Ben Chehida, Jochen G. Hofstaetter, Franz Grill, Rudolf Ganger, and Susanne Gerit Kircher. “Can Multiple Hereditary Exostoses Overlap with Mesomelic Dysplasia?” *Journal of Clinical Medicine Research* 8, no. 8 (2016): 605–9. https://doi.org/10.14740/jocmr2593w.

Baines, John. "Merit by Proxy: The Biographies of the Dwarf Djeho and His Patron Tjaiharpta." *The Journal of Egyptian Archaeology* 78 (1992): 241. https://doi.org/10.2307/3822075.

Beckett, Ronald G., and Gerald J. Conlogue. "The Importance of Pathophysiology to the Understanding of Functional Limitations in the Bioarchaeology of Care Approach." *International Journal of Paleopathology* 25 (2019): 118–28. https://doi.org/10.1016/j.ijpp.2018.06.006.

Binder, Gerhard. "Short Stature Due to SHOX Deficiency: Genotype, Phenotype, and Therapy." *Hormone Research in Paediatrics* 75, no. 2 (2011): 81–89. https://doi.org/10.1159/000324105.

Bohling, Solange, Karina Croucher, and Jo Buckberry. "The Bioarchaeology of Disability: A Population-Scale Approach to Investigating Disability, Physical Impairment, and Care in Archaeological Communities." *International Journal of Paleopathology* 38 (2022): 76–94. https://doi.org/10.1016/j.ijpp.2022.05.006.

Bower, Bruce. "Care-Worn Fossils." *Science News* 162, no. 21 (2002): 328. https://doi.org/10.2307/4013860.

Brown, Emma L., and Andrew S. Wilson. "Using Evidence from Hair and Other Soft Tissues to Infer the Need for and Receipt of Health-Related Care Provision." *International Journal of Paleopathology* 25 (2019): 91–98. https://doi.org/10.1016/j.ijpp.2018.08.008.

Budka, Julia. "Addressing the Gods Home Away from Home: Case Studies from New Kingdom Nubia." In *Across the Mediterranean – Along the Nile. Studies in Egyptology, Nubiology and Late Antiquity Dedicated to László Török on the Occasion of His 75th Birthday*, edited by Tamás A. Bács, Adám Bollók, and Tivadar Vida. Budapest: Institute of Archaeology, Research Centre for the Humanities, and Hungarian Academy of Sciences and Museum of Fine Arts, 2018.

Bunyan, David J., Maria Baffico, Lucia Capone, Silvia Vannelli, Lorenzo Iughetti, Sébastien Schmitt, Emma-Jane Taylor, Adam Herridge, Deborah Shears, Antonino Forabosco, and Domenico Coviello. "Duplications Upstream and Downstream of *Shox* Identified as Novel Causes of Leri-Weill Dyschondrosteosis or Idiopathic Short Stature." *American Journal of Medical Genetics Part A* 170, no. 4 (2015): 949–57. https://doi.org/10.1002/ajmg.a.37524.

Buzon, Michele R. "Health of the Non-Elites at Tombos: Nutritional and Disease Stress in New Kingdom Nubia." *American Journal of Physical Anthropology* 130, no. 1 (2006): 26–37. https://doi.org/10.1002/ajpa.20303.

Buzon, Michele R., and A. Bombak. "Dental Disease in the Nile Valley during the New Kingdom." *International Journal of Osteoarchaeology* 20, no. 4 (2009): 371–87. https://doi.org/10.1002/oa.1054.

Buzon, Michele R., and Rebecca Richman. "Traumatic Injuries and Imperialism: The Effects of Egyptian Colonial Strategies at Tombos in Upper Nubia." *American Journal of Physical Anthropology* 133, no. 2 (2007): 783–91. https://doi.org/10.1002/ajpa.20585.

Buzon, Michele R., Stuart Tyson Smith, and Antonio Simonetti. "Entanglement and the Formation of the Ancient Nubian Napatan State." *American Anthropologist* 118, no. 2 (2016): 284–300. https://doi.org/10.1111/aman.12524.

Byrnes, Jennifer F., and Jennifer Lynn Muller. *Bioarchaeology of Impairment and Disability: Theoretical, Ethnohistorical, and Methodological Perspectives.* Cham, Switzerland: Springer Publishing International, 2018.

Cormier, Aviva A., Jane E. Buikstra, and Anna Osterholtz. "Overlapping Genetic Pathways in the Skeletal Dysplasias of a Middle Woodland Individual: A Case Study." *International Journal of Paleopathology* 18 (2017): 98–107. https://doi.org/10.1016/j.ijpp.2017.06.001.

Cummings, C., and E. Rega. "A Case of Dyschondrosteosis in an Anglo-Saxon Skeleton." *International Journal of Osteoarchaeology* 18, no. 4 (2008): 431–37. https://doi.org/10.1002/oa.948.

Dasen, Véronique. "Dwarfism in Egypt and Classical Antiquity: Iconography and Medical History." *Medical History* 32, no. 3 (1988): 253–76. https://doi.org/10.1017/s0025727300048237.

Dasen, Véronique. *Dwarfs in Ancient Egypt and Greece.* Oxford: Clarendon Press, 1993.

Dettwyler, Katherine A. "Can Paleopathology Provide Evidence for 'Compassion'?" *American Journal of Physical Anthropology* 84, no. 4 (1991): 375–84. https://doi.org/10.1002/ajpa.1330840402.

Dittmar, Jenna M., Bram Mulder, Anna Tran, Piers D. Mitchell, Peter D. Jones, Sarah A. Inskip, Craig Cessford, and John E. Robb. "Caring for the Injured: Exploring the Immediate and Long-Term Consequences of Injury in Medieval Cambridge, England." *International Journal of Paleopathology* 40 (2023): 7–19. https://doi.org/10.1016/j.ijpp.2022.07.004.

Felman, Alvin H., and John A. Kirkpatrick. "Madelung's Deformity: Observations in 17 Patients." *Radiology* 93, no. 5 (1969): 1037–42. https://doi.org/10.1148/93.5.1037.

Frayer, David W., William A. Horton, Roberto Macchiarelli, and Margherita Mussi. "Dwarfism in an Adolescent from the Italian Late Upper Palaeolithic." *Nature* 330, no. 6143 (1987): 60–62. https://doi.org/10.1038/330060a0.

Frayer, David W., Roberto Macchiarelli, and Margherita Mussi. "A Case of Chondrodystrophic Dwarfism in the Italian Late Upper Paleolithic." *American Journal of Physical Anthropology* 75, no. 4 (1988): 549–65. https://doi.org/10.1002/ajpa.1330750412.

Halcrow, Siân E., Melanie J. Miller, Anne Marie Snoddy, Wenquan Fan, and Kate Pechenkina. "Growing Up Different in Neolithic China: A Contextualised Case Study and Differential Diagnosis of a Young Adult with Skeletal Dysplasia." *International Journal of Paleopathology* 28 (2020): 6–19. https://doi.org/10.1016/j.ijpp.2019.11.001.

Hawass, Zahi. "The Statue of the Dwarf Pr-n(j)-'nẖ(w) Recently Discovered at Giza." *Mitteilungen des Deutschen Archäologischen Instituts Abteiling Kairo* 47 (1991): 157–62.

Hawkey, Diane E. "Disability, Compassion and the Skeletal Record: Using Musculoskeletal Stress Markers (MSM) to Construct an Osteobiography from Early New Mexico." *International Journal of Osteoarchaeology* 8, no. 5 (1998): 326–40. https://doi.org/10.1002/(sici)1099-1212(19980 90)8:5<326::aid-oa437>3.0.co;2-w.

Heath, Karen. "Leri-Weill Dyschondrosteosis." *National Organization for Rare Disorders,* Last modified February 18, 2020. https://rarediseases.org/rare-diseases/leri-weilldyschondrosteosis/.

Jeffreys, David, and John Tait. "Disability, Madness, and Social Exclusion in Dynastic Egypt." In *Madness, Disability and Social Exclusion: The Archaeology and Anthropology of 'Difference'*, edited by Jane Hubert, 87–95. London: Taylor and Francis, 2013.

Kozin, Scott H., and Dan A. Zlotolow. "Madelung Deformity." *The Journal of Hand Surgery* 40, no. 10 (2015): 2090–98.

Kozma, Chahira. "Dwarfs in Ancient Egypt." *American Journal of Medical Genetics Part A* 140A, no. 4 (2006): 303–11. https://doi.org/10.1002/ajmg.a.31068.

Kozma, Chahira. "Skeletal Dysplasia in Ancient Egypt." *American Journal of Medical Genetics Part A* 146A, no. 23 (2008): 3104–12. https://doi.org/10.1002/ajmg.a.32501.

Kozma, Chahira. "The Ancient Egyptian Dwarfs of the Walters Art Museum." *American Journal of Medical Genetics Part A* 152A, no. 10 (2010): 2556–62. https://doi.org/10.1002/ajmg.a.33616.

Kozma, Chahira, Azza Mohamed Sarry El Din, Rokia Abd El Shafy El Banna, Wafaa Abd El Samie Kandeel, and Ralph Lachman. "The Ancient Egyptian Dwarfs of the Pyramids: The High Official and the Female Worker." *American Journal of Medical Genetics Part A* 155, no. 8 (2011): 1817–24. https://doi.org/10.1002/ajmg.a.34038.

Lichtheim, Miriam. *Ancient Egyptian Literature: The New Kingdom.* Berkeley: University of California Press, 1984.

McKenzie, Catriona J., Eileen M. Murphy, and Iain Watt. "Considering Care: A Traumatic Obturator Fracture Dislocation of the Hip in a Middle-Aged Man from Gaelic Medieval Ballyhanna, Co. Donegal, Ireland." *International Journal of Paleopathology* 38 (2022): 115–22. https://doi.org/10.1016/j.ijpp.2022.07.003.

Molto, Joseph E., and Casey L. Kirkpatrick. "How Short is Short, and Why? A Probable Case of Proportionate Dwarfism from Egypt's Third Intermediate Period in the Dakhleh

Oasis, Egypt." *International Journal of Osteoarchaeology* 28 (2018):3–17. https://doi.org/10.1002/oa.2625.

Nerlich, Andeas G., Stephanie Panzer, Estelle Hower-Tilmann, and Sandra Lösch. "Paleopathological-Radiological Evidence for Cerebral Palsy in an Ancient Egyptian Female Mummy from a 13th Dynasty Tomb." *BAR International Series* 2141 (2010): 113–16.

Olney, Robert C. "Acromesomelic dysplasia." *National Organization for Rare Disorders,* Last modified May 29, 2012. https://rarediseases.org/rare-diseases/acromesomelic-dysplasia/.

Palma Málaga, Martha R., and Krzysztof Makowski. "Bioarchaeological Evidence of Care Provided to a Physically Disabled Individual from Pachacamac, Peru." *International Journal of Paleopathology* 25 (2019): 139–49. https://doi.org/10.1016/j.ijpp.2018.08.002.

Powell, Lindsay, William Southwell-Wright, and Rebecca Gowland. *Care in the Past: Archaeological and Interdisciplinary Perspectives.* Oxford: Oxbow Books, 2017.

Raxter, Michelle H., Christopher B. Ruff, Ayman Azab, Moushira Erfan, Muhammad Soliman, and Aly El-Sawaf. "Stature Estimation in Ancient Egyptians: A New Technique Based on Anatomical Reconstruction of Stature." *American Journal of Physical Anthropology* 136, no. 2 (2008): 147–55. https://doi.org/10.1002/ajpa.20790.

Roberts, Charlotte. "Disability in the Skeletal Record: Assumptions, Problems and Some Examples." *Archaeological Review from Cambridge* 15, no. 2 (1999): 79–97.

Ross, Judith L., Karen Kowal, Charmian A. Quigley, Werner F. Blum, Gordon B. Cutler, Brenda Crowe, Karine Hovanes, Frederick F. Elder, and Andrew R. Zinn. "The Phenotype of Short Stature Homeobox Gene (SHOX) Deficiency in Childhood: Contrasting Children with Leri-Weill Dyschondrosteosis and Turner Syndrome." *The Journal of Pediatrics* 147, no. 4 (2005): 499–507. https://doi.org/10.1016/j.jpeds.2005.04.069.

Schrader, Sarah A. "Activity Patterns in New Kingdom Nubia: An Examination of Entheseal Remodeling and Osteoarthritis at Tombos." *American Journal of Physical Anthropology* 149, no. 1 (2012): 60–70. https://doi.org/10.1002/ajpa.22094.

Schrader, Sarah A. "Bioarchaeology of the Everyday: Analysis of Activity Patterns and Diet in the Nile Valley." PhD diss., Purdue University, 2013.

Schrader, Sarah A., and Michele R. Buzon. "Everyday Life After Collapse: A Bioarchaeological Examination of Entheseal Change and Accidental Injury in Postcolonial Nubia." *Bioarchaeology International* 1, no. 1–2 (2017): 19–34. https://doi.org/10.5744/bi.2017.1000.

Smith, Stuart Tyson. *Wretched Kush: Ethnic Identities and Boundaries in Egypt's Nubian Empire.* London: Routledge, 2003.

Smith, Stuart Tyson, and Michele R. Buzon. "The Fortified Settlement at Tombos and Egyptian Colonial Strategy in New Kingdom Nubia." In *From Microcosm to Macrocosm: Individual Households and Cities in Ancient Egypt and Nubia,* edited by Julia Budka and Auenmüller Johannes. Leiden, Netherlands: Sidestone Press, 2018.

Spikins, Penny, Andy Needham, Lorna Tilley, and Gail Hitchens. "Calculated or Caring? Neanderthal Healthcare in Social Context." *World Archaeology* 50, no. 3 (2018): 384–403. https://doi.org/10.1080/00438243.2018.1433060.

Sullivan, Richard. "Deformity-A Modern Western Prejudice with Ancient Origins." *Proceedings-Royal College of Physicians of Edinburgh* 31, no. 3 (2001): 262–66.

Tilley, Lorna. "Accommodating Difference in the Prehistoric Past: Revisiting the Case of Romito 2 from a Bioarchaeology of Care Perspective." *International Journal of Paleopathology* 8 (2015a): 64–74. https://doi.org/10.1016/j.ijpp.2014.10.003.

Tilley, Lorna. *Theory and Practice in the Bioarchaeology of Care.* London: Springer International Publishing, 2015b.

Tilley, Lorna, and Tony Cameron. "Introducing the Index of Care: A Web-Based Application Supporting Archaeological Research into Health-Related Care." *International Journal of Paleopathology* 6 (2014): 5–9. https://doi.org/10.1016/j.ijpp.2014.01.003.

Tilley, Lorna, and Marc F. Oxenham. "Survival against the Odds: Modeling the Social Implications of Care Provision to Seriously Disabled Individuals." *International Journal of Paleopathology* 1, no. 1 (2011): 35–42. https://doi.org/10.1016/j.ijpp.2011.02.003.

Tilley, Lorna, and Alecia A. Schrenk. *New Developments in the Bioarchaeology of Care Further Case Studies and Expanded Theory.* Cham, Switzerland: Springer International Publishing, 2018.

Whitmore, Katie M., and Michele R. Buzon. "Two Cases of Skeletal Dysplasia from New Kingdom (c. 1400–1050 BCE) Tombos, Sudan." *International Journal of Paleopathology* 26 (2019): 135–44. https://doi.org/10.1016/j.ijpp.2019.07.006.

World Health Organization. *International Classification of Impairments, Disabilities, and Handicaps: A Manual of Classification Relating to the Consequences of Disease.* Geneva: 29th World Health Assembly, January 1, 1980. https://apps.who.int/iris/handle/10665/41003.

Worne, Heather. "Bioarchaeological Analysis of Disability and Caregiving from a Nineteenth-Century Institution in Central Kentucky." *Bioarchaeology International* 1, no. 3–4 (2017): 116–30. https://doi.org/10.5744/bi.2017.1010.

Zakrzewski, Sonia R. "Palaeopathology, Disability and Bodily Impairments." In *Palaeopathology in Egypt and Nubia: A Century in Review*, edited by Ryan Metcalfe, Jenefer Cockitt, and Rosalie David, 57–68. Oxford: Archaeopress, 2014.

Zakrzewski, Sonia R. "'Behind Every Mask There is a Face, and Behind that a Story'. Egyptian Bioarchaeology and Ancient Identities." In *Egyptian Bioarchaeology: Humans, Animals, and the Environment*, edited by Salima Ikram, Jessica Kaiser, and Roxie Walker, 157–67. Leiden, Netherlands: Sidestone Press, 2017.

13 *Talipes cavus* in Mummified Egyptian Human Remains

Michael R. Zimmerman

In 1992, an expedition by the Royal Ontario Museum and Canadian Institute for the Study of Egyptian Antiquities Archaeologic expedition invited me to examine mummified human remains found during the excavation of the ancient city of Kellis, in the Dakhleh Oasis in the western desert of Egypt.[1] The Dakhleh Oasis Project is jointly sponsored by the Royal Ontario Museum and the Society for the Study of Egyptian Antiquities, Toronto, Ontario, Canada and is largely funded by the Social Sciences and Humanities Research Council of Canada. The project has been engaged since 1978 in an interdisciplinary study of the relationship between human activity and environmental change in the site in the western desert of Egypt. The time frame under study for this project is mid-Pleistocene to the present (some 500,000 years) and the team consists of prehistorians, historical archeologists, geologists, zoologists, botanists, physical anthropologists, paleopathologists and others.

The Kellis site was occupied from the first to the third century CE, the time of transition in Egypt from the traditional religion to Christianity.[2] Egypt remained Christian until the Moslem conquest of 641 CE, but Kellis had been abandoned some 300–400 years earlier, presumably because the water ran out (wells in the area, now referred to as the New Valley, are as much as 300 meters deep). Mud-brick buildings are buried in the sand, including the remains of a church. The town covers a square kilometer and the population was probably several thousand. Surrounding the town are numerous low hills, 20–30 m high. At their bases are tombs, visible as sand-filled depressions. It was here that I discovered one of the more interesting case studies from the Dakhleh Oasis project: a man with clubfoot, whom I will examine in detail in this chapter.

Clubfoot or *talipes cavus*, variously referred to as idiopathic congenital (unknown cause, present at birth) *talipes equinovarus* (ICTEV), is a range of foot abnormalities usually present at birth, in which the baby's foot is twisted. Tendons connecting the muscles to the bone are typically shorter. This fairly common congenital disability (1 in 1,000 babies born in the United States of America each year) is usually an isolated case for an otherwise healthy newborn.[3] The foot may curl sideways with the toes bent at an angle, or it might have an odd shape and point in the wrong direction, with 40% of cases being bilateral.[4]

DOI: 10.4324/9781003440369-16

Clubfoot was depicted in Egyptian hieroglyphs and was described by Hippocrates around 400 BCE.[5] Hippocrates advised treatment with gentle manipulation and bandages and was the first to provide a hypothesis to explain the etiology (cause) of congenital *talipes cavus*.[6] Today several hypotheses remain, and research findings do not clearly support any particular argument. Proposed mechanisms are uterine restriction, abnormalities of joint and/or bone formation, connective tissue, distal limb vasculature, neurological development, muscle migration or an underlying developmental abnormality or developmental arrest.[7]

For modern cases, there is a very effective treatment for clubfoot, the Ponseti method. The treatment is named for Ignatio Ponseti, MD (1914–2009), who developed the technique over a number of years at the University of Iowa.[8] The Ponseti method has three phases: casting, minimal surgery (Achilles tenotomy) and bracing.[9] What is interesting is that this more modern method is reminiscent of the methodology Hippocrates proposed thousands of years ago, especially the casting and bracing phases of the treatment. Both Hippocrates and the Ponseti method also note the importance of initiating treatment shortly after the child is born. The casting phase in the Ponseti method is initiated shortly after birth. The casts are changed weekly until all elements of the impairment are corrected except a tight Achilles tendon. The first phase is complete after 5–7 casts. The second phase is a very minor surgical procedure on the Achilles tendon, required in 90% of cases. Tenotomy is performed by incisions in the Achilles tendon, resulting in inflammation and increased blood flow, which is followed by healing. Next is a final prolonged period of bracing, for three months after casting and then nighttime only until the child is 4 to 5 years old. Treatment is usually initiated shortly after birth, well before the child is walking.[10] Despite modern treatment, many cases still require surgery and disability often persists despite treatment. If untreated, the condition will result in lifelong difficult and painful walking.[11]

In my 1992 visit, I examined 14 mummified bodies, noting externally gross pathology and taking samples of all organs and structures identified in these individuals. Tissue samples were rehydrated, paraffin embedded and examined by light microscopy.[12] Previous paleopathological findings on this project have included evidence of hyperparathyroidism, trephination, fluorochrome labeling in bone and leprosy.[13]

One of the individuals, labeled 31/420-C5-1/2-M Tomb 2 Body M, was without the cranium, but otherwise a complete body of an adult male. Since he dated from a later time period, internal organs were still present in the body's interior as part of the standard practice of the time. Anterior bowing of the right mid-tibia was noted, with marked shortening of the right lower leg, which measured 40 cm from the lower border of the patella to the heel, 6 cm shorter than the left. The anterior bowing was approximately 1.5 cm. There was a marked variation of the right foot, in a *talipes cavus* configuration, with elevation of the arch and curling of the lateral 4 toes. The right heel pad was markedly thickened, measuring 2 cm in external thickness as compared to 1 cm for the left pad. Samples were taken of the skin and subcutis of both heels.

In antiquity, the anterior thoracic and abdominal walls had been removed and I noted the body cavities to be completely filled with dirt, sand and small pebbles. The right lung was grey tan, suggesting anthracosis (the deposition of carbon pigment). Impressions of the ribs were noted on the posterior aspect of the lung, suggestive of emphysema (pathologic swelling of the air sacs and scarring of the walls). The left lung was partially adherent to the lateral chest wall. With rehydration, microscopy revealed severe diffuse anthracosis, in the lung and in lymph nodes adjacent to blood vessels and bronchi. This meant that this man may have experienced symptoms such as shortness of breath, labored breathing, and coughing and the production of phlegm. Some of the enlarged peribronchial lymph nodes contained sclerotic areas, old necrotizing granulomas, evidence of a long-standing infectious process. A special acid-fast stain revealed several acid-fast positive rods, diagnostic of tuberculosis.

The superficial layer of the skin of the right heel shows fragments of thickened hyperkeratotic material, cells of the superficial layer which no longer have nuclei. Within underlying fibroadipose tissue are seen several cystic structures lined by dense fibrous membranes, apparently dilated lymphatics. The left heel showed a lesser degree of hyperkeratosis. These are all the result of extreme stress while walking, and would have occurred due to the man's altered gait as caused by his condition.

This individual, presenting with *talipes cavus* of his right foot, with shortening and bowing of his right lower leg, had a number of other impairments, including aortic atherosclerosis (narrowing of the arteries in the heart), lumbar osteophytosis (bone spurs), mild scoliosis (spinal curvature), papillary transitional cell carcinoma of the bladder (cancer) and pulmonary tuberculosis.[14] The liver showed identifiable portal areas (containing blood vessels and bile ducts), with numerous fine fibrous bands extending into the surrounding liver tissue and encircling individual liver cells. While the parasitic worm disease schistosomiasis can involve the liver and was common in ancient Egypt (and remains so in the present), no parasite ova were seen in the portal areas. The general centrilobular pattern of the fibrosis and the absence of ova suggest an alcoholic pathogenesis (alcoholism). One can speculate that the resultant discomfort of these various disorders, primarily the *talipes cavus*, led to self-medication by alcohol and the subsequent alcoholic cirrhosis observed in this man.[15] It is known that the western oases had a well-developed wine industry.[16] While this man did have these various impairments, he was buried in the cemetery at the Dakleh Oasis with everyone else, in one of the three tombs that were examined during my study.[17] It seems he was a man of some financial means, since he could afford a burial, and the cost of the wine he was using to presumably treat his impairments. This points to societal integration and care of those with physical disability in ancient Egypt in both life and death. What is also particularly interesting about this man is that he lived long enough to develop bladder cancer. As I have previously elaborated, the diagnosis of cancer in Egyptian mummified remains is rare. At this point, only two examples of cancer have been diagnosed histologically in Egyptian mummified remains, cancer of the rectum and of the urinary bladder in two c. 200 CE mummies from the Dakhleh Oasis.[18] Therefore, he is, to date, one of only two examples of individuals with histologically diagnosed cancer from ancient Egypt.[19]

The hand is never affected in *talipes cavus* and explanation of its pathology may lead to identification of genes whose effects are exclusive to the foot and lower limb. What this particular case also reveals is the importance of remembering "that we are in fact studying deceased humans."[20] While examinations of ancient pathology are indeed valuable, what they ultimately reveal is the variation of the human experience in both the past and the present. This individual with *talipes cavus* in the distant past, combined with advances in genetic mapping techniques, development of mouse models, improved understanding of the control of developmental processes and genetic epidemiology studies are all likely to further the study of idiopathic congenital *talipes equinovarus*. Therefore, the deceased can be considered to help the modern world in better understanding of the full variation present in the human past, including that of disabled individuals.

Notes

1 M. R. Zimmerman (1977, 33–36).
2 Michael R. Zimmerman (2017, 85–91).
3 Paul J. Gibbons and Kelly Gray (2013), E434–E437. https://doi.org/10.1111/jpc.12167.
4 Ibid., E434–E437.
5 Douglas W. Owsley and Robert W. Mann (1990, 97), James Longrigg (1998, 182).
6 James Longrigg (1998, 182).
7 Zosia Miedzybrodzka (2003, 37–42). https://doi.org/10.1046/j.1469-7580.2003.00147.x.
8 Jennie McKee (December 2007: Clinical 6).
9 Ibid., Clinical 6.
10 Ibid., Clinical 6.
11 Ibid., Clinical 6.
12 It should be noted that this is debatable whether this is still accepted best practice, since advances in technology have allowed for less invasive methods of examination like MRIs to be used.
13 A. C. Aufderheide et al. (1999, 197–211).
14 M. R. Zimmerman and J. Mirro (June 1983, 6–7).
15 M. R. Zimmerman and A. C. Aufderheide (2010, 16–23).
16 Michael R. Zimmerman (2017, 85–91).
17 Ibid., 85–91.
18 Michael R. Zimmerman (2019, 47).
19 A. R. David and M. R. Zimmerman (September 3, 2010).
20 Michael R. Zimmerman (2019, 48).

Bibliography

Aufderheide, A. C., M. Zlonis, L. L. Cartmell, M. R. Zimmerman, P. Sheldrick, M. Cook, and J. E. Molto. "Human Mummification Practices at Ismant El-Kharab." *Journal of Egyptian Archeology* 85 (1999): 197–211.

David, A. R., and M. R. Zimmerman. "Cancer: A New Disease, an Old Disease, or Something in Between?" *Invited Paper, Nature Reviews Cancer* 10 (September 3, 2010): 728–33.

Gibbons, Paul J., and Kelly Gray. "Update on Clubfoot." *Journal of Paediatrics and Child Health* 49, no. 9 (September 2013): E434–E437. https://doi.org/10.1111/jpc.12167.
Longrigg, James. *Greek Medicine from the Heroic to the Hellenistic: A Source Book.* New York: Routledge, 1998.
McKee, Jennie. "Ponseti Method Revolutionizes Clubfoot Care." *Bulletin of the American Academy of Orthopedic Surgeons (AAOS Now)* 1, no. 10 (December 2007): Clinical 6.
Miedzybrodzka, Zosia. "Congenital Talipes Equinovarus (Clubfoot): A Disorder of the Foot but Not the Hand." *Journal of Anatomy* 202, no. 1 (January 2003): 37–42. https://doi.org/10.1046/j.1469-7580.2003.00147.x.
Owsley, Douglas W., and Robert W. Mann. "An American Indian Skeleton with Clubfoot from the Cabin Burial Site (A1184), Hemphill County, Texas." *Plains Anthropologist* 35, no. 128 (May 1990): 97.
Zimmerman, Michael R. "The Mummies of the Tomb of Nebwenenef: Paleopathology and Archeology." *Journal of the American Research Center in Egypt* 14 (Fall 1977): 33–36.
Zimmerman, Michael R. *My Patients Were Mummies*. New York: Nova Science Publishers, 2017.
Zimmerman, Michael R. "Journey into the Human Body: Studying Mummies to Understand Ancient Disease." *Expedition* 61, no. 1 (Spring 2019): 47.
Zimmerman, Michael R., and A. C. Aufderheide. "Seven Mummies of the Dakhleh Oasis, Egypt: Seventeen Diagnoses." *Paleopathology News* l, no. 150 (June 2010): 16–23.
Zimmerman, Michael R., and J. Mirro. "The Paleopathology of the Human Remains from Nebwenenef's Tomb, Part II: Histologic Findings." *Paleopathology News* l, no. 42 (June 1983): 6–7.

14 Siptah's Leg and Other Stories

Aidan Dodson

The study of disability in the pre-modern times may be hampered by problematic diagnoses of conditions visible in human remains or artistic depictions. This may be the result of a lack of awareness of particular conditions, even among those with professional medical or pathological knowledge, leading to "loose" diagnoses that pass into the literature as "fact." It is in this context that archaeologists who themselves are subject to disabilities can bring their own lived experience into the evaluation of conditions visible, or potentially visible, in the archaeological record. In my case, I have spastic cerebral palsy, a result of birth trauma, resulting in a degree of hemiplegia of the right side.

On the other hand, in bringing one's own lived experience into the study of the ancient world, it is important to beware of imposing on the ancient world modern Western notions regarding what it means to be a member of the non-normative group with which one feels affiliated. Otherwise, there is always a danger of interpreting data through an inappropriate lens, thus creating what may turn out to be a house of cards that can do more harm than good to the understanding of the non-normative past individuals in question. Thus, in the context of the present volume, one has to be wary of positing a "disabled community" as such in ancient Egypt, or even a broad category of "disabled" that could be generally recognised by a member of the country's ancient society. One strongly suspects that the reality was that much depended on the degree of impairment, the nature of the local community and also how that impairment was perceived, not only by others, but by the individual in question.

In recent years, there has been considerable discussion of whether the remains of Tutankhamun display indications of physical impairment, and if so to what degree,[1] but there is a striking lack of unanimity over diagnoses.[2] However, there is another youthful king whose mummified remains show that he was unequivocally subject to physical impairment. This is Siptah, of the late 19th Dynasty.

The king's antecedents are less than clear, and his chancellor, Bay, boasts that he "placed the king on the seat of his father." This unique claim is especially interesting when placed in the context of the six years that directly preceded Siptah's accession. During these six years, the apparently-legitimate king, Sethy II, had been displaced from the rule of Nubia and the south of Egypt by a rival pharaoh, Amenmeses (seemingly his own son), before being restored, albeit not long before

DOI: 10.4324/9781003440369-17

Sethy's own death.[3] It was following Sethy's death that we find Bay claiming to have acted as "king-maker" for the approximately nine-year-old Siptah, and then apparently directing Egypt's affairs in concert with Sethy II's widow, Tawosret, until he was executed as a traitor on the order of "Pharaoh," in Siptah's Year 5. It is possible that the "father" on whose "seat" Siptah had been placed by Bay was none other than the rebel Amenmeses.

Siptah himself only survived Bay's demise by a year, after which Tawosret was elevated to female king, continuing the year-count of Siptah, and erasing the latter's names in his tomb (KV47) and elsewhere. These circumstances inevitably lead to a suspicion that Siptah's death was not natural. However, none of the examinations of his mummified remains, which was reburied in the tomb of Amenhotep II (KV35) during the 21st Dynasty, and found there in 1898,[4] have reported anything regarding the cause of death.

However, what was clear from the moment the body was unwrapped at the end of August 1905 by Grafton Elliot Smith[5] was that the king had been subject to an impairment of his left leg. Smith himself noted that during the unwrapping process, "the left foot, distorted in the manner known as talipes equino-varus, was exposed in its original wrappings" (Figure 14.1).[6] Smith makes no further comment on the nature of the condition, and his statement was subsequently generally taken as

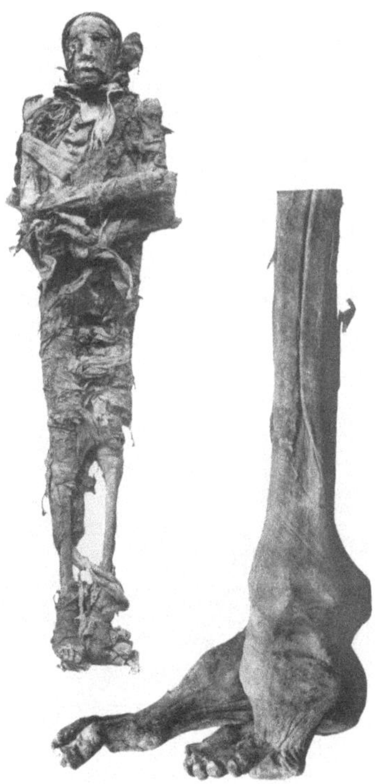

Figure 14.1 The mummified remains of King Siptah (Cairo CG61080), showing the distortion of his left leg (Smith, Royal Mummies, pl. lxii).

meaning that Siptah had the condition known colloquially as "club foot." This is a condition in which one or both feet are rotated inward and downward at birth, usually without any obvious cause.[7]

This diagnosis was seemingly not questioned until Siptah, along with most of the other royal mummified remains, then in the Egyptian Museum, Cairo, was the subject of x-ray examination in 1967, by a mission from the Universities of Michigan and Alexandria. In the publication of this work, the following assessment was made:

> The deformity of the left lower extremity of Siptah has in the past been described as clubfoot or talipes equinovarus. In both its external appearance and radiographic appearance, however, it strongly resembles a postpoliomyelitis deformity with underdevelopment of the entire extremity and hyperextension of the foot and ankle to compensate for the resulting inequality in leg length. Accordingly this is thought to represent the results of poliomyelitis or a similar neuromuscular disease occurring earlier in life. The deformity is well seen in the specimen photograph from Smith (1912) and the x-rays of the leg.[8]

The report also notes an earlier diagnosis of polio in an Old Kingdom body from Deshasha (Figure 14.2). In this case, the examining physician stated

> that the left leg is considerably shorter than the right, and at first sight the femur of the left side seems heavier and thicker than the right one. Measurement, however, makes it evident that the left femur's apparent greater circumference is only due to its shortening, and to strongly marked ridges at the site of the muscular attachments, which suggest that the muscles may have been hypertrophied on that side. With this exception the left femur is imperfectly developed in all directions. . . . So far as can be told the bones of the feet are unaffected, but as the terminal phalanges have crumbled almost entirely away, nothing can be stated with certainty about them.[9]

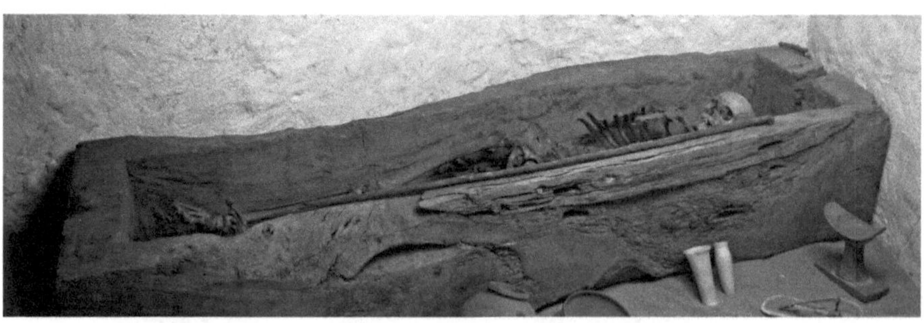

Figure 14.2 Skeletonised Old Kingdom mummified remains from Deshasha, with a distorted left leg (University of Pennsylvania Museum of Anthropology and Archaeology, Philadelphia, E2552). Photograph by Aidan Dodson.

However, another comment in the volume publishing the Michigan-Alexandria team's results notes that "in [Siptah's] case, in spite of the considerable shortening and thinning of the bones of the left lower limb, the hypertrophy of the muscular processes throws some doubt on the [polio] diagnosis."[10]

While the new analysis quite rightly pointed out that the condition of Siptah's leg and foot is not compatible with a club foot, it is curious that only polio is considered as an alternative diagnosis, particularly since polio produces muscle weakness, rather than the muscular tightness displayed by the locking of Siptah's foot in a downward position. Such a result is, however, a regular result of spastic cerebral palsy (CP).

CP is caused by damage to or abnormal development in parts of the brain that control movement, balance, and posture. These may be of indeterminate cause during pregnancy, or by trauma at or shortly after birth. In the case of spastic CP, this can result in the atrophy of the muscles of the lower leg, over-tightening the Achilles tendon, and locking the foot in a downward position. This then leads to an undergrowth of the leg in question – all producing exactly the effect seen with the leg of Siptah.

It is unclear why this explanation for the state of Siptah's leg was seemingly long ignored by medical practitioners when considering the cause of the king's disability. My own awareness of the possibility came about through my personal experience of spastic CP, which resulted in a right leg that would have, had it not been for corrective surgery, been indistinguishable from Siptah's left leg. This led to me making, in 1998, what may have been the first suggestion in print that CP may be the cause of the condition of Siptah's leg.[11] The proposal received a positive assessment in a 2013 paper from the Professor of Paediatrics and Paediatric Neurology, University of Thessaloniki[12] and also in discussion with my own university's Professor of Neonatal Neuroscience.[13]

The failure by earlier writers to consider CP as a diagnosis for Siptah's leg should not be taken as an implicit criticism of the professionalism of those involved. However CP expertise tends to lie with paediatricians, since its effects become manifest in early life, with diagnoses of the type experienced by Siptah and myself made when a child could not walk at the expected age. As such, it may not immediately occur as a solution to more "generalist" practitioners, or be something that will be included in the training of bioarchaeologists. Secondly, polio has been a high-profile disease for many years, with its potential for causing a wasting-based disability well known, including causing superficially similar effects to the lower limbs. As such, it might seem the most "obvious" diagnosis for anyone without a detailed knowledge of CP.[14]

A case in which CP has been diagnosed in the publication of ancient Egyptian remains in more recent years is that of a 13th-Dynasty individual named Geheset, buried at Dra Abu'l-Naga, Western Thebes.[15] In this case, there were also clear issues with the individual's arm and dentition, underlining the existence of hemiplegia, something very much associated with CP.

The significance of a diagnosis of Siptah's leg (and also probably the Deshasha remains) as being something *other* than polio is that it potentially removes ancient

Egypt from any history of that disease. I say "potentially," since it *may* have been present – but Siptah's leg does not provide evidence in favour of the proposition. As a result, modern histories of the disease[16] which trace polio back beyond its first description by Underwood[17] are not actually based on substantive evidence.

In addition to Siptah's leg and the Deshasha skeleton, one other piece of evidence has been put forward in support of polio in ancient Egypt. This is the stela of the Doorkeeper Roma, datable to the reign of Amenhotep III (Figure 14.3).[18] Its provenance is unknown, all that is known being that it was acquired in Egypt during the 1890s. However, an origin at or near Saqqara is indicated by its *ḥtp-di͗-nsw* formula calling for Roma's goodly burial in the "desert to the west of Memphis."

The piece shows the principal figure with a withered right leg, with the foot flexed in a downward position, and leaning on a staff. Such an overt depiction of a non-perfect physique, especially of a high-status Egyptian, is unusual in Egyptian art.[19] This might be seen as an assertion by Roma of a significant part of his identity, or be linked with the stela's dedication to the goddess Astarte, who had healing attributes.[20] It is interesting that she is also invoked in the piece's *ḥtp-di͗-nsw* formula.

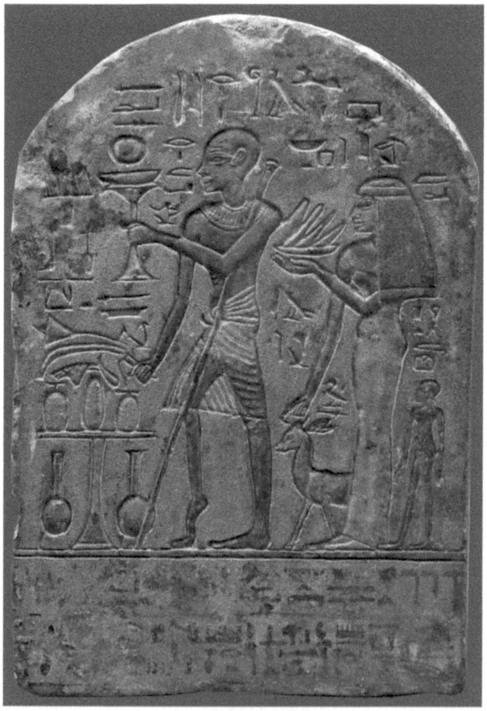

Figure 14.3 Stela of the Doorkeeper Roma (Ny Carlsberg Glyptotek, Copenhagen, ÆIN 134). Photograph by Aidan Dodson.

Diagnoses from art works can be problematic at best (cf. the vast, but inconclusive, literature on the possible pathologies of Akhenaten), but in Roma's case it is clear that a real condition is being depicted in some detail. As with Siptah, Roma's condition has been all but universally attributed to polio,[21] but in his case as well the gross appearance of the affected leg seems wholly consistent with spastic CP. The identification of CP in ancient Egypt is hardly surprising. A major cause of CP is trauma at birth, and in pre-modern times this will have been even more prevalent than today. Indeed, the surprise is that so few examples have been highlighted in the literature to date.

The case of Siptah's leg (and that of Roma) is an instructive one, especially in how our picture of the past may be distorted by the limitations of the lenses applied to its study. As an Egyptologist, I am very much reliant on the professional expertise of those whose fields lie beyond mine, and I would probably have been content to accept the diagnosis of polio, had it not been for my own lived experience. Thus, from the moment that I saw a photograph of Siptah's leg in my early teens it seemed to me that CP had to be at the very least another option for its diagnosis. As already noted, one has to be very careful to not to privilege such a personally derived hypothesis over others, but it does emphasise how a scholar needs to maintain the widest possible awareness of "stuff" to supplement that derived from more typically academic sources.

Notes

1 While there are principled objections to retrospective diagnoses, it may be argued that a rounded understanding of an historical figure is only possible if there is an awareness of any physical challenges they may have had to face.
2 Rühli and Ikram 2014, 51–63.
3 Dodson 2016.
4 Cairo CG61080, now in the National Museum of Egyptian Civilization, Fustat, Cairo.
5 Smith 1912, 70–73, pl. lx–xiii.
6 Smith 1912, 71.
7 Gibbons and Gray 2013, 434–37.
8 Whitehouse 1980, 293–94; see also Harris and Weeks 1973, 45, 159.
9 Pennsylvania University Museum of Anthropology & Archaeology E2552 (Mitchell 1900, 914).
10 Ghalioungui 1980, 69.
11 Ikram and Dodson 1998, 326.
12 Panteliadis, Panteliadis, and Vassilyadi 2013, 285–86.
13 I am most grateful to Marianne Thoreson for her time, and a most enlightening discussion of CP in its broadest terms.
14 See Panteliadis, Panteliadis, and Vassilyadi 2013, 288–89 for a long-standing confusion between CP and polio.
15 Nerlich et al. 2010, 113–16.
16 E.g. Paul 1971.
17 Underwood 1789, 88–91.
18 Copenhagen-Ny Carlsberg ÆIN 134: see Jørgensen 1998, 118–19, with previous bibliography.
19 Robinson 2017, 6–33.
20 Ranke 1932, 412–18.

21 E.g. Hamburger 1911, 1914; Moro 1932; Slomann 1927, 62–86; Jørgensen (1998, 118), comments, "There is a general consensus that this deformity was caused by polio."

Bibliography

Dodson, Aidan. *Poisoned Legacy: The Decline and Fall of the Nineteenth Egyptian Dynasty*. Revised ed. Cairo: American University in Cairo Press, 2016.

Ghalioungui, Paul. "Medicine in Ancient Egypt." In *An X-ray Atlas of the Pharaohs*, edited by James E. Harris and Edward F. Wente, 52–79. Chicago: University of Chicago Press, 1980.

Gibbons, Paul J., and K. Gray. "Update on Clubfoot." *Journal of Paediatrics and Child Health* 49, no. 9 (2013): 434–37.

Hamburger, Ove. "Un cas de paralysie infantile dans l'antiquité." *Bulletin de la Société Française d'Histoire de la Médecine* 10 (1911): 407–12.

Hamburger, Ove. "Zwei Darstellungen von Krankheiten aus dem alten Ägypten." *Janus* 19 (1914): 241–45.

Harris, James E., and Kent R. Weeks. *X-Raying the Pharaohs*. London: Macdonald, 1973.

Ikram, Salima, and Aidan Dodson. *The Mummy in Ancient Egypt: Equipping the Dead for Eternity*. London: Thames & Hudson, 1998.

Jørgensen, Mogens. *Catalogue Ny Carlsberg Glyptotek: Egypt II (1550–1080 BC)*. Copenhagen: Ny Carlsberg Glyptotek, 1998.

Mitchell, John K. "Study of a Mummy Affected with Anterior Poliomyelitis." *Philadelphia Medical Journal* 6 (1900): 914–15.

Moro, Ernst. "Zur Vorgeschichte der Poliomyelitis." *Medizinische Klinik* 28 (1932): 1333–34.

Nerlich, A. G., S. Panzer, E. Hower-Tilmann, and S. Lösch. "Palaeopathological-Radiological Evidence for Cerebral Palsy in an Ancient Egyptian Female Mummy from a 13th Dynasty Tomb." In *Pharmacy and Medicine in Ancient Egypt: Proceedings of the Conferences Held in Cairo (2007) and Manchester (2008)*, edited by Jenefer Cockitt and Rosalie David, 113–16. Oxford: Archaeopress, 2010.

Panteliadis, Christos, Panos Panteliadis, and Frank Vassilyadi. "Hallmarks in the History of Cerebral Palsy: From Antiquity to Mid-20th Century." *Brain & Development* 35 (2013): 285–92.

Paul, J. R. *A History of Poliomyelitis*. Yale Studies in the History of Science and Medicine. New Haven: Yale University Press, 1971.

Ranke, Hermann. "Istar als Heilgöttin in Ägypten." In *Studies Presented to F. Ll. Griffith*, 412–18. London: Egypt Exploration Society, 1932.

Robinson, Joanne-Marie. " 'Your Mouth Speaks, Your Feet Walk': Representations of Physical Abnormalities and Perceptions of the Human Body in Ancient Egyptian Funerary Iconography." *Archaeological Review from Cambridge* 32, no. 1 (2017): 6–33.

Rühli, Frank J., and Salima Ikram. "Purported Medical Diagnoses of Pharaoh Tutankhamun." *Homo – Journal of Comparative Human Biology* 65 (2014): 51–63.

Slomann, H. C. "Contribution à la paléo-pathologie égyptienne." *Bulletins et Mémoires de la Société d'anthropologie de Paris, 7th Series* 8, part 1 (1927): 62–86.

Smith, Grafton Elliot. *The Royal Mummies*. Cairo: Imprimerie de l'institut français d'archéologie, 1912.

Underwood, Michael. *A Treatise on the Diseases of Children, with General Directions for the Management of Infants from the Birth*. Vol. II. London: J. Mathews, 1789.

Whitehouse, Walter M. "Radiologic Findings in the Royal Mummies." In *An X-ray Atlas of the Pharaohs*, edited by James E. Harris and Edward F. Wente, 286–97. Chicago: University of Chicago Press, 1980.

15 And the Children Shall Lead

Harpocrates, Harpocratis, and Cerebral Palsy

Alexandra F. Morris

Harpocrates was considered one of the major deities of the Ptolemaic and Greco-Roman periods of the ancient world, especially in Egypt. He was considered a child iteration of the sun god Horus, and was associated with both the solar cult of Ptah-Sokaris and the mortuary cult. He was further recognised as the god of secrets, confidentiality, and silence; the embodiment of hope; and the representative of the newborn sun.[1] Later, Harpocrates was recognised as a protector of mothers and children.[2] He also has a feminine form known as Harpocratis.[3] He is described in literature by Plutarch, as being "prematurely delivered and weak/lame in his lower limbs."[4] I have previously established that the ancient Egyptians deliberately depicted the god Harpocrates, and by extension his feminine form Harpocratis, as having cerebral palsy, and that depictions of both gods with cerebral palsy seemed to extend to other periods besides the Ptolemaic period.[5]

Cerebral palsy is a disability/group of disorders which affects movement, balance, posture, coordination, and motor skills.[6] It is often, but not always, caused by brain damage occurring in utero or during or shortly after birth, and is often associated with premature birth.[7] This impairment is one of the most common congenital disabilities today, and is the most common childhood physical disability, affecting 4 out of every 1,000 births worldwide.[8] I have also previously theorised that this was most likely a common impairment in the ancient world since pregnancy and childbirth difficulties existed and were probably more common at that time.[9] Additionally, it should be noted that Plutarch's life and work briefly overlapped with that of the Roman emperor Claudius, who is also believed by historians such as Barbara Levick and medical professionals to have had cerebral palsy.[10] However, what this chapter addresses are the larger implications of what these depictions mean through a disability paradigm. I examine this material from the context of experience of my own embodiment with cerebral palsy. This methodology of using my own embodied understanding of this impairment to further clarify, identify, and think through possible societal implications in the historical record has been used prior in other disability history and Disability Studies scholarship.[11] I examine the possible societal implications of this physically impaired god, as well as depictions of Harpocrates in more depth, particularly those in which he is depicted with other physically impaired gods. Artefacts examined date from the New Kingdom through Roman-period Egypt, with

DOI: 10.4324/9781003440369-18

additional examples from other ancient civilisations, when relevant. In examining these artefacts more closely, I argue that there appears to be a gendered aspect to depictions of both the deities Harpocrates and Bes, and posit what this can tell us about both gender and disability in ancient Egypt.

Harpocrates and Harpocratis are typically depicted in set poses. These poses include but are not limited to the following: Harpocrates or Harpocratis standing as depicted on Greek or Egyptian style statues, amulets, beads, and cameos; there are others in which they are either in a sitting or half-crawling position, statues in which they are sitting or riding on the back of animal, and depictions of Harpocrates breastfeeding from the goddess Isis.[12] These representations are often made from copper, bronze, terracotta, or glass, and some were mould made, indicating that these were popular items in the ancient world.[13]

What Can Art Tell Us About Embodied Experience of Disability?

Standing Depictions

Both Harpocrates and Harpocratis are depicted in standing poses (Figure 15.1). Some of these just depict them as holding a finger to their lips.[14] Some of them are

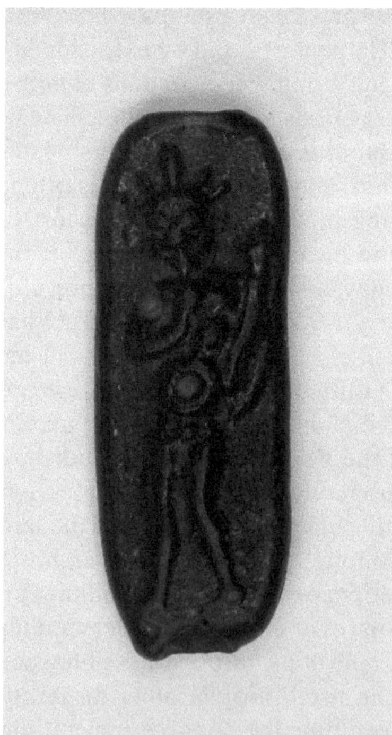

Figure 15.1 Amulet of the God Harpocrates. Roman Period. 30 BCE–395 CE. Glass. Art Institute of Chicago. 1894.840. Photo by the Art Institute of Chicago.

clothed, and some of them show Harpocrates as nude, another trait in Egyptian iconography that indicates childhood. This gesture, along with depicting him with the sidelock of hair, were recognised by the ancient Egyptians as meaning that the subject was a child, and stems from the hieroglyph determinative for child (𓀔).[15] These varied representations were popular items in the ancient world.[16] Others depict Harpocrates and Harpocratis holding a cornucopia, a symbol of fertility. Some also depict both masculine and feminine forms of the deity as leaning against a column or other architectural feature typically placed to one side, rather than behind them.[17] Both Harpocrates and Harpocratis are frequently shown wearing the crown of Upper and Lower Egypt, which is another symbol of their connections to the pharaohs as heir of Osiris and son/daughter of Serapis.[18] Interestingly on some of these depictions, the crowns are framed by lotus flowers. The lotus flowers are a reference to the god Nefertum, who was another solar deity. It is also accepted by scholars that lotuses were used by the ancient Egyptians as a source of pain relief, and pain is something commonly seen in some who have cerebral palsy, especially the spastic cerebral palsy subtype.[19]

One figure depicts a standing terracotta female Harpocratis with right index finger to her mouth, holding a cornucopia in her hand, and dressed in a Greek-style tunic dress.[20] She has curly hair, and wears crescent-shaped earrings, a wreath, and double crown of Egypt. She is also resting her arm, the one holding the cornucopia, against an altar upon which a falcon (the animal sign of Horus) sits, possibly with the altar meant to give her extra stability. This figure is inscribed with hieroglyphs, which are a partial copy of the *Instructions of Khety* dating to the Middle Kingdom. However, the inscription seems to have been added after the piece was fired, and there is no clear reason for why this inscription appears on this piece. *The Instructions of Khety* is considered a satirical piece that extolls the advantages of being a scribe while disparaging various forms of manual labour.[21] However, taking the possible mobility impairment into account may give us a clue for the inscription's purpose: a scribe was a sedentary job, whereas most forms of manual labour were not.

The statues were often located in temples and shrines as well as private household shrines, and were used for religious purposes relating to both the living and the dead.[22] During the Greco-Roman period, their use as votives for domestic shrines increased, as did their roles in a domestic/protective function.[23] These statues more specifically are believed to have had either an apotropaic or healing function.[24] This may mean the statues were also literally depicting their function as protective and healing objects through the reading of pain relief as shown by the lotuses. That these lotuses can also be read as a societal accommodation and therefore societal care for the deities is another bonus. It also means that a congenitally impaired god and goddess were expected to aid in both protection and the healing process, meaning that society viewed those deities with the impairment as fulfilling a role within the universe and society and more importantly not associating the impairment with stigmatisation. Instead, disability and impairment in this instance were associated with protection and healing, thus with hope. This connection is more captivating when one remembers that one of Harpocrates'/Harpocratis' roles was as the embodiment or symbol of hope, especially as related to ill health or injury in humanity, after Harpocrates was cured of a poisonous snake bite by Ra.[25]

Group Depictions and Supported Standing Figures

Harpocrates and Harpocratis are also sometimes depicted on amulets and wall paintings as standing or sitting, sometimes standing with no aid, sometimes with the help of a cane which doubles as a ceremonial cane, and sometimes physically being supported in a triad of gods which can include either Isis and Nephthys, Isis and Osiris, Isis and Hathor, Hathor and Khnum, or Khnum and Heket (Figure 15.2).[26] In these depictions, especially those in which Harpocrates or Harpocratis is standing while being physically supported, the signs of cerebral palsy are again present. These depictions reveal societal accommodation and care since the deity is being physically supported in their attempts to stand either with a mobility aid or the physical support of the deities around them. One particularly interesting Ptolemaic example from the temple of Philae depicts a nude Harpocrates standing, while being formed on a potter's wheel by the god Khnum. The goddess Heket looks on, providing assistance and protection in the form of an ankh.[27] As noted by Egyptologist Sandra Sandri, this

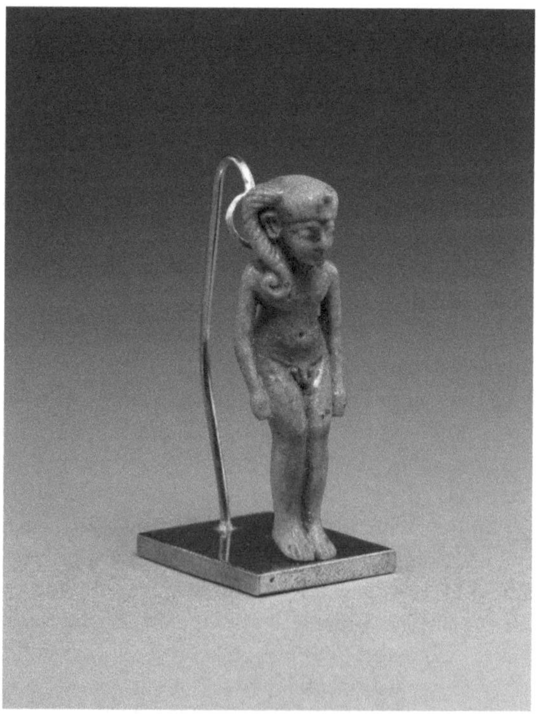

Figure 15.2 *Harpocrates.* Late-Ptolemaic period, 664–30 BCE, Faience. New York, Metropolitan Museum of Art. 44.4.29. Photo by the Metropolitan Museum of Art, New York.

example ties into the local birth myth and local gods, but the Ptolemies have changed the local god's myth to be Harpocrates.[28] What is interesting about this example is that we know from the myth that Khnum formed humanity on his potter's wheel with the help of Heket. In this example, although he is standing unaided, Harpocrates does appear to have one leg that is slightly twisted and less muscular than the other, and his arms also display uneven musculature, again displaying symptoms of cerebral palsy. It is representative of this impairment and shows that both the artists and the Ptolemies were deliberately representing Harpocrates to be disabled from the moment of his creation. In other words, Khnum is shown as making the deliberate choice to make Harpocrates disabled from the time of conception. This depiction therefore emphasises that disability and impairment were perceived as part of the necessary natural variation and order of the universe.

Seated and Crawling Figures

Both Harpocrates and Harpocratis are also depicted in seated or half-crawling poses. In these positions, they are typically shown in a half-crouched position with legs off to one side.[29] They clutch either a cornucopia, a goose, or a jar in these figures, and are depicted primarily in Greek-style clothing, although some sculptures do show them nude.[30] In some figures, the genitals are visible as well, most likely referencing their fertility aspect. In some of these depictions Harpocrates also appears seated directly on a lotus flower, occasionally with that lotus flower placed on a papyrus boat framed by other gods such as Isis, Nephthys, and Anubis. In these depictions there again appear to be references to the lotus as both being representative of the sun (the boat in these instances literally becomes a solar barge), and as pain relief: in being directly seated on it, Harpocrates brings it into direct contact with his affected limbs, again meaning this is a societal accommodation for his pain.

Like the statues discussed earlier, these figures were also used for religious purposes for both the living and dead. However, here the focus seems to be abundance, fertility, and their roles as protective deities, rather than a focus on healing. Again, instead of disability and impairment being associated with stigma or negativity, they are associated here with abundance and fertility. It may be that the Egyptians and Greeks associated fertility with cerebral palsy because the more children a family had, the more chances of cerebral palsy presenting itself, and the more chances of having a child who was the physical manifestation of Harpocrates or Harpocratis. In that sense, the children could be linked to Khnum's creations upon his potter's wheel and were therefore a natural and expected part of the variation of the universe.

Seated While Riding Animals

Finally, both Harpocrates and Harpocratis are sometimes depicted riding animals. These depictions include animals such as horses, geese, elephants, or rams.[31] These depictions are typically made from terracotta, painted faience, or bronze, and are mostly mould made, signalling their widespread popularity and use. They would

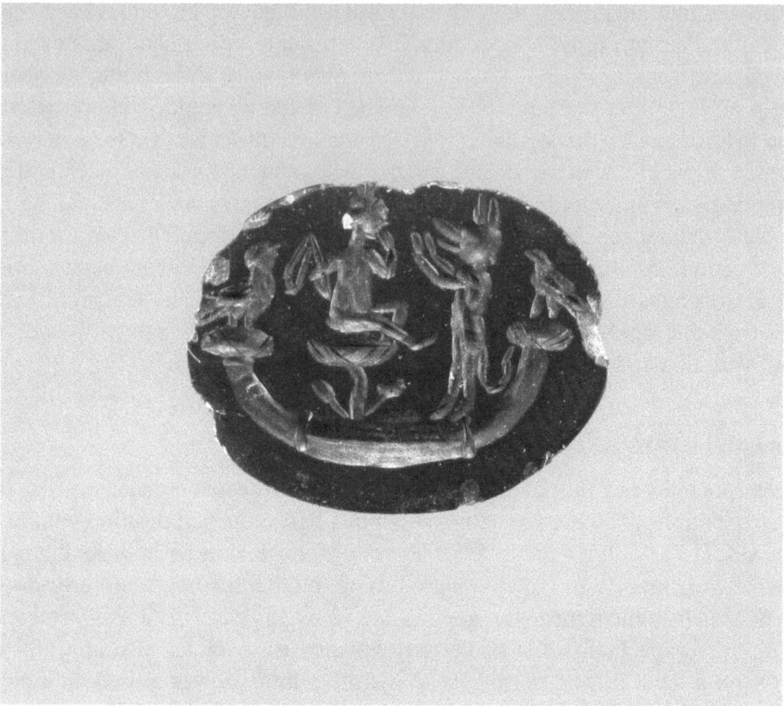

Figure 15.3 Jasper intaglio: Harpocrates seated on Lotus in Papyrus Boat. Roman period. Second to third century CE. Green Jasper. New York, Metropolitan Museum of Art. 81.6.295. Photo by the Metropolitan Museum of Art, New York.

have been used as votive offerings in a religious context. In some of the depictions of Harpocrates riding on horses, he is dressed in the military gear of a Macedonian solider. In some cases, the horse is seen trampling a prisoner.[32] This is most likely a continuation of the traditional Egyptian motif of pharaohs trampling or crushing enemies.[33] It is also a visual example of order triumphing over chaos, with prisoners representing chaos and Harpocrates taking the place of the pharaoh representing order.

These examples show cross cultural influence from ancient Greece and Egypt. The Harpocrates figures that depict him riding on geese and elephants show cross-cultural influence from Greece and India, namely from the Seleucid Empire. Figures that depict Harpocrates riding an elephant are very similar to the figures that show him as a Macedonian soldier riding a horse. The artists extended this motif to include what became another animal used by the ancient Greeks in war. Similarly, Harpocratis riding a ram can be seen as a reference to the god Zeus-Ammon, another Greek-Egyptian hybrid deity, as well as Amun the Egyptian equivalent, or to Serapis, the father of this deity. Amun, Zeus-Ammon, and Serapis were seen as solar/sky deities, creator and fertility gods, and associated with kingship. Harpocratis, in this case, is representing the power and connection to the pharaohs, as well as fertility and abundance, since she also clutches a cornucopia. In many of these examples, the crowns of Upper and Lower Egypt are again framed by lotus flowers, once more linking cerebral palsy with pain relief, as well as the deities with the sun. Impairment and disability are again associated with abundance and fertility, rather than anything stigmatising or negative. More importantly in these examples, impairment and disability are associated with power, and the triumph of order over chaos, and perhaps makes a deliberate allusion or connection of disability with power, and the ability to rule. In other words, Harpocrates and Harpocratis are not holding this power in spite of their impairment: instead, it is part of what qualifies them to wield political power, since it was part of the natural variation of the universe, and therefore part of the natural order or *Ma'at* of that universe.

Therefore, disability and impairment were essential to help contain chaos or *Set/Isfet*. This seems to be especially true in those depictions of Harpocrates as a soldier, particularly when he is dressed as a Macedonian, and may be a reference to the disabled war veterans who held political, religious, and societal power during the Ptolemaic period.[34] It should also be noted that another physically impaired god, Bes, who will be discussed in further detail later, was also sometimes shown dressed as a soldier.[35] For both gods, it seems to suggest that disability and impairment were an expected part of *Ma'at* and that all those who were capable were expected to function in protective roles as soldiers in society, regardless of their actual impairment status. It again possibly points to art being created that would have mass societal appeal, partially because it may have reminded the buyers of themselves. It also points to gender roles within Egypt and the Classical world since only the male versions of both deities were depicted as soldiers, despite the Egyptians also having a female goddess of warfare (Sekhmet).

The depictions of Harpocrates riding a goose have a different origin. Historian Attilio Mastrocinque has noted that the Harpocrates goose figures were directly modelled from Greek figures of the Greek god Eros riding a goose, and the goose was also associated with the Greek goddess Aphrodite.[36] Eros was the god of love who was sometimes depicted as a child and was also considered a fertility symbol.[37] This makes yet another example of the cultural fusion which existed in the Greco-Roman period. To the Egyptians, these Harpocrates figures also became literal hieroglyphs: the word for "son," *sA/zA*, was a goose followed by a child determinative (𓅭𓀔).[38] However, these examples also provide a direct connection of the concept of disability and impairment with beauty as well as fertility, since Aphrodite was the goddess of both. Overall, all the foregoing examples emphasise that disability and impairment were seen as a part of everyday life, and a part of the natural variation of the universe, something that was expected to be lived with and dealt with: not an aberration or societal tragedy. The examples of the deities riding animals can also point to societal accommodation of disability. Discussed in my previous research, as well as elsewhere in this book, mobility aids and other societal accommodations were in use, and it is not a stretch to consider an animal as a mobility aid, particularly when there was already a history of mobility aids being used and depicted in an artistic context in both ancient Egypt and ancient Greece.[39]

Harpocrates Breastfeeding

Harpocrates is depicted as breastfeeding or being carried, mainly by his mother Isis, but also occasionally with other goddesses.[40] The other goddesses Harpocrates is shown with include Hathor (goddess of love, beauty, and music), Wadjet (the official goddess of the office of the king), and the mother of the Apis bull (a bull sacred to ancient Egyptians, who was believed to be an intermediary between humans and Hathor, Ptah, Osiris, and Atum); Harpocrates was also believed to be a manifestation of the pharaoh.[41] In all of these images, Harpocrates shows all the physical manifestations of cerebral palsy. Additionally, he does not seem to be interested in breastfeeding, instead sitting passively, leaning to one side, on his mother's or another female goddess's lap. The physical manifestations of the cerebral palsy do not disappear when the goddess changes. Additionally, when one compares these images to other sculptures of Egyptian women breastfeeding infants, both divine and mortal, the other examples show a child or deity who is actively engaged in breastfeeding.[42] These suggest that there was an active societal investment in the care of disabled infants in ancient Egypt. They additionally link kingship with both disability and impairment in ancient Egypt. One must wonder if both were seen as an essential part of *Ma'at*, and therefore somewhat necessary to be associated with the king, and his struggle to keep the universe in a state of *Ma'at* in ancient Egypt, either through his own manifestation or through his care of others. We have biological evidence for at least three disabled pharaohs in ancient Egypt (Tutankhamun, Siptah, and Philip III Arrhidaeus), as well as multiple disabled individuals appearing in the pharaoh's court throughout Egyptian history.[43] Additionally, *Ma'at* could be an explanation as to why all these figures depict a male manifestation of the deity: it needed to be a male manifestation to counterbalance Isis' feminine energy, and therefore ensure the continuation of *Ma'at*. Pharaohs in ancient Egypt were also traditionally male with only seven female kings throughout Egypt's history, and Harpocrates here is associated with kingship in these figures.

Harpocrates and Bes

Besides being depicted with his mother Isis, Harpocrates is also depicted with the god Bes. Significantly, Bes is also a physically impaired god who functioned in a protective capacity, and more specifically is known to have been a protector of women during childbirth.[44] More interestingly, Bes is also one of the only other Egyptian gods who has a female counterpart known as Beset.[45] When they do appear together it appears that the pairing of Harpocrates and Bes include only the male versions of both. There are no pairings to my knowledge of Harpocratis with Beset, Harpocrates with Beset, or Harpocratis with Bes. There appear to be two main contexts in which the two are shown together. One is on healing cippi and the other is on small metal figures in which Harpocrates is seated with multiple versions of Bes.[46] Water was poured over the healing cippi and then collected to be given to patients for various ailments as part of medical treatment.[47] On the healing cippi, Harpocrates is typically depicted standing nude on the backs of crocodiles (as few as one and as many as six), strangling snakes in each hand. In some of these images papyrus canes or standards appear on either side of him, almost giving the appearance of crutches or mobility aids. Some of the canes also feature a seated falcon resting at the top. Bes is typically depicted as a partial image, with only his head appearing, directly above Harpocrates, giving the impression that Bes is encircling the Harpocrates figure, while magical hieroglyphic texts and other gods appear in the backgrounds and on the backs of these cippi.[48] Some Egyptologists, such as Nora Scott, have suggested that the two deities appearing together means that they are supposed to be interpreted as different manifestations of the same god with Harpocrates representing childhood, and Bes representing an old man.[49] Marc Coenen has theorised that they were united to link and strengthen as many different apotropaic elements as possible.[50] If either of these theories is true, then both gods would have been implicitly understood by the ancient Egyptians and Greeks as being congenitally physically impaired, which, as discussed later, creates an intriguing connection between disability, physical impairment, and healing. Interestingly, we do have a few statues in which a standing Harpocrates is wearing a Bes mask.[51] These particular statues were most likely made for apotropaic purposes, but further demonstrate the link between the two congenitally impaired gods. It also challenges Scott's theory that they represent different aspects of the same god.

On the metal statues of Harpocrates, he typically appears nude in a clearly seated position, seated on a high-backed throne, with one finger to his lips.[52] The thrones typically feature lions and *sema-tawy* or lotus and papyrus imagery, alluding to Harpocrates' roles as a sun god and association with kingship in ancient Egypt.[53] In some cases the lotuses appear making up the entire back of the piece. However, the lotuses could also be read secondarily as providing pain relief, something that is not atypical for a physically impaired body as caused by cerebral palsy. Bes appears in these images in pairs (multiple versions of the same god) standing in front of the throne holding a club in one hand, sometimes with other gods or worshippers, so that he is in essence framing Harpocrates and his legs, the throne, and the other gods or worshippers, and acting as a physical barrier to anyone who approaches. It seems clear that from both types of examples, Bes is meant to be acting in a protective role, and in the cippi examples also participating in the healing process. In both examples, Harpocrates and Bes are acting in their roles as protective and/or healing deities. This means that two congenitally physically impaired gods were expected to assist in the healing process or be able to provide protection to the owners or users of these artefacts. There was a societal expectation that congenitally physically impaired gods could and should assist in healing and/or protection. This also reveals a rather interesting duality, and perhaps underscores an important point: how the ancients possibly viewed those with congenital impairments in ancient Egypt. Both Harpocrates and Bes in their masculine and feminine versions were seen as healing and protective deities. Therefore, while both deities were recognised by the ancients as having a bodily difference, they were also understood as being complete, rather than broken or defective. There seems to have been no stigma or negative connotation to these bodily differences, which may be precisely because these were congenital disabilities. Harpocrates and Bes were given the power to heal others possibly because they themselves were viewed as being fine as they were and part of the natural variation of the universe akin with *Ma'at*. It is entirely possible that they, and people like them, were viewed as being necessary to help sustain *Ma'at* as well and that this healing ability was seen as part of a cycle to help keep the universe from descending into *Set/Isfet*.

What is particularly fascinating about these figures is that Bes appears by the two main areas which Harpocrates' cerebral palsy is described by Plutarch as having affected him: Bes frames his legs, and his head. We know now that cerebral palsy is a disability caused by damage to the brain (i.e. head) in utero or during or shortly after birth, and Plutarch states that Harpocrates was born "weak in his lower limbs."[54] Therefore, there are multiple depictions of Bes with Harpocrates in which we know both legs were affected. It should also be noted that in all examples of lotuses discussed in this chapter, they appear either by the deity's head in the form of a wreath, crown, or framing the pharaoh's crown, or again by his legs, i.e. on the base or backs of the thrones, or underneath so that the deity is seated directly on them; there are no known examples in which the deity simply holds the lotuses. It is widely accepted that the ancient Egyptians had a different understanding of the function of the brain, believing instead that the cognitive and emotive areas of a person were located in the heart; however the Greeks did have an understanding of the brain as being the centre of consciousness and physical function.[55] We have to remember that Harpocrates is a hybrid deity, so it is possible that this understanding could have been passed on to the artists who made these artefacts. Another possible interpretation is that Bes is also acting in a secondary protective and supportive function to Harpocrates himself, besides also offering that same protective and healing function to the user of these artefacts. Therefore, the protective functions of these cippi and statues are being depicted both literally (i.e., through Harpocrates' conquering of chaos in the form of dangerous animals), and figuratively through the support Bes offers. Knowing the ancient Egyptians' love of dualism, and often depiction of art that can be read on both a literal and a figurative level, this should not be a surprise, and is representative of the care and thought these ancient people took in creating these artefacts.

Lastly, something needs to be stated about these depictions only being of the male embodiments of these two congenitally impaired deities. Indeed, it strikes me as strange, but it can possibly tell us something about how gender, disability, and impairment were viewed in ancient Egypt. We have already seen that certain depictions of Harpocrates seem to be of his male version only: that of the soldier, and that of him breastfeeding. It is interesting that within a purely medical/healing context, again only the male versions of both Harpocrates and Bes are shown. This could be because of established societal norms that influenced the market for these objects, and the ancient Egyptian need for balance. While the ancient Egyptians and Greeks did have female doctors and midwives, physician roles were primarily male.[56] Priests and priestesses associated with healing temples tended to be of both genders, but they had specific roles within those temples.[57] Additionally, it is believed that these particular objects were associated with fertility cures, along with being a cure for more general ailments such as snakebites and scorpion stings, and protection for women and children during childbirth.[58] It is possible that the

Egyptians saw the need for more male energy to balance out the female energy of those they were treating (or in essence create a state of *Ma'at* in order for things to work), especially if these were paired with other figures of Bes, or with the female goddess Tawaret. It is also possible that because the market was trying to appeal to people familiar with both Egyptian and Greek culture, they used the male representation because people from both cultures were used to seeing men in a medical context; it was only the Egyptians who had female physicians.

Conclusions

These representations of Harpocrates and Harpocratis depict what may have been a common birth occurrence in the ancient world. As illustrated in this chapter, there are potential dangers in approaching art from a default nondisabled perspective, resulting in ableist bias. Signs of impairment can be ignored or missed, effectively erasing these people and gods from the historical narrative, or resulting in their being re-written as nondisabled.[59] This leads to an incomplete and inaccurate picture of the ancient world. When one examines Harpocrates and Harpocratis more fully in terms of both their societal implications and a paradigm of the physical embodiment of disability, it reveals a great deal about ancient Greco-Roman and Egyptian culture and society, creating a much better understanding of the ancient world. Also, this analysis has revealed that both deities had some roles that seemed to have been gender-specific, and that gender specificity was linked to how these roles were perceived in society.

This chapter demonstrates that the ancient Egyptians viewed congenital disability and impairment as being part of the natural order of the universe, linking it explicitly with *Ma'at*, and therefore had no reason within society for it to be stigmatised. Instead, it appears in the case of Harpocrates and Bes to have been linked with healing and protection, and this link with healing and protection may have been these deities' function specifically to maintain *Ma'at*. We also have gained further possible insight into both the Greek and Egyptian understanding of the bodily differences associated with the physical embodiment of cerebral palsy, as evidenced by their placement of both lotuses and the god Bes in relation to Harpocrates. Both seem to be clustered around areas that would have been affected by Harpocrates' and Harpocratis' embodiments of cerebral palsy. This also allows us to reflect on the possibility of pain as being seen as part of the embodiment of this condition, and therefore an expected part of the lived experience as well. Finally, this analysis has revealed the extent of the many different levels at which ancient Egyptian art was made to be viewed and understood, since all examples discussed have multiple layers of meaning. Some of these layers can be read as specific societal care or adjustments for this particular impairment (i.e. lotuses for pain or the papyrus reeds which can also be read as canes), while also connecting to the religious and political aspects associated with these disabled and congenitally impaired deities. Egyptian art was complex and multi-faceted, and it is only by looking at it in its complete context with disability included that we gain a fuller understanding of this ancient civilisation.

Notes

1 László Török (1995, 19–21).
2 Ibid., 19–21.
3 Ibid., 19–21.
4 Plutarch (1936, 154).
5 Alexandra F. Morris (2022, 145–209).
6 Centers for Disease Control and Prevention "What is Cerebral Palsy?" last updated April 30, 2019. https://www.cdc.gov/ncbddd/cp/facts.html.
7 Ibid.
8 Ibid.
9 Morris (2022).
See Aidan Dodson's chapter, "Siptah's Leg and Other Stories," in this book for more historical examples of cerebral palsy. Additionally for more historical examples see Kyle Lewis Jordan's talk on Geheset, "Disability in Ancient Egypt: The Case of Geheset," *Unlimited Access Symposium, Allaird Pierson Museum*, June 25, 2021, https://www.youtube.com/watch?v=fMBMdbpE-qM&t=12s and Sandra Losch, Stefanie Panzer, and Andreas G. Nerlich, "Cerebral Paralysis in an Ancient Egyptian Female Mummy from a 13th Dynasty Tomb- Paleopathological and Radiological Investigations," in *Behinderungen und Beeintrachtigungen,* ed. Rupert Breitwieser (Oxford: Archaeopress, 2012), 37–40.
10 Panteliadis, Panteliadis, and Vassilyadi (2013, 286), Barbara Levick (1990, 13–15).
11 Virdi (2020), Williams and Bendelow (1998, i), Gillespie-Sells, Hill, and Robbins (1998, v), Campbell and Oliver (1996, i, 1).
12 Morris (2023, 1–28), Morris (2022, 145–209).
13 Morris (2022, 159).
14 *Figure; Amulet* (AN1896-1908-EA.616), Late-Ptolemaic Period, 6th Century–2nd Century BC, Copper Alloy, H: 3.70 cm, W: 0.90 cm, D: 0.50 cm, London, British Museum, accessed February 2020, https://research.britishmuseum.org/research/collection_online/search.aspx; *Figure* (EA49137), Late-Ptolemaic Period, 664–31 BC, Copper Alloy, H: 2.95 cm, W: 0.80 cm, D: 0.85 cm, London, British Museum, accessed February 2020, https://research.britishmuseum.org/research/collection_online/search.aspx; *Amulet; Figure* (9,9,86,105.b), Late-Ptolemaic Period, 6th Century–1st Century BC, Copper Alloy, H: 6.80 cm, T: 2 cm, W: 2 cm, London, British Museum, accessed February 2020, https://research.britishmuseum.org/research/collection_online/search.aspx; *Amulet; Figure* (H1029.3), Late-Ptolemaic Period, 4th Century–1st Century BC, Copper Alloy, L: 5.30 cm, T: 1.40 cm, W: 1.70 cm, London, British Museum, accessed February 2020, https://research.britishmuseum.org/research/collection_online/search.aspx; *Amulet; Figure* (H1029.2), Late-Ptolemaic Period, 4th Century–1st Century BC, Copper Alloy, H: 3.15 cm, W: 1.15 cm, D: 1 cm, London, British Museum, accessed February 2020, https://research.britishmuseum.org/research/collection_online/search.aspx; *Figure* (EA60975), Late-Ptolemaic Period, 6th Century–1st Century BC, Copper Alloy, H: 8.10 cm, W: 2.30 cm, London, British Museum, accessed February 2020, https://research.britishmuseum.org/research/collection_online/search.aspx; *Figure* (EA64487), Late-Ptolemaic Period, 6th Century–1st Century BC, Copper Alloy, Electrum, H: 15 cm, W: 4.80 cm, London, British Museum, accessed February 2020, https://research.britishmuseum.org/research/collection_online/search.aspx; *Standing Statuette of Harpocrates in the Greek Style*, Ptolemaic Period, 305–30 BC, Bronze, H: 14.8 cm, New York, Brooklyn Museum, accessed February 2020, https://www.brooklynmuseum.org/opencollection/objects/60259; *Figure* (86.252), Late-Ptolemaic Period, 6th Century–2nd Century BC, Copper Alloy, H: 8.50 cm, London, British Museum, accessed February 2020, https://research.britishmuseum.org/research/collection_online/search.aspx; *Figure of Harpocrates,* Ptolemaic Period, 305–30 BC, Painted Pottery, H: 19.3 cm, W: 3.1 cm, D: 6.6 cm, New York, Brooklyn Museum, accessed February 2020, https://www.brooklynmuseum.org/opencollection/

objects/118147; *Figure* (EA67198), Late-Ptolemaic Period, 6th Century–1st Century BC, Copper Alloy, H: 15.40 cm, W: 4.20 cm, D: 6 cm, London, British Museum, accessed February 2020, https://research.britishmuseum.org/research/collection_online/search.aspx; *Figure* (EA60992), Late- Ptolemaic Period, 6th Century–1st Century BC, Copper Alloy, H: 22.30 cm, W: 5.40 cm, London, British Museum, accessed February 2020, https://research.britishmuseum.org/research/collection_online/search.aspx; *Glass Pendant in the Shape of Harpokrates* (17.194.419), Hellenistic Period, late 2nd Century–1st Century BC, Moulded Glass, H: 2.5 cm, New York, Metropolitan Museum of Art, accessed February 2020, https://www.metmuseum.org/art/collection/search/249656; *Glass Pendant in the Shape of Harpokrates* (17.194.421), Hellenistic Period, 1st Century BC–1st half of 1st Century AD, Moulded Glass, H: 2.8 cm, W: 0.7 cm, D: 0.9 cm, New York, Metropolitan Museum of Art, accessed February 2020, https://www.metmuseum.org/art/collection/search/249658; *Glass Pendant in the Shape of Harpokrates* (17.194.420), Hellenistic Period, late 2nd Century–1st Century BC, Moulded Glass, H: 2.8 cm, New York, Metropolitan Museum of Art, accessed February 2020, https://www.metmuseum.org/art/collection/search/249657; *Figure; Amulet* (E20829), Ptolemaic Period, 3rd Century BC, Glazed Composition, H: 9.80 cm, W: 4.50 cm, London, British Museum, accessed February 2020, https://research.britishmuseum.org/research/collection_online/search.aspx; *Pendant* (1879,0522.33), Ptolemaic Period, 2nd Century BC–1st Century AD, Glass, Gold, L: 2.60 cm, London, British Museum, accessed February 2020, https://research.britishmuseum.org/research/collection_online/search.aspx; *Figure* (1982,0301.1), Ptolemaic Period, 2nd Century–1st Century BC, Terracotta, H: 16.50 cm, London, British Museum, accessed February 2020, https://research.britishmuseum.org/research/collection_online/search.aspx; *Alabastron* (2011,5016.6), Ptolemaic Period, 3rd Century BC, Terracotta, L: 11.70 cm, London, British Museum, accessed February 2020, https://research.britishmuseum.org/research/collection_online/search.aspx; *Figure* (1886.31.60.a), Late-Ptolemaic Period, 664–31 BC, Copper Alloy, H: 4.30 cm, W: 1.60 cm, D: 1.10 cm, London, British Museum, accessed February 2020, https://research.britishmuseum.org/research/collection_online/search.aspx.

15 Kozma (2005, 307).

16 *Glass Pendant in the Shape of Harpokrates* (17.194.421), Hellenistic Period, 1st Century BC–1st half of 1st Century AD, Moulded Glass, H: 2.8 cm, W: 0.7 cm, D: 0.9 cm, New York, Metropolitan Museum of Art, accessed February 2020, https://www.metmuseum.org/art/collection/search/249658; *Figure* (EA60975), Late-Ptolemaic Period, 6th Century–1st Century BC, Copper Alloy, H: 8.10 cm, W: 2.30 cm, London, British Museum, accessed February 2020, https://research.britishmuseum.org/research/collection_online/search.aspx; *Standing Statuette of Harpocrates in the Greek Style*, Ptolemaic Period, 305–30 BC, Bronze, H: 14.8 cm, New York, Brooklyn Museum, accessed February 2020, https://www.brooklynmuseum.org/opencollection/objects/60259; *Figure* (1982,0301.1), Ptolemaic Period, 2nd Century–1st Century BC, Terracotta, H: 16.50 cm, London, British Museum, accessed February 2020, https://research.britishmuseum.org/research/collection_online/search.aspx.

17 *Standing Statuette of Harpocrates in the Greek Style*, Ptolemaic Period, 305–30 BC, Bronze, H: 14.8 cm, New York, Brooklyn Museum, accessed February 2020, https://www.brooklynmuseum.org/opencollection/objects/60259; *Figure of Harpocrates* Ptolemaic Period, 305–30 BC, Painted Pottery, H: 19.3 cm, W: 3.1 cm, D: 6.6 cm, New York, Brooklyn Museum, accessed February 2020, https://www.brooklynmuseum.org/opencollection/objects/118147; *Figure; Amulet* (E20829), Ptolemaic Period, 3rd Century BC, Glazed Composition, H: 9.80 cm, W: 4.50 cm, London, British Museum, accessed February 2020, https://research.britishmuseum.org/research/collection_online/search.aspx; *Figure* (1982,0301.1), Ptolemaic Period, 2nd Century–1st Century BC, Terracotta, H: 16.50 cm, London, British Museum, accessed February 2020, https://research.britishmuseum.org/research/collection_online/search.aspx.

18 László Török, *Hellenistic and Roman Terracottas from Egypt* (Rome: L'Erma di Bretschneider, 1995), 19–21.
19 Benson Harer Jr. (1985, 49–54), Rosso (2010, 83–84).
20 *Votive Figure* (EA27333), Ptolemaic Period, 2nd Century–1st Century BC, Terracotta, H: 18.70 cm, W: 7.68 cm, D: 3.40 cm, London, British Museum, accessed February 2020, https://research.britishmuseum.org/research/collection_online/search.aspx.
21 Lichtheim (1980, 184–93).
22 Török (1995, 19–21).
23 Cristea (2013, 76–77).
24 Ibid., 75–77.
25 Pinch (2004, 146), Cristea (2013, 75).
26 Sandri (2006, 129–35, 140–42, 145–47, 151, 231).
27 Ibid., 231, Plate 100.
28 Ibid., 56–57.
29 *Figure* (1990,0601.2), Ptolemaic Period, 3rd Century–2nd Century BC, Terracotta, H: 9 cm, London, British Museum, accessed February 2020, https://research.britishmuseum.org/research/collection_online/search.aspx; *Figure* (AN1888.176), Ptolemaic Period, 300–100 BC, Terracotta, H: 10.20 cm, L: 10.80 cm, W: 3.80 cm, London, British Museum, accessed February 2020, https://research.britishmuseum.org/research/collection_online/search.aspx; *Figure* (1845,0705.1), Ptolemaic Period, 245 BC, Silver, H: 9.20 cm, London, British Museum, accessed February 2020, https://research.britishmuseum.org/research/collection_online/search.aspx; *Figure-Mould* (EA46702), Ptolemaic-Roman Period, 1st Century BC–1st Century AD, Pottery, H: 17 cm, W: 16 cm, London, British Museum, accessed February 2020, https://research.britishmuseum.org/research/collection_online/search.aspx; Figure (1972,0125.8), Ptolemaic Period, 3rd Century–2nd Century, Terracotta, H: 15 cm, London, British Museum, accessed February 2020, https://research.britishmuseum.org/research/collection_online/search.aspx; *Figure* (E20832), Ptolemaic Period, 300–100 BC, Terracotta, H: 5.60 cm, T: 2.90 cm, W: 4.80 cm, London, British Museum, accessed February 2020, https://research.britishmuseum.org/research/collection_online/search.aspx; *Figure* (86.397), Ptolemaic Period, 300–100 BC, H: 4 cm, London, British Museum, accessed February 2020, https://research.britishmuseum.org/research/collection_online/search.aspx.
30 *Figure* (86.397), Ptolemaic Period, 300–100 BC, H: 4 cm, London, British Museum, accessed February 2020, https://research.britishmuseum.org/research/collection_online/search.aspx.
31 *Figure* (NA490), Ptolemaic Period, 2nd Century–1st Century BC, Terracotta, H: 9.60 cm, T: 3.60 cm, W: 7.50 cm, London, British Museum, accessed February 2020, https://research.britishmuseum.org/research/collection_online/search.aspx; *Figure* (NA489), Ptolemaic Period, 2nd Century–1st Century BC, Terracotta, H: 11.30 cm, T: 3.70 cm, W: 6.20 cm, London, British Museum, accessed February 2020, https://research.britishmuseum.org/research/collection_online/search.aspx; *Figure* (1972,0125.6), Ptolemaic Period, 1st Century BC, Terracotta, H: 12 cm, London, British Museum, accessed February 2020, https://research.britishmuseum.org/research/collection_online/search.aspx; *Figure* (EA37559), Ptolemaic-Roman Period, 1st Century BC–1st Century AD, Terracotta, H: 17.50 cm, W: 10.75 cm, D: 4.33 cm, London, British Museum, accessed February 2020, https://research.britishmuseum.org/research/collection_online/search.aspx; *Figure* (EA22159), Ptolemaic Period, 2nd Century BC, Terracotta, H: 13.90 cm, W: 8.20 cm, D: 4.33 cm, London, British Museum, accessed February 2020, https://research.britishmuseum.org/research/collection_online/search.aspx; *Figure* (1814,0704.1649), Hellenistic or Ptolemaic Period, 3rd Century–1st Century BC, Lead, H: 3.70 cm, W: 3.90 cm, D: 0.40 cm, London, British Museum, accessed February 2020, https://research.britishmuseum.org/research/collection_online/search.aspx; *Figure* (EA24372), Ptolemaic Period, 2nd Century BC, Pottery, H: 15.30 cm,

W: 8.37 cm, D: 4.30 cm, London, British Museum, accessed February 2020, https://research.britishmuseum.org/research/collection_online/search.aspx; *Figure; Plaque* (A.1832), Ptolemaic, 330–250 BC, Terracotta, H: 7.70 cm, T: 2 cm, W: 7.80 cm, London, British Museum, accessed February 2020, https://research.britishmuseum.org/research/collection_online/search.aspx; *Figure; Plaque* (GR.11.1885), Ptolemaic Period 330–250 BC, Terracotta, H: 7 cm, T: 1.40 cm, W: 7.40 cm, London, British Museum, accessed February 2020, https://research.britishmuseum.org/research/collection_online/search.aspx; *Figure* (1886,0401.1450), Ptolemaic Period, 2ndCentury–1st Century BC, H: 9.80 cm, T: 3.90 cm, W: 8.80 cm, London, British Museum, accessed February 2020, https://research.britishmuseum.org/research/collection_online/search.aspx; *Figure* (86.410), Ptolemaic Period, 330–250 BC, Terracotta, H: 8 cm, L: 11.50 cm, London, British Museum, accessed February 2020, https://research.britishmuseum.org/research/collection_online/search.aspx; *Figure; Plaque* (E20831), Ptolemaic Period, 330–250 BC, Terracotta, H: 11.30 cm, W: 10.10 cm, London, British Museum, accessed February 2020, https://research.britishmuseum.org/research/collection_online/search.aspx; *Figure; Plaque* (NA499), Ptolemaic Period, 4th Century BC, Terracotta, H: 7.70 cm, T: 2.20 cm, W: 8 cm, London, British Museum, accessed February 2020, https://research.britishmuseum.org/research/collection_online/search.aspx; *Figure; Amulet* (7624), Ptolemaic-Roman Period, 2nd Century–1st Century BC, Glazed Composition, H: 4.80 cm, L: 5 cm, W: 2.40 cm, London, British Museum, accessed February 2020, https://research.britishmuseum.org/research/collection_online/search.aspx; *Plaque; Figure* (GR.10.1885), Ptolemaic Period 330–250 BC, Terracotta, H: 7.40 cm, T: 1.35 cm, W: 5.40 cm, London, British Museum, accessed February 2020, https://research.britishmuseum.org/research/collection_online/search.aspx.

32 *Figure* (86.410), Ptolemaic Period, 330–250 BC, Terracotta, H: 8 cm, L: 11.50 cm, London, British Museum, accessed February 2020, https://research.britishmuseum.org/research/collection_online/search.aspx; *Figure; Plaque* (E20831), Ptolemaic Period, 330–250 BC, Terracotta, H: 11.30 cm, W: 10.10 cm, London, British Museum, accessed February 2020, https://research.britishmuseum.org/research/collection_online/search.aspx.

33 Luiselli (2011, 12–16).

34 Morris (2022, 15–16), Fischer-Bovet (2014, 13, 151–52, 200).

35 Ibid., 93; *Pottery Flask* (EA15477), Ptolemaic Period, 2nd Century BC, Pottery, H: 7.3 cm, W: 6.6 cm, D: 3.2 cm, London, British Museum, accessed December 2019, https://research.britishmuseum.org/research/collection_online/search.aspx; *Bes Figure* (EA12745), Ptolemaic Period, 2nd Century–1st Century BC, Terracotta, H: 24.8 cm, W: 12.5 cm, D: 4.6 cm, London, British Museum, accessed December 2019, https://research.britishmuseum.org/research/collection_online/search.aspx; *Bes Figure* (1888,0601.96), Ptolemaic Period, 2nd Century–1st Century BC, Terracotta, H; 12.7 cm, London, British Museum, accessed January 2020, https://research.britishmuseum.org/research/collection_online/search.aspx.

36 Mastrocinque (2016, 220–22).

37 Ibid., 220–22.

38 Ibid., 220–22.

39 Morris (2023, 1–28), Morris (2022, 209, 241, 246), Draycott (2019).

40 *Figure* (1888,0601.107), Ptolemaic Period, 3rd Century–2nd Century BC, Terracotta, H: 15.50 cm, T: 4.40 cm, W:7.70 cm, London, British Museum, accessed February 2020, https://research.britishmuseum.org/research/collection_online/search.aspx; *Figure* (1888,0601.108), Ptolemaic Period, 3rd Century–2nd Century BC, Terracotta, H: 16.50 cm, T: 4.30 cm, W: 6.30 cm, London, British Museum, accessed February 2020, https://research.britishmuseum.org/research/collection_online/search.aspx; *Figure* (EA63797), 30th Dynasty-Ptolemaic Period, 3rd Century–2nd Century BC, Glazed Composition, H: 12.20 cm, W: 3.13 cm, D: 5.94 cm, London, British Museum, accessed February 2020, https://research.britishmuseum.org/research/collection_online/search.aspx.

41 *The Goddess Wadjet with the Horus Child*, Late-Ptolemaic Period, 664–30 BCE, Cupreous Metal, H: 12 cm, W: 4.8 cm, D: 6.2 cm, New York, Metropolitan Museum of Art, accessed March 2023, https://www.metmuseum.org/art/collection/search/570707.
42 *Amulet of Mut with Khonsu* (1892.52), Third Intermediate-Late Period, 1070–332 BCE, Faience, H: 6.1 cm, W: 1.7 cm, D: 3.4 cm, Chicago, Art Institute of Chicago, accessed December 2022, https://www.artic.edu/artworks/135832/amulet-of-mut-with-khonsu; *Group of Two Women and a Child* (22.2.35), Middle-Early New Kingdom, 1981–1500 BCE, Limestone, New York, Metropolitan Museum of Art, https://www.metmuseum.org/art/collection/search/544225.
43 Morris (2022, 38–39, 66–74, 139), Callendar (2006, 52), Plutarch (1919, 250–51, 439), Justin (1853, 13.2), Siculus (1947, 15, 20, 53–72).
44 Dasen (1993, 55–56).
45 Ibid., 59–60.
46 Special thanks to Julia Windrich for sharing her examples of these statues with me.
47 *Cippus of Horus on the Crocodiles*, Ptolemaic Period, 3rd Century BC, Steatite, H: 23.2 cm, W: 13.5 cm, D: 5.6 cm, New York, Brooklyn Museum, accessed February 2020, https://www.brooklynmuseum.org/opencollection/objects/3684.
48 Cristea (2013, 75).
49 Scott (1951, 201–17).
50 Sandri (2006, 157–60).
51 Roeder (1937, 20–21), Roeder (1956, Tafel 15, plates l, m, n).
52 Grimm-Stadelmann (2012, 152), Pieke (2021, 151).
53 Grimm-Stadelmann (2012, 152), Pieke (2021, 151).
54 Plutarch (1936, 154).
55 Crivellato and Ribatti (2007, 327–36).
56 Nunn (2002, 127–35), Theocharis (2020), http://nrs.harvard.edu/urn3:hlnc.essay:TheocharisDN.Women_in_Medicine.2020.
57 Lang (2012, 45–100), Nunn (2002, 127–35).
58 Swan Hall (1977, 55–56).
59 Morris (2022, 209–10).

Bibliography

Callendar, Gae. "The Cripple, the Queen, and the Man from the North." *KMT* 17, no. 1 (2006): 46–61.

Campbell, Jane, and Mike Oliver. *Disability Politics: Understanding Our Past, Changing Our Future.* London: Routledge, 1996.

Centers for Disease Control and Prevention. "What is Cerebral Palsy?" Last updated April 30, 2019. https://www.cdc.gov/ncbddd/cp/facts.html.

Cristea, Stefana. "Egyptian, Greek, Roman Harpocrates – A Protecting and Saviour God." In *Angels, Demons, and Representation of Afterlife within the Jewish, Pagan, and Christian Imagery,* edited by Iulian Moga. Iasi: Editura Universității Alexandru Ioan Cuza, 2013.

Crivellato, Enrico, and Domenico Ribatti. "Soul, Mind, Brain: Greek Philosophy and the Birth of Neuroscience." *Brain Research Bulletin* 71, no. 4 (2007): 327–36.

Dasen, Veronique. *Dwarfs in Ancient Egypt and Greece.* Oxford: Oxford University Press, 1993.

Draycott, Jane. *Prostheses in Antiquity.* London: Routledge, 2019.

Fischer-Bovet, Christelle. *Army and Society in Ptolemaic Egypt.* New York: Cambridge University Press, 2014.

Gillespie-Sells, Kath, Mildrette Hill, and Bree Robbins. *She Dances to Different Drums: Research into Disabled Women's Sexuality.* London: King's Fund, 1998.

Grimm-Stadelmann, Isabel. *Aesthetic Glimpses: Masterpieces of Ancient Egyptian Art the Resandro Collection.* Munich: Resandro, 2012.

Harer Jr, W. Benson. "Pharmacological and Biological Properties of the Egyptian Lotus." *Journal of the American Research Center in Egypt* 22 (1985): 49–54.

Justin, Marcus Junianus. *Epitome of the Philippic History of Pompeius Trogus.* Translated by John Selby Watson. London: Henry G. Bohn, 1853.

Kozma, Chahira. "Historical Review: Dwarfs in Ancient Egypt." *American Journal of Medical Genetics Part A* 140 (2005): 303–11.

Lang, Phillipa. *Medicine and Society in Ptolemaic Egypt.* Boston: Brill, 2012.

Levick, Barbara. *Claudius.* New Haven: Yale University Press, 1990.

Lichtheim, Miriam. *Ancient Egyptian Literature: A Book of Readings.* Berkeley: University of California Press, 1980.

Losch, Sandra, Stefanie Panzer, and Andreas G. Nerlich. "Cerebral Paralysis in an Ancient Egyptian Female Mummy from a 13th Dynasty Tomb-Paleopathological and Radiological Investigations." In *Behinderungen und Beeintrachtigungen*, edited by Rupert Breitwieser. Oxford: Archaeopress, 2012.

Luiselli, Maria Michela. "The Ancient Egyptian Scene of 'Pharaoh Smiting His Enemies': An Attempt to Visualize Cultural Memory?". In *Cultural Memory and Identity in Ancient Societies,* edited by Martin Bommas, 10–25. New York: Continuum International Publishing Group, 2011.

Mastrocinque, Attilio. "Birds and Love in Greek and Roman Religion." In *Animals in Greek and Roman Religion and Myth*, edited by Patricia A. Johnston, Attilio Mastrocinque, and Sophia Papaioannou, 213–26. Newcastle upon Tyne: Cambridge Scholars Publishing, 2016.

Morris, Alexandra F. "Let that Be Your Last Battlefield: Tutankhamun and Disability." *Athens Journal of History* 6, no. 1 (2020): 53–72.

Morris, Alexandra F. "Plato's Stepchildren: Disability in the Ptolemaic Egypt and the Hellenistic World (332–30 BCE)." PhD thesis, Teesside University, 2022.

Morris, Alexandra F. "Cerebral Palsy in Ancient Egypt." *Pediatric Stroke* 5 (2023): 1–28.

Nunn, John. *Ancient Egyptian Medicine.* Norman: University of Oklahoma Press, 2002.

Panteliadis, Christos, Panos Panteliadis, and Frank Vassilyadi. "Hallmarks in the History of Cerebral Palsy: From Antiquity to the Mid-20th Century." *Brain & Development* 35 (2013): 286.

Pieke, Gabrielle. "Egypt in Mannheim: New Visions for an Old Collection." Edited by Caroline M. Rocheleau and Tom Hardwick. *Offerings to Maat. Essays in Honour of Emily Teeter CIPEG* 5 (2021): 151.

Pinch, Geraldine. *Egyptian Mythology: A Guide to the Gods, Goddesses, and Traditions of Ancient Egypt.* Oxford: Oxford University Press, 2004.

Plutarch. *Loeb Classical Library: The Parallel Lives.* Translated by Bernadotte Perrin. Cambridge: Harvard University Press, 1919.

Plutarch. *Loeb Classical Library: Moralia.* Translated by Frank Cole Babbitt. Cambridge: Harvard University Press, 1936.

Roeder, Günther. *Ägyptische Bronzewerken.* Glückstadt, Hamburg, and New York: J.J. Augustin, 1937.

Roeder, Günther. *Ägyptische Bronzefiguren.* Vol. 6.2. Berlin: Staatliche Museen Zu Berlin Mitteilungen Aus Der Ägyptischen Sammlung, 1956.

Rosso, Ana Maria. "Poppy and Opium in Ancient Times: Remedy or Narcotic?" *Biomedicine International* 1 (2010): 81–87.

Sandri, Sandra. *Har-Pa-Chered (Harpokrates): Die Genese eines ägyptischen Götterkindes.* Leuven: Peeters Publishers, 2006.

Scott, Nora E. "The Metternich Stela." *The Metropolitan Museum of Art Bulletin* 9, no. 8 (1951): 201–17.

Siculus, Diodorus. *Loeb Classical Library: Library of History.* Translated by Russell M. Geer. Cambridge: Harvard University Press, 1947.

Swan Hall, Emma. "Harpocrates and Other Child Deities in Ancient Egyptian Sculpture." *Journal of the American Research Center in Egypt* 14 (1977): 55–58.

Theocharis, Dimitrois N. "Women in Medicine: An Epigraphic Research." *CHS Research Bulletin* 8 (2020). http://nrs.harvard.edu/urn3:hlnc.essay:TheocharisDN.Women_in_Medicine.2020.

Török, László. *Hellenistic and Roman Terracottas from Egypt.* Rome: L'Erma di Bretschneider, 1995.

Virdi, Jaipreet. *Hearing Happiness: Deafness Cures in History.* Chicago: University of Chicago Press, 2020.

Williams, Simon J., and Gillian Bendelow. *The Lived Body: Sociological Themes, Embodied Issues.* London: Routledge, 1998.

16 On Deafness in Ancient Egyptian Literary and Para-literary Texts

Ilaria Cariddi

Introduction: Outlines of the Approach, and the Lexicon Related to Deafness

The subject of deafness in ancient Egypt has received limited scholarly attention, despite the profound cultural significance attributed to auditory faculties. A probable cause lies in the scarcity of sources: as indicated in the concise entry "Taubheit" in the *Lexikon der Ägyptologie*, deafness and other aural ailments are featured significantly less frequently than blindness in medical and literary texts.[1] Nevertheless, despite the complexity of the topic, and the challenge of studying a disability that is often 'invisible', both on the societal level and in bioarchaeological remains, investigations in written corpora reveal substantial data for evaluating the subject, even within the constraints of a text-centric approach.

The lexicon regarding deafness and hardness of hearing comprises:

- ***ỉmr*** – "to be deaf", WB I, 87.18, Faulkner, *Concise Dictionary,* 21 (TLA lemma-no. 26370). *Wörterbuch* reports a possible connection with the Assyrian *"ameru"*.
- ***ỉdỉ*** – "to be/become deaf", WB I, 151.13–15 (TLA lemma-no. 33890). Takács has proposed Afroasiatic correlations for *ỉdỉ*, *s<u>h</u>ỉ*, and *dng*.[2]
- ***n<u>d</u>s*** – "dull (of ears)", Faulkner, *Concise Dictionary,* 145.
- ***hhỉ*** – "to deafen, to benumb, to be unheard (of words)", WB II, 502.10; Lesko, *Dictionary* II, 88 (TLA lemma-no. 99290).
- ***sḫỉ*** – "to be deaf", Faulkner, *Concise Dictionary,* 239; Lesko, *Dictionary* II, 66; ***sḫy*** – "to be deaf", "deaf person", Lesko, *ibid.*
- ***s<u>h</u>ỉ*** – "to be deaf, deafen", Wb III, 473.16–474.10, Lesko, *Dictionary* III, 92 (TLA lemma-nos. 874802 (root), 143400, 550303, 854862); ***s<u>h</u>ỉ ḥr*** "deaf of face, neglectful", WB III, 474.5–10; Faulkner, *Concise Dictionary,* 244; ***s<u>h</u>y*** "deaf person", Wb III, 474.11–12 (TLA lemma-no. 143410).
- ***sḫ̂*** – "deaf person", in Demotic (TLA lemma-no. dm3125).
- ***dng*** – "deafness, illness of the ear", WB V, 470.2–3 (TLA lemma-no. 179970); ***dnrg*** in Late Egyptian, Lesko, *Dictionary* II, 251.

Most lemmas are determined with the ear-classifier. The word "*ms<u>d</u>r*", "ear", attested since the 4th Dynasty, is written with the sign of a cattle ear (F21); an

DOI: 10.4324/9781003440369-19

alternative spelling with the human ear (D18) emerges in the 19th Dynasty. Bovine ears might have been emblematic of the auditory sensation for their size and ability to move towards sound sources.[3] The second most common designation for ears, documented from the 18th Dynasty, is "*ꜥnḫwy*", "the two living ones":[4] a testimony to the value placed on sound perception in cultivating a virtuous, prosperous existence.

A study of deafness, in fact, necessarily rests upon the well-known premise of the role of 'hearing' in life, as presented in numerous sources, mainly paraenetic and autobiographical, from the early Middle Kingdom onwards.[5] Hearing is regarded as the primary means of acquiring knowledge and elevating the ethos: as summarized by the *Teaching of Ptahhotep*, "useful is hearing to one who hears, hearing is better than everything that is; he who hears well, speaks well . . . one who hears is loved by the god; does not hear, one whom the god hates . . . failure follows him who hears not".[6] Egyptian wisdom literature constantly advocates for 'communicative solidarity', emphasizing the importance of language in fostering social cohesion. At the heart of this notion lies attentive listening, complemented by truthful speech and righteous actions, as encapsulated by Assmann's concept of the "*homo auditor*":

> The aim of Egyptian education is the man who knows how to listen, *homo auditor*, the one who hears and obeys, the attentive, benevolent, docile individual who bows before the speaker and accepts the given advice. The entire Egyptian civilization seems to be founded on, and animated by, this ability to listen to one another.[7]

Hence, Egyptian court society displays a distinct, culturally specific correlation between physical hearing, cognitive apperception, and living a successful life, thereby implying potentially severe limitations associated with deafness. The verb "*sḏm*" covers a wide range of meanings related to hearing, paying attention, understanding, obeying, and communication with both the living and the divine sphere.[8] Therefore, hearing difficulties may hinder these abilities, and metaphorical uses of the concept of 'deafness' encompass all these subtle nuances.

Hearing Impairments in Para-literary Sources

To gain insights into the perception and attitudes regarding this disability in Egyptian society, medical sources can serve as an initial reference, although this chapter aims to minimize reliance on a medical perspective. Ear-related syndromes are described in scientific texts, which provide the nomenclature of parts of the organ[9] and detail certain ailments.

The Edwin Smith Papyrus (16th–17th Dynasty), among its 48 cases of head and torso injuries, discusses acquired hearing loss. Case 21 (Smith 8, 6–9) describes a man wounded to the temple "bleeding from one nostril and ear . . . and it is hard for him to hear speech from it (*iw ḳsn sḏm.f mdt ḫr.s*)"; case 23 (Smith 8, 18–28) illustrates a severe wound of the ear. Both are classified as treatable conditions ("an ailment I will fight with").[10] Case 22 (Smith 8, 9–17) considers a compound fracture of the temple, with blood discharge from nostrils and ear: "if you call to him and he is speechless and he cannot speak (*ỉw.f dgm.y n mdw.n.f*) . . .: an ailment not to be treated". Gloss C details the patient's unresponsiveness: "As for 'he is speechless', it means that he is silent, in sadness, without speaking (*gr m dgꜣw nn mdt*), like one suffering from feebleness (*dgy*) because of something that entered from the outside."[11] This possibly describes trauma-related neurological deafness and/or aphasia.[12]

Papyrus Ebers (18th Dynasty) has a short section on otology, providing examination of different ear discharges (Eb. 764, 91, 2–770, 92, 6).[13] In the chapters regarding the heart, its author displays a unique interest in hearing-related issues. Multiple aetiologies are proposed, ranging from vascular pathologies to external forces that penetrate the organ and abide inside it.

> Eb. 854e (99, 14–17): As for that through which the two ears are deaf (*ỉr ỉddt msḏrwy ẖr.s*): two vessels/arteries (*mtw*) leading to the root of the eye are the ones causing it. Another formulation: . . . the two temples (*mꜣꜥy*) of a man are affected with *nssw*-air. This means that a beheading demon (*ḥsḳ*) is causing (it) inside the man; so, he (*scil.* the demon) receives his (*scil.* the man's) breaths for himself.[14]
>
> Eb. 854f (100, 2–5): There are four vessels (*mtw*) to his ears, two vessels on his right shoulder, two on his left shoulder. The wind of life enters the right ear (*ꜥḳ ṯꜣw n ꜥnḫ m msḏr wnmy*); the wind of death enters the left ear (*ꜥḳ ṯꜣw n mwt m msḏr ỉꜣby*).[15]

The last statement has generally been interpreted in connection with the position of the body in the coffin on the left side, especially in Middle Kingdom burials: the right ear is the one 'free' to receive the benefits of prayers, offering formulas and vivifying rituals.[16] In 854e, deafness is attributed to a demon, as is often the case with diseases whose pathology was not understood.[17] Ears and their syndromes are notably interconnected with the eyes, as will be observed throughout the study.

> Eb. 854c – 855d (99, 21–100, 1): As for the fact that he is deaf and he cannot open his mouth (*ỉr ỉd.f m wnn rꜣ.f*), all his body-parts are weak in consequence of that (thing) of which the heart receives. As for the anger (*ꜣd*) that has arisen in the heart, it is a torsion (*ẖꜣsf*; *scil.* of the *mtw*-vessels) . . . . It follows that he has become deaf, his vessels sagging after their twisting has heated (*hh*) them. Then it will unravel.

It is unclear whether the initial segment proposes an aetiology of deaf-muteness, or for pathologies resulting in the patient's unresponsiveness. The phrase "that of which the heart receives" likely refers to the "breath (*ṯꜣw*)" at the outset of the section (855a, 99, 12); the heart may inappropriately absorb it, leading to general feebleness, and hindering the reception of sounds. The latter portion incorporates deafness into a clinical depiction of an individual whose heart is overtaken by "anger (*ꜣd*)", derived from the twisting and heating of blood vessels. As elucidated by Nyord, "unlike many humorological traditions, Egyptian medical texts do not seem to regard the temperature of the body as an equilibrium of forces . . . rather, heat in various forms is portrayed as a sign or cause of illness".[18] Several Egyptian lexemes denoting anger and confrontation stem from the semantic domain of 'heat', and from medical terminology. The conceptual metaphor associating emotions and temperature, while well attested cross-linguistically, holds particular significance in Egyptian ethical discourse, especially concerning verbal violence.[19] Bardinet observes that "*ꜣd*", with the classifier of the sparrow (G37), may indicate not common rage, but a pathological attack; he suggests Meniere's syndrome, or apoplectiform deafness.[20]

The Berlin Medical Papyrus (P. Berlin 3038, 19th Dynasty) prescribes fumigations "to drive out deafness that comes from the outside (*hhyt nt ꜥḳ m rwt*(*y*))" (Bln. 70, 6, 10–11); "another (fumigation) to remove a dead man inside the ear (*kt nt sḥrw mt m msḏr*)" (Bln. 71, 6, 11). The *mwt*, roaming, unjustified dead, are often causes for illnesses in medical and magical texts.[21] Bln. 200–3 (*v* 2, 6–12) also deal with hearing diseases, prescribing remedies to unblock ears from "heaviness (*dns*)?" and "*stt*", one of the main pathogens in medical treatises, perceived as traveling infective entities that could enter any body part, particularly in certain periods of the year.[22]

The second-century CE Manual of the Priest of Sekhmet from the Tebtynis temple library (PSI inv. I 73+P. Carlsberg 463) addresses the notorious "pestilence of the year (*iꜣdt rnpt*)"; it states about the infirm that "his face is blind and deaf as a newborn dog (*iw ḥr.f ḫp sḫ mi ḥm ꜣm ṯsm*)", but, presumably after the cure, he will say: "I have freed myself from the binding of the god, I have opened my eyes . . . my deaf ears (*ꜥnḫwy.i sḫy*)".[23]

The investigation of disease identification, remedies, and incidence through histological analysis lies outside the purview of this study.[24] To conclude this section, it is significant to note that, in contrast to Mesopotamian medical traditions, which lack therapeutic interventions for such profound sensory impairments as deafness and blindness, Egyptian texts offer explanations and treatments for at least certain types of disabilities. It is also pertinent to acknowledge the existence of medically substantiated occurrences of hearing pathologies. Khufu's western cemetery at Giza has yielded cases of cholesteatoma and mastoiditis, which may have led to deafness;[25] the mummified remains PUM II (Penn Museum, Philadelphia) of a first-century CE man present a pathological tympanic membrane perforation, suggesting a middle ear infection.[26] An historical testimony of a deaf individual is also provided by the mummy-label BM EA24471, attributed to a second-century CE woman from Psonis (Bassuna) named, in Demotic and Greek, "Senpsais, daughter of Psais the deaf (*Šr-šyt tꜣ Pꜣ-šyt sḫ*/Σενψαϊς Ψαϊτος κωφοῦ)".[27]

Auditory impairments are also documented because of punitive measures. Mutilation of ears and nose (usually in pair) is attested especially in the New Kingdom for several crimes, mainly trespassing/alteration of boundaries, appropriation of temple resources, office abuse, theft and false testimony.[28] It was the 'standard' penalty referenced in legal oaths: "If I speak falsehood, may my nose and ears be cut off, me being (banished) to Kush."[29] Such punishment was probably restricted to courts operating under royal jurisdiction,[30] but evidence suggests its rather frequent implementation.[31] The oath formula, royal decrees, and trial proceedings imply that survival was expected after the trauma. While the lived experience of mutilated persons is not preserved in written sources, it is probable that they did not face complete deafness, but rather diminished hearing, confusion when receiving sounds from multiple sources, ear infections, and chronic maladies.[32] Furthermore, mutilation marks, especially on the face, would have posed significant challenges to social interactions, also for the probable stigma stemming from knowledge of the injuries' source. Supra-functional significances of such maiming are discussed in the next paragraph.

Magical and Divine Influence on Hearing Ailments

Deafness and related afflictions are also recurrent within magical texts and funerary formulae for the restoration of bodily functions. Given the extensive evidence, this section presents a curated collection of salient instances to provide insights on culturally perceived impairments.

The Pyramid Texts frequently allude to liberation of the pharaoh's auditory faculties: "he opens his ears" (Pyr. 712b), "his ears are opened" (Pyr. 788c), "disclose for him his mouth, open his ears" (Pyr. 1673b), "Unis is not blind, even if you place him in darkness; he is not deaf, even if he does not hear your voice (*n šp Wnỉs dỉ.k sw m kkw n ỉd.f tm.f sḏm ḥrw.k*)" (Pyr. 499b-c). Similarly, in the Coffin Texts it is said: "O Hearer, o Unstopper (of ears), hear me, unstop (me?) (*smtt sšnt smt ỉm.ỉ sšn.ỉ*)" (CT III, 13b-14a), "my eyes are opened for me by the Eyeless one . . . my ears are opened for me by this Falcon to whom men do not speak, and I hear with them (*ỉw wn n.ỉ msḏrwy.ỉ sḏm.ỉ ỉm sny ỉn bỉk pw n tw mdw n.f*)" (CT II, 117f-h), "I am not blind, I am not deaf (*n šp.ỉ n ỉd.ỉ*)" (CT V, 233g).

Several formulae related to our subject are found in the Book of the Dead among those aimed to reverse the processes of death. For example, BD 178: "Formula for raising the body, opening the eyes, strengthening the ears (*sḫm ꜥnḫwy*)", and BD 154 "my eye is not swollen . . . my ear is not deaf (*n ỉd msḏr.ỉ*)". In BD 190, the deceased is initiated into "mysteries no one knows for the treatment of the transfigured spirit . . . to drive deafness out of him (*dr ỉdt ḥr.f*), to open his face along with the god".

Distance from such deathly impediments is also wished to the fictional addressee of the epistolary *Tale of Woe* (21st-23rd Dynasties): "Your ears should escape the hindrances of your body and its parts (*ỉw smty.k sšsꜣ ḥr ỉtnt ḏt.k ỉry.sn*)".[33] The desired result is described poetically in the invocation to Mut of the cattle accountant for Amun Samut-Kyky (Ramesses II): "May you keep me safe, until my end . . . let my eyes see the rays . . ., (let my) ears hear without deafness (*ꜥnḫwy sḏm nn ỉd*) . . ., all my [limbs] complete, as (in) life".[34]

Conversely, the same faculties are negated to demons: "I have blinded his eyes and annihilated his hearing . . . rendering it non-existent (*ỉw nḥm.n.ỉ sḏm ỉr.f . . . ỉr.ỉ sw m tm wn*)".[35] In the Book of Gates, quoting Morenz, "Apophis appears as the . . .

embodiment of anticommunication. Language endows meaning and relation, and Apophis is the negation of precisely these ideas. . . . 'One without its eyes is this snake, without its nose, without its ears (*ỉwty msḏrwy.fy*)'".[36]

The Opening the Mouth ritual and associated liturgies serve the same objectives, (re)activating all the sensory and cognitive capabilities of a deceased, or a statue, through 'opening' their mouths, eyes, and ears, thus facilitating their role as mediums for cultic communication. In view of this principle, the punitive cutting of ears carries profound supra-practical consequences. It is plausible that the incapacitation of the organs during lifetime was believed to persist post-mortem; therefore, the act could disrupt divine judgment upon the deceased, their ability to receive vivifying formulas, and their interaction with the divine sphere, in both lifetime and the hereafter.[37] Systematic disfigurements of statues and paintings, particularly concentrated on the face, are attested since the Old Kingdom. Although the interpretation of certain cases, such as the renowned 'reserve heads', continues to present challenges, the deliberate aim of impeding the image's performativity is evident.[38]

For safeguarding vital senses during life, reference can be made to the corpus of oracular amuletic decrees for the protection of children, dated between the late New Kingdom and the Third Intermediate Period. While safety against blindness is attested in virtually all papyri, hearing ailments feature in 8 of 21 examples of Edwards's compendium; the formulae are "I shall keep her/him safe from an ailment of the eye, from an ailment of the ear (*ỉw šd st/sw šnw msḏr*)",[39] "I shall keep his/her ears healthy (*ỉw.ỉ snb ꜥnḫwy.f/.st*)",[40] "I/we shall cause her/his eye to see, her/his ears to hear (*ỉw.ỉ/.n rdỉt . . . sḏm ꜥnḫwy.st/.f*)",[41] "I shall keep healthy her/his left ear [and right ear] (*ỉw.ỉ snb msḏrꜣꜥ.st/.f ỉꜣby*)".[42] Ocular and auditory problems are, again, paired, with eyes typically preceding. P. Turin 1983*v* displays specifications resonating with medical nomenclature: "We shall keep healthy her ears . . . and the arteries of her ears (*nꜣ mt*(*w*) *ꜥnḫwy.st*). We shall keep her safe from any constriction (?) of the ear, from any deafness of the ear, from any ineffectiveness of the ear (*ỉw.n šd st r sbn nb n msḏr r sḫ nb n msḏr r tm nb n msḏr*). We shall cause it to hear and not allow it to be deaf (*ỉw.n rdỉt sḏm.f ỉw bn ỉw.n rdỉt sḫ.f*)".[43]

Hearing Impairments in Literary Texts

In the prologue of the *Teaching of Ptahhotep,* dated to late 11th–early 12th Dynasties but copied at least until the 20th,[44] the eponymous vizier famously laments the ailments of old age, offering a record of socially acknowledged disabilities. Hearing loss occurs in pair with failing eyesight:

> "*ỉrty nḏs.w ꜥnḫwy ỉmr.w . . .*
> *rꜣ gr*(*.w*) *n mdw.n.f*"
> "Eyes are weak, ears have become deaf . . .
> the mouth is silent, it does not speak.[45]

For "be/become deaf", the Middle Kingdom P. Prisse (4.4=11) has the *hapax legomenon* "*ỉmr*",[46] later copied in the Carnarvon tablet (C, 2),[47] the earliest New

Kingdom manuscript (17th-18th Dynasties).[48] The sense is, however, assured by the fact that other New Kingdom copies, P. BM EA10509 (L2, 1,4), P. Turin 54014 (T, 2) and O. DeM 1233 (3) have "*ỉd.w*".[49] This does not necessarily imply that copyists were unacquainted with this verb, since the tendency to replace uncommon words in more recent redactions of *Ptahhotep* is not absolute, and may result from aesthetic preferences.[50] The prologue thus poses an immediate focus on the importance of 'hearing', to be echoed in the epilogue's portrait of the perceptive reader/listener who has internalized the advice: "his eyes seeing, his ears complete at hearing what is beneficial for his son".[51]

Deaf persons are mentioned in the eulogy of the king's performative and transformative authority in the *Teaching of a Man to His Son*, commonly attributed to the late 12th Dynasty.[52]

> He turns the ignorant into the wise. . .,
> he enables the least to be like the great. . . .
> He teaches the mute to speak (*ỉw.f sbꜣ.f ꜣbb r mdt*),
> he opens the ears of the deaf (*swbꜣ.f ꜥnẖwy ỉdw*).[53]

Notwithstanding the lexical difficulties, the meaning is perspicuous: the king possesses the ability to accomplish seemingly impossible feats, on a social level, and even in physical terms. Deafness is juxtaposed with mutism, as in *Ptahhotep* (though with a more specific term, "*ꜣbb*", instead of "*grw*"[54]), and they serve as 'tangible' examples of the miraculous and pervasive royal power. While hyperbolic in nature, this acknowledgment represents a rare inclusion of disabilities within a catalogue of the underprivileged members of society, alongside the poor, the struggling, the lowliest. The pair deaf-mute is rooted in reality, as observed in medical literature; however, within the present context, the conceptual emphasis on the relationship between speaking and hearing supersedes the traditionally more prominent blindness. A fragmentary document of Thutmose III seems to paint a similar scenario: "Royal decree . . . to protect the blind (?), to chase away pathogens, to cure he who [suffers] from his illness, after His Majesty had read a book of protection from the ancestors' [time]."[55]

Meyer-Dietrich has instead suggested that "mute" and "deaf" in the *Teaching* could indicate the deceased, whose senses are reawakened by the king when entering the Duat.[56] Presumably interpreting such renovation within the framework of the Amarnian concept of afterlife, she substantiates the hypothesis citing the aforementioned BD 190: "secrets of the god's land . . . to drive deafness out of him (*dr ỉdt ḥr.f*), to cause his face/sight to be opened with the god", underlining the usage of "*ỉdt*" for deafness.[57] However, "*ỉdi*" is also present in corpora related to earthly life, such as P. Ebers 854c and 854e. The passage rather appears to emphasise the role of the king's instruction in improving worldly existence, as well as the social centrality of discourse, wherein even individuals who are deaf and mute can be incorporated: as remarked by Worthington, "It is also interesting that the head of the state . . . – the 'linchpin of society' – should be presented as a promoter, an enabler, of speech".[58] Disabled persons can become recipients of royal propaganda, and be transformed into propagandists themselves.

From a philological perspective, a noteworthy wordplay can be discerned between "*sbꜣ*", "teach" and "*swbꜣ*", "make open": deafness is here visualised not as an inability, but as an obstruction of the auditory canals (the aforementioned "*mtw*", which, also in Egyptian, share the same designation as waterways), that can be removed to 'clear the way'. Lastly, it is interesting to observe that "*ỉdw*" is employed for "deaf", as in New Kingdom manuscripts of *Ptahhotep*; however, an examination of the sources reveals that scribes encountered difficulties with the orthography of this word. Fischer-Elfert ponders whether it has to do with its supposed antiquity and/or rareness, though recognising its presence in the 'more modern' copies of *Ptahhotep*. He suggests that the confusion may have arisen due to the usage of "*ꜥnḫwy*" for "ears", whereas other texts, such as P. Ebers, employ "*ỉdỉ*" with the more customary "*msḏrwy*".[59] The possible unfamiliarity of scribes with this lemma is, in any case, remarkable.

An overturning of this motive of the almighty power of the ruler is staged in the *Tale of the Eloquent Peasant.* As it is known, the text mobilises several key cultural values of Egyptian society, particularly the one of 'hearing' (or lack thereof). The deliberate impassiveness of the High Steward Rensi, who remains silent before the peasant's pleas to protract his brilliant orations, sets the plot in motion, yet also constitutes the crucial misunderstanding. Readers are provided with the motives behind the choice, while the unaware protagonist perceives it as indifference and injustice: "Judge (*lit.* "listener"), you just not hear! So why do you not hear (*sḏmw n ꜣ sḏm.n.k tm.k tr sḏm ḥr m*)?"[60] Hence, he accuses Rensi of being the antithesis of the 'renovating authority' eulogised by the *Teaching of a Man*:

> *pr mꜣw špw sḏmw sḫw ssmw ḫpr*(*w*) *m stmnw*
> For the watcher has turned out blind, the hearer deaf, the leader became a misleader![61]

Since "*mꜣꜣ*", "to see", also carries the connotation of "concerning oneself with something", "*šp*", "be blind", can allude to moral disregard.[62] This observation carries even greater significance for "*sḫỉ*", "be deaf", which, as we will discuss, possesses a powerful metaphorical implication when combined with the object of the peasant's discourses, *maat.* His yearning for a "good hearing" and for justice lends great weight to the topic of 'deafness' in the *Tale*. The third petition expands upon these themes:

> The son of Meru is astray. His face is blind to what he sees, deaf to what he hears (*ḥr.f šp*(*w*) *r mꜣꜣt.f sḫ*(*w*) *r sḏmt.f*), his heart drifting from what he is reminded of (*th-ỉb ḥr sḫꜣyt n.f*).[63]

The peasant employs imageries of ailments (even "*thỉ*", the "malfunctioning" of the heart is mentioned as "perishing and forgetfulness" of the organ in P. Ebers[64]) for their figurative overtones. Rensi is capable of seeing, but he cannot perceive; he hears, but he fails to listen. Inattentiveness, inertia, deliberate deficiency in 'seeing, hearing, and remembering' are the offences against *maat* of which the protagonist accuses his interlocutor, held responsible for disrupting the principles of communicative and factual solidarity emphasized in wisdom texts. The non-response of Rensi not only violates decorum, as seen in *Ptahhotep*'s exhortation to listen attentively and allow petitioners to relieve their hearts,[65] but also constitutes an unacceptable behaviour for a judge. A comparison can be drawn with the Nauri decree of Sethi I: "As for the officer (?) . . . to [whom] anyone . . . goes complaining to, and his face is deaf towards him (*sẖ ḥr r.f*), . . . the law shall be executed against him".[66]

Middle Kingdom literature also attests cases of temporary loss of hearing, or incapacity to receive/process discourse. In the *Tale of the Shipwrecked Sailor*, upon the clamour of the theophany of the Snake in "a roar of thunder"[67] and his menacing inquiry, the protagonist reacts as follows:

> *ỉw mdw.*[*n.f*] *n.ỉ nn wỉ ḥr sḏm st ỉw.ỉ m bꜣḥ.*[*f*] *ẖm.n.*(*ỉ*) *wỉ*
> He spoke to me, but I did not hear it; I was in his presence, but I did not know myself.[68]

The last expression is idiomatic for "losing consciousness"; shock, and perhaps loudness, temporarily disrupt the ability to engage with verbal communication. A similar formulation will reappear in the New Kingdom *Longing for Memphis* (P. Anastasi IV), in which the protagonist thus describes nostalgia: "My heart is not in my body, evil has seized all my limbs, my eye is faint through looking, my ear hears not (*tꜣy.ỉ msḏr bw mḥ*)".[69]

A difficult case is found in the *Dispute of a Man with His Ba*, in the second 'parable' narrated by the *ba* to illustrate the imponderability of life. A man asks his wife for a meal (before due time, possibly), then walks out "for a moment only";

> *ʿnn.f sw r pr.f ỉw.f mỉ ky ḥmt.f ḥr sšꜣ n.f n sḏm.n.f n.s sṯ n.f* (?) *wš ỉb n wpwtyw*
> When he turns back to his house, he is like another man; his wife pleads to him, but he does not hear her, offended (?) and unreceptive to those of the household.[70]

Due to rare words and unclear spellings, there is no consensus on what happens to the man, if a sudden strike of an infirmity, of mental illness, or a fit of rage, and therefore whether he "cannot hear" or "doesn't listen". Allen interprets the *hapax* "*wš ỉb*" as "emotional barrenness, hence, lack of receptivity".[71] A noteworthy analogy can be drawn with the case of P. Ebers 855d describing deafness resulting from a pathological outburst of wrath: "anger that has arisen in the heart . . . he has become deaf". The convergence of cardiac distress, auditory impairment, and rage suggests a connection, potentially indicating a psychosomatic ailment.

As for classical literature, the information, quoted by Cicero,[72] Pliny the Elder and Seneca,[73] that dwellers of the Nile cataracts regions were deaf due to the thunderous waters, consequently leading a difficult existence, is not supported by pharaonic sources. A more plausible explanation is that locals were inclined to raise their voices against the loud background sound, creating a mistaken perception of deafness. Nonetheless, it is likely that certain occupations experienced hardness of hearing because of high-noise working and living conditions.[74]

Metaphorical Deafness: Negligence and Disinterest

While contemporary studies and modern disability community discourage metaphorical uses of disability language,[75] it remains necessary to concisely examine the matter within this study, as it offers understanding on certain perspectives of disabled and nondisabled bodies.[76] The occurrences of figurative uses of 'deafness' can be understood in the framework of Conceptual Metaphor Theory (CMT), which posits that abstract concepts are represented in terms of more concrete sensorimotor and bodily experiences.[77] Because a D/deaf person may be unable to hear an auditory input, individuals deemed 'deaf' to commands or advice are symbolically portrayed as unresponsive, unwilling to hear and act upon the message. The lexicon of 'deafness' is thus used to describe nonsensory processes, in particular, 'moral deafness'. As discussed earlier, the *Eloquent Peasant* accuses Rensi of such a crime:

> Do not blind your face (*m šp ḥr.k*) against one who looks to you! . . . There is no yesterday for the negligent, no friend for him who is deaf to truth (*nn ḫnms n sẖ mꜣꜥt*).[78]

The excerpt revolves around metaphors of disability, regarded as deliberate, reprehensible behaviours, with 'deafness' outweighing 'blindness' in significance within the *Tale*. As highlighted by the peasant's injunction to "speak maat, do maat (*ḏd mꜣꜥt ỉr mꜣꜥt*)",[79] refusing to hear and speak truth is as grave as refusing to act on it, and Rensi's conduct is a violation of 'communicative solidarity and justice', to employ Assmann's definitions.

It is significant that the avoidance of this crucial fault will feature in the 'negative confession' of BD 125: "I have not deafened my face to words of truth (*n sẖ.ỉ ḥr.ỉ ḥr mdt nt mꜣꜥt*)". After passing judgement, the illuminated spirit exclaims: "How beautiful it is to see with two eyes, (having) two ears for hearing *maat* (*nfr.wy mꜣꜣ m ỉrty ꜥnḫwy m sḏm mꜣꜥt*)!" (BD 133)

The locution "*sẖ ḥr*", literally "deaf of face",[80] assumes a connotation of "unwillingness to hear/heed", evolving into "turning a deaf ear", "be neglectful". Also, "it is used in reference to criminal negligence concerning a legal provision, endowment, or upkeep of an institution".[81] The following occurrences illustrate its connection to the auditory domain, emphasising how it involves 'lack of listening', rather than simple inattentiveness.

- *Eloquent Peasant*, B1 219 (12th Dynasty): "his face . . . deaf to what he hears (*ḥr.f . . . sẖ(w) r sḏmt.f*)".
- Sehel graffito n°76 of Antef (Senwosret III), address to visitors: "do not be neglectful of what is on (my) mouth (*m sẖ ḥrw.ṯn r nt(t) ḥr rꜣ*)".[82]

- Stela of User, Grenoble Inv.1954 (Thutmose III), address to visitors: "do not be neglectful concerning what I have said (*m sẖ ḥrw.ṯn r ḏdi*)".[83]
- Nauri decree of Sethi I: "As for the officer (?) . . . to [whom] anyone . . . goes complaining to, and his face is deaf towards him (*sẖ ḥr r.f*)".[84]
- Wadi Mia decree of Sethi I: "as for anyone who shall be deaf to this decree (*ir pꜣ nty nb iw.f r sẖ ḥr r wḏt tn*), Osiris will pursue him".[85]

Remarkably, "*sẖ ḥr*" also carries a positive connotation, a 'necessary deafness' against verbal aggression and litigation. The theme of non-intervention is recurrent in paraenetic literature, often presenting silence as the preferred course of action.[86] However, the counsel to 'be deaf' precedes even silence, as a responsible act of rendering oneself impervious to damaging words. In wisdom literature, this connotation is found in two passages ascribed to the *Teaching of a Man*, but recently confirmed as part of the *Teaching of Hordjedef*:[87]

> § 17, 2: "*m sḏm sḏw r ky*", "heed not slanders against another."
> § 24, 7: "*ḳb sẖ ḥr.f tm štm*", "tranquil is he who deafens his face and does not provoke."[88]

A comparable example features in the self-presentation of Amenhotep son of Hapu (Amenhotep III), effectively combining the requirements of hearing and non-hearing: "There is no man called near me whose words I do not listen . . . I do not give my face to listen to falsities discrediting another (*n rd.i ḥr.i r sḏm iwms r sḏw ky*)".[89]

Another metaphorical use of 'deafness' involves disinterest and obduracy, particularly in the reproach of idle students in New Kingdom 'scholastic miscellanies'.

> P. Anastasi V, 17,3–5: "I heard that you whirl around in pleasures and have neglected what I said (*mkḥꜣ.k iḏdt.i*). You pay no attention to any words: pleasures have deafened your hearing (*bw rdi.k ib.k n mdwt nbt hhi ꜣbw mꜣꜥ.k*)".[90]

The last phrase, literally "pleasures have deafened your temple",[91] employs medical terminology: "*hhi*" as in "*hhyt*", the "deafness coming from outside" of Bln. 70, and "*mꜣꜥ*(y)", the "temple" of Eb. 854e, affected by poor distribution of air caused by a demon. Once more, the origin of auditory insensitivity lies outside the body, but here it is represented by distracting leisure. In an analogous text, such pleasures have aural connotations: "singing to the pipe, chanting to the flute, intoning to the lyre".[92]

> P. Anastasi IV, 2,4–8: "I am told that you have abandoned writing . . . your ear is deaf (*msḏr.k dnrg*). . . . Yet you are not one who is deaf and cannot hear, to whom they make (signs) with the hand (*nn mntk sḫy iw bw ir.f sḏm ir.tw n.f m ḏrt*)."[93]

The passage's most intriguing aspect lies in its deliberate deconstruction of the metaphor, with the distinction between the heedless scribe and actual deaf individuals, who genuinely "cannot hear" and bear no responsibility for it. Yet they are integrated into conversations and actively engaged in life, with a notable reference to communication through hands – possibly alluding to the existence of a form of sign language, or simply to communication with gestures. The idle student, instead, willingly isolates himself from beneficial advice, and thus, from life.

Conclusions: Hypotheses on the Lived Experience of Deafness

The presented catalogue has illustrated a complex landscape that, while offering insights into certain aspects, also sparks unresolved questions about our understanding of the daily existence of deaf individuals in Pharaonic and Graeco-Roman Egypt. For example, deafness was not found where perhaps one expected it. Exemplary acts of benevolence in élite autobiographies do not seem to include mentions of caring for "the deaf"; similarly, the *Teaching of Amenemope* recommends not to ridicule a blind person, a dwarf person, a paralyzed person, because "man is clay and straw, and god is his creator".[94] We have observed how scribes were occasionally unfamiliar with the terminology of hearing loss. Was deafness 'overlooked'?

Hearing impairments, whether congenital or acquired, were certainly not uncommon throughout Egyptian history, and both medical and magical texts, in fact, offered related protections and cures; yet it is conceivable that deafness, if not rarer, may have been (or perceived as) less impactful than other conditions. The absence of provisions for deaf persons amongst the moral duties in advice literature and autobiographies might suggest that they required less (or no) support, or experienced less (or no) marginalisation. However, it is also possible that hearing difficulties were not specifically mentioned because they were not as 'visible' as other disabilities. Deafness might have been attributed an in-between, singular status, akin to how some members of the Deaf community today do not consider themselves disabled.[95]

It has been reasonably assumed that disabilities were more common and had greater lifelong effects in the ancient world,[96] a notion that holds several implications for societal studies. For instance, the Edwin Smith Papyrus describes injuries, and acquired impairments, that might have occurred during labour or battle; the anthology may have targeted the battlefield, or its aftermath. As a corollary, amongst the élites, particularly military figures of the New Kingdom, there must have been a significant number of disabled individuals, as estimated for later periods.[97] The mentioned second-century CE woman "Senpsais, daughter of Psais the deaf"[98] testimonies that Psais was probably a man not without means (since his daughter could afford mummification), known in the community as "the deaf", therefore not unacknowledged as a disabled person; on the other hand, his designation implies infrequency of deaf individuals in his village.

The question of social acceptance of hearing-related disabilities remains partially ambiguous. Multiple sources concur in portraying an overall inclusive attitude in Egyptian society, wherein most illnesses and physical differences, albeit attributed to divine agency, were not generally perceived as punishments, and not stigmatised.[99] While literary passages may use figurative deafness derogatorily, some differentiate between the metaphor and the actual impairment, acknowledging the potential harmfulness or inaccuracy of the comparison, and engaging in its deconstruction. Ear mutilations probably carried a degree of stigma, but also due to the visible reminder they provided of the committed crime.

The aspect of employment opportunities for individuals with aural disabilities lacks direct sources of information. In a society such as that of ancient Egypt, wherein 'hearing' was regarded as a crucial aspect of individual and communal well-being, a deaf person may have faced significant challenges. Building on textual materials, it seems conceivable that profound hearing impairments could hinder full participation in society, particularly in élite roles that emphasized speech and listening. Nevertheless, we do not possess definitive evidence to confirm or disprove this assessment. Our understanding of Egyptian attitudes towards deafness remains limited, and it is plausible that deaf persons were treated differently based on status and individual circumstances.

Textual sources present a dual prospect on deafness: one that is non-judgemental and non-stigmatising, potentially perceiving it as a condition with limited reliance on assistance, and accepted as part of life, especially for old age. On the other hand, it is, comprehensibly, regarded as something to safeguard against and find remedies for. Due to impaired hearing, elderly Ptahhotep is considered inapt to vizier duties. However, his disabilities do not overshadow his skills and experience, nor do they exclude him from society; instead, he can fulfil a new, key role in providing life guidance. Likewise, as observed in the *Teaching of a Man* and in scholastic miscellanies, deaf people can be integrated into collective communication.

Within the eschatological dimension, religious beliefs determine a shift in perspective regarding disability, undoubtedly driven by the significance of possessing an intact body for a successful transition into the netherworld. Thus, post-mortem concerns for bodily integrity may have obscured actual lived experiences of deafness; reasons of decorum, and the performative power ascribed to writing, have probably prevented its mention in the élites' autobiographical narrations.

It is the author's hope that the evidence hereby presented will serve as a foundation to delve into additional dimensions of the topic, to expand our comprehension of the material and socio-cultural intricacies concerning deaf individuals in ancient Egypt.

Notes

1 Grieshammer (1986, 241).
2 Takács (1999, 176).
3 Emerit (2011, 63).
4 Störk (1982, 559).
5 Schlichting (1977, 1232–33).
6 539–41, 545–46, 572; Zăba (1956, 58–60).
7 Assmann (2003, 44); translation by the present author.
8 WB IV, 384–87; Schlichting (1977).
9 Störk (1982, 559).
10 Bardinet (1995, 506–7). All transliterations and translations are by the present author.
11 Ibid., 560.
12 Pahor (1992b, 686).
13 Bardinet (1995, 358–59), Pahor (1992a, 684–85).

14 Bardinet (1995, 92).
15 Ibid., 97.
16 Meyer-Dietrich (2017, 85).
17 Lucarelli (2010, 3).
18 Nyord (2018, 25–26).
19 Shupak (2009, 245–60).
20 Bardinet (1995, 95–96).
21 Lucarelli (2010, 2).
22 Bardinet (1995, 125–28).
23 A1, 2, 9; Rosati (1998, 197–98, 204, 206).
24 For these topics, refer to Bardinet, Pahor, and related bibliography.
25 Pahor (1992a, 685).
26 Benitez (1988, 490).
27 Arlt (2011, n. 24, 18). "*ꞽd/ꞽdt*", "The De af" (and possibly "*ḏꜣg/ḏꜣgt*", "*8nrg/8ngt*"), are attested as personal names in pharaonic times: Ranke PN I, 14; 16; 180; 400; II, 11; 27; 178; 332.
28 Lorton (1977, 25–26, 28, 35, 38, 40, 42), Loktionov (2017, 263–91), Matić (2019, 35–36).
29 Loktionov (2017, 264–65).
30 Ibid., 273.
31 Loktionov (2019, 10).
32 Loktionov (2017, 275–78).
33 I, 1,14–2,2; Caminos (1977, 11, 21–22). The passage is difficult, and could refer to earthly life or to the hereafter; see discussions in Caminos and in TLA https://thesaurus-linguae-aegyptiae.de/sentence/IBUBdxsec91viEjlghK7rzv3cho.
34 TT409; KRI III, 337, 9.
35 P. Bremner-Rhind 27, 11; Faulkner (1933, 62).
36 Morenz (2004, 204).
37 Loktionov (2017, 284–85).
38 Ibid., 266, 278–79.
39 Edwards (1960, L.2*v*, 40–41).
40 Ibid., L.5*r*, 12–13; L.6*r*, 23; T.1*v*, 59–60; P.4, 45–46.
41 Ibid., T.1*r*, 51–52; C.1*r*, 24–26.
42 Ibid., B*r*, 75–76.
43 Ibid., T.1*v*, 59–65. The nominal use of "*tm n msḏr*" for "ear ineffectiveness/failure" is a *unicum*.
44 Hagen (2012, 129, 187).
45 Zăba (1956, 16).
46 WB I, 87, 18; Grieshammer (1986, 241).
47 Hagen (2012, 228).
48 Ibid., 174.
49 Ibid., 251.
50 Ibid., 228.
51 528–31; ibid., 208–19.
52 Alternative proposals suggest an early 18th Dynasty dating, yet evidence remains inconclusive: see Stauder (2013, 508).
53 §4, 1–10; Fischer-Elfert (1999, 68).
54 For the term, see Posener (1965, 192–93).
55 P. Berlin 3049, as quoted in Lhoyer (2021, 18).
56 Meyer-Dietrich (2017, 125).
57 Ibid.
58 Worthington (2013, 285).
59 Fischer-Elfert (1999, 77).

60 B1 211; Parkinson (1991, 31).
61 B1 144–45; ibid., 24.
62 Parkinson (2012, 122–23).
63 B1 218–20; Parkinson (1991, 31).
64 Eb. 855u, col. 102, 4–5; Bardinet (1995, 110–11).
65 264–76; Zăba (1956, 36–47).
66 KRI I, 58, 7–10.
67 56; Golénischeff (1912, 3).
68 73–76; ibid., 4.
69 Gardiner (1937, 39, 5, 3–4).
70 83–85; Allen (2010, 76–78).
71 Ibid., 78.
72 Cic., *Rep.,* 6, 18–19.
73 Plin., *HN* VI, 181; Sen., *QNat.,* 4, 2, 5.
74 Pahor (1992a, 686–87).
75 E.g. Morris (2021).
76 The subject will be discussed in full by the present author in a forthcoming paper.
77 Lakoff and Johnson (1980).
78 B2 105–10; Parkinson (1991, 46–47).
79 B1 351; Parkinson (1991, 45).
80 WB III 474, 5–10.
81 Morschauser (1987, 60).
82 Habachi (1953, 51–53).
83 Urk. IV, 1033, 6.
84 KRI I, 58, 7–10.
85 KRI I, 70, 3–4.
86 Cariddi (2024), esp. 40–54.
87 Verhoeven (2023).
88 Fischer-Elfert (1999, 174–76, 248, 250–51).
89 Statue CG42127; Urk. IV 1828,2; Varille (1968, 5–6).
90 Gardiner (1937, 7–8, 65).
91 For the extended meaning "hearing" for "temple", see Caminos (1954, 251).
92 Anastasi IV, 12,2; ibid., 182.
93 Gardiner (1937, 5, 6–37).
94 24, 9–14; Laisney (2007, 210–11). Deafness is also absent in comparable passages of other Teachings: ibid., 213–14.
95 See, e.g., Harvey (2013, 42).
96 See, e.g., Pudsey (2017, 22–34).
97 Morris (2022, 14–15, 262–63).
98 Arlt (2011, n. 24, 18), TM Per 81905.
99 Volokhine (2015, 139–41), David (2017, 84–86), Lhoyer (2021). Interpretations on the renowned Deir el-Medina supplications to alleviate divine-imposed 'blindness' vary, and they may not even pertain to a physical ailment: see Assmann (1994, 13–29), Galán (1999, 18–30). Conversely, evidence from the Graeco-Roman period attests to some skin conditions being perceived as divine punishment, resulting in exclusion from specific positions and banishment: Volokhine (2015), Jacob (2018, 65–69).

Bibliography

Allen, James P. *The Debate Between a Man and His Soul.* Leiden: Brill, 2010.
Arlt, Carolin. *Deine Seele möge leben für immer und ewig: die demotischen Mumienschilder im British Museum.* Leuven: Peeters, 2011.

Assmann, Jan. "Ocular Desire in a Time of Darkness. Urban Festivals and Divine Visibility in Ancient Egypt." *Jahrbuch Für Religiöse Anthropologie* 1 (1994): 13–29.

Assmann, Jan. *Maât, l'Égypte pharaonique et l'idée de justice sociale.* Paris: La Maison de Vie, 2003.

Bardinet, Thierry. *Les Papyrus Médicaux de l'Égypte Pharaonique: Traduction Intégrale et Commentaire.* Paris: Fayard, 1995.

Benitez, Jaime T. "Otopathology of Egyptian Mummy Pum II: Final Report." *The Journal of Laryngology & Otology* 102, no. 6 (1988): 485–90.

Caminos, Ricardo A. *Late-Egyptian Miscellanies.* London: Oxford University Press, 1954.

Caminos, Ricardo A. *A Tale of Woe.* Oxford: Griffith Institute, 1977.

Cariddi, Ilaria. "Discourses on Ethics and Ethics of Discourse in Ancient Egyptian Wisdom Literature." In *Wisdom Discourse in the Ancient World*, edited by Sara De Martin and Anna Lucia Furlan, 34–63. London: Routledge, 2024.

David, Rosalie. "Egyptian Medicine and Disability. From Pharaonic to Greco-Roman Egypt." In *Disability in Antiquity,* edited by Christian Laes, 75–89. London: Routledge, 2017.

Edwards, I. E. Stephen. *Hieratic Papyri in the British Museum: Fourth Series. Oracular Amuletic Decrees of the Late New Kingdom.* London: British Museum, 1960.

Emerit, Sibylle. "Listening to the Gods: Echoes of the Divine in Ancient Egypt." In *Laut und Leise: der Gebrauch von Stimme und Klang in Historischen Kulturen,* edited by Erika Meyer-Dietrich, 61–89. Bielefeld: Transcript, 2011.

Faulkner, Raymond O. *The Papyrus Bremner-Rhind: British Museum No. 10188.* Bruxelles: Édition de la Fondation Égyptologique Reine Elisabeth, 1933.

Fischer-Elfert, Hans-Werner. *Die Lehre eines Mannes für seinen Sohn: eine Etappe auf dem 'Gottesweg' des loyalen und solidarischen Beamten des Mittleren Reiches.* Wiesbaden: Harrassowitz, 1999.

Galán, José. "Seeing Darkness." *Chronique d'Egypte* 74, no. 147 (1999): 18–30.

Gardiner, Alan H. *Hieratic Papyri in the British Museum. Third Series: Chester Beatty Gift.* London: British Museum, 1935.

Gardiner, Alan H. *Late-Egyptian Miscellanies.* Bruxelles: Édition de la Fondation Égyptologique Reine Elisabeth, 1937.

Golénischeff, Vladimir. *Le Conte Du Naufragé.* Cairo: IFAO, 1912.

Grieshammer, Reinhard. "Taubheit." In *Lexikon Der Ägyptologie VI*, 241–42. Wiesbaden: Harrassowitz, 1986.

Habachi, Labib. "Graffito of the Chamberlain and Controller of Works Antef at Sehēl." *The Journal of Egyptian Archaeology* 39 (1953): 50–59.

Hagen, Fredrik. *An Ancient Egyptian Literary Text in Context: The Instructions of Ptahhotep.* Leuven: Peeters, 2012.

Harvey, Erica. "Deafness: A Disability or a Difference." *Health Law and Policy Brief* 2, no. 1 (2013): 42–56.

Jacob, Amber. "Demotic Pharmacology: An Overview of the Demotic Medical Manuscripts in the Papyrus Carlsberg Collection." In *Parlare la medicina: fra lingue e culture, nello spazio e nel tempo,* edited by Nicola Reggiani and Francesca Bertonazzi, 57–79. Milano: Le Monnier, 2018.

Laisney, Vincent Pierre-Michel. *L'Enseignement d'Aménémopé.* Roma: Pontificio Istituto Biblico, 2007.

Lakoff, George, and Mark Johnson. *Metaphors We Live By.* Chicago: University of Chicago Press, 1980.

Lhoyer, Bénédicte. "Le différent, l'infirme et le marginal en Égypte ancienne." *Les nouvelles de l'archéologie* 165 (2021): 15–20.

Loktionov, Alexandre. "May My Nose and Ears Be Cut off: Practical and 'Supra-Practical' Aspects of Mutilation in the Egyptian New Kingdom." *Journal of the Economic and Social History of the Orient* 60, no. 3 (2017): 263–91.

Loktionov, Alexandre. "Tortured, Banished, Forgotten (and Frequently Ripped Off)? Experience of Ancient Egyptian Criminal Judgment and Its Consequences through the 2nd Millennium BCE." In *Invisible Archaeologies: Hidden Aspects of Daily Life in Ancient Egypt and Nubia,* edited by Loretta Kilroe, 6–16. Oxford: Archaeopress, 2019.

Lorton, David. "The Treatment of Criminals in Ancient Egypt through the New Kingdom." *Journal of the Economic and Social History of the Orient* 20 (1977): 2–64.

Lucarelli, Rita. "Demons (Benevolent and Malevolent)." *UCLA Encyclopedia of Egyptology* (2010), 1–10.

Matić, Uroš. *Body and Frames of War in New Kingdom Egypt: Violent Treatment of Enemies and Prisoners.* Wiesbaden: Harrassowitz, 2019.

Meyer-Dietrich, Erika. *Auditive Räume des alten Ägypten: Die Umgestaltung einer Hörkultur in der Amarnazeit.* Leiden: Brill, 2017.

Morenz, Ludwig D. "Apophis: On the Origin, Name, and Nature of an Ancient Egyptian Anti-God." *Journal of Near Eastern Studies* 63, no. 3 (2004): 201–5.

Morris, Alexandra F. "Blog: A Brief Guide to Disability Terminology and Theory in Ancient World Studies." 2021. https://classicalstudies.org/scs-blog/alexandra-morris/blog-brief-guide-disability-terminology-and-theory-ancient-world-studies.

Morris, Alexandra F. "Plato's Stepchildren: Disability in Ptolemaic Egypt and the Hellenistic World (332–30 BCE)." PhD thesis, Teesside University, 2022.

Morschauser, Scott. *Threat Formulae in Ancient Egypt.* Baltimore: Johns Hopkins University Press, 1987.

Nyord, Rune. "Analogy and Metaphor in Ancient Medicine and the Ancient Egyptian Conceptualisation of Heat in the Body." In *The Comparable Body – Analogy and Metaphor in Ancient Mesopotamian, Egyptian, and Greco-Roman Medicine,* edited by John Z. Wee, 12–42. Leiden: Brill, 2018.

Pahor, Ahmes L. "Ear, Nose and Throat in Ancient Egypt – Part I." *The Journal of Laryngology & Otology* 106, no. 8 (August 1992a): 677–87.

Pahor, Ahmes L. "Ear, Nose and Throat in Ancient Egypt – Part III." *The Journal of Laryngology & Otology* 106, no. 10 (October 1992b): 863–73.

Parkinson, Richard B. *The Tale of the Eloquent Peasant.* Oxford: Griffith Institute, 1991.

Parkinson, Richard B. *The Tale of the Eloquent Peasant: A Reader's Commentary.* Hamburg: Widmaier, 2012.

Posener, Georges. "'Muet, Mutité' en Égyptien." *Revue d'Égyptologie* 17 (1965): 192–93.

Pudsey, April. "Disability and Infirmitas in the Ancient World: Demographic and Biological Facts in the Longue Durée." In *Disability in Antiquity,* edited by Christian Laes, 22–34. London: Routledge, 2017.

Rosati, Gloria. "PSI inv. I 73 + pCarlsberg 463: Manuale del sacerdote di Sakhmet." In *Papiri geroglifici e ieratici da Tebtynis,* edited by Jürgen Osing and Gloria Rosati, 189–215. Firenze: Istituto Papirologico 'G. Vitelli', 1998.

Schlichting, Robert. "Hören." In *Lexikon Der Ägyptologie II*, 1232–35. Wiesbaden: Harrassowitz, 1977.

Shupak, Nili. "Positive and Negative Human Types in the Egyptian Wisdom Literature." In *Homeland and Exile. Biblical and Ancient Near Eastern Studies in Honour of B. Oded,* edited by Gershon Galil, Markham Geller, and Alan Millard, 245–60. Leiden: Brill, 2009.

Stauder, Andréas. *Linguistic Dating of Middle Egyptian Literary Texts.* Hamburg: Widmaier, 2013.

Störk, Lothar. "Ohr." In *Lexikon Der Ägyptologie IV*, 559–62. Wiesbaden: Harrassowitz, 1982.

Takács, Gábor. "Materials for the Semantic Opposition in Egyptian and Afrasian." *Folia Orientalia* 33 (1997): 143–62.

Takács, Gábor. *Etymological Dictionary of Egyptian I.* Leiden and Boston: Brill, 1999.

Varille, Alexandre. *Inscriptions concernant l'architecte Amenhotep, fils de Hapou.* Cairo: IFAO, 1968.

Verhoeven, Ursula. "The Second Half of the 'Teaching of Hardjedef' -in Fact Well Known." In *ICE XII. Proceedings of the Twelfth International Congress of Egyptologists, 3rd–8th November 2019, Cairo, Egypt.* Vol. VI, edited by Ola El-Aguizy and Burt Kasparian, 887–92. Cairo: IFAO, 2023.

Volokhine, Youri. "Colère et châtiment divin en Égypte ancienne: la question des maladies cutanées." In *Colères et repentirs divins,* edited by Jean-Marie Durand, Lionel Marti, and Thomas Römer, 139–52. Fribourg: Academic Press, 2015.

Worthington, Martin. "Literatures in Dialogue: A Comparison of Attitudes of Speech in Babylonian and Middle Egyptian Literature." In *Ancient Egyptian Literature: Theory and Practice,* edited by Roland Enmarch and Verena Lepper, 261–92. Oxford: Oxford University Press, 2013.

Zăba, Zbyněk. *Les Maximes de Ptaḥḥotep.* Prague: Éditions de l'Académie Tchécoslovaque des Sciences, 1956.

17 Impairments as Biometric Modalities in Graeco-Roman Papyri, 241 BCE–299 CE

Ella Karev

Ἀπολλόδοτος ὡς (ἐτῶν) μ μέσος μελίχρως στρογγυλοπρ(όσωπος) χωλαίνων τὸ δεξιὸν σκέλος.

Apollodotus: forty years old, medium height, honey-toned skin, round-faced, and paralyzed in his right leg.

– Loan (*CPR* 18.24, 232 BCE)[1]

Introduction

Biometric identification systems (the determination of identity through physiological characteristics) are familiar to us today in the form of fingerprint or retina scanners, but these systems are modern. Before the advent of digital tools, biometric identification had taken the form of simple lexical descriptions of the physical characteristics of an individual. Although often considered an invention of the nineteenth century CE,[2] this form of biometric identification was in use as early as the Ptolemaic period in Egypt.[3]

Beginning in the early Ptolemaic period (c. 300 BCE),[4] Greek-language documentary texts[5] in Egypt included detailed physical descriptions (*eikones*)[6] alongside the names and patronyms of contracting parties. The texts in which such descriptions appear amount to nearly 1,300 documents recording the physical characteristics of nearly 4,000 people. The *eikones* were highly standardized in their order and terminology, including details such as the height, skin tone, and face shape. In certain cases, these descriptions included other identifiers like tattoos,[7] pierced ears,[8] attached earlobes[9] – and impairments.

The impairments appearing most frequently in this corpus were visual: blindness in one or both eyes, missing eyes, poor eyesight, and cataracts. Bodily impairments were recorded for the limbs, paralysis, limping, and kyphosis ("bent"). Deafness/muteness is attested twice, and a stammer in one instance. Because audio-visual impairments are difficult to detect in physical remains, these are of particular importance for Disability Studies. Certain impairments, as well as impairment-related traits (i.e. assistive aids), are absent from the *eikones*.

The corpus of *eikones* in general demonstrates how the population of Graeco-Roman Egypt saw and identified themselves and each other, adding another

DOI: 10.4324/9781003440369-20

dimension to artistic depictions and physical remains. Artistic representations, even when aiming for realism, incorporated some degree of idealization and standardization. Physical remains are neither standardized nor idealized, but also do not provide insight into the perception impairments. Human remains are also limited in their preservation. The physical descriptions in these *eikones* were necessarily true to life; otherwise, they would not have served their purpose as identifiers.

This chapter examines the distribution and nature of the impairments present in documentary Greek papyri from Egypt, from the third century BCE to the third century CE. Alongside these data, I include a discussion of the impairments not noted in the *eikones*, in comparison with physical remains and contemporary artistic depictions, as well as the more general reception of impairments. This study therefore fulfills two goals: firstly, to evaluate impairments as present in the Greek-speaking[10] population of Graeco-Roman Egypt; secondly, to highlight the role of impairments as non-stigmatizing identifying markers (or *biometric modalities*) within a biometric system.

Introduction to the Data Set

The data under examination here is a subset of a much larger corpus: the collection of the 3,868 physical descriptions (*eikones*) evident in Greek documentary papyri from Egypt dating roughly from the early Ptolemaic Period (c. 300 BCE) through to the Roman Era (c. 299 CE).[11] In this period, contractual agreements such as sales and loans included physical descriptions of the individuals involved, which provided a physical portrait of an individual for identification purposes.

The *eikones* can be split into two chronological phases. In the first phase (c. 300 BCE to first century CE) the descriptions were highly detailed. Over the course of the first century CE and until the end of the Roman Empire in the fourth century CE, the descriptions shorten to note only an unspecified identifying marker (*oulē*).

The identifying description employed in the *eikones* could include a permanent[12] physical impairment. However, such notation was uncommon, and likely optional if the individual had a more distinctive identifying marker. The identification of a person as able-bodied is only through absence of an impairment.[13] The use of the word "impairment" rather than "disability" here is intentional: the definition set forth by Disabled People International (DPI) distinguishes between the two, defining an impairment as a functional limitation of the body whereas disability is the loss or limitation of opportunities within a community as a result of physical impairment.[14] As argued later in this paper, the impairments in the *eikones* were not disabilities because they were not representative of loss of opportunities. Rather, they were a practical notation for the purpose of identification.

In the complete corpus of *eikones*, the notation of impairment was far from common. Out of a total of 1,273 texts describing 3,868 individuals, only 81 texts describing 87 individuals[15] note a physical impairment. These impairments, tabulated in the appendix (Table 17.1) include the following: blindness (including cataracts and glaucoma), poor eyesight (including squinting), trachoma, missing an eye, partial paralysis, a stammer, a limp, and deafness/muteness.

Types, Frequency, and Distribution of Impairments in the Papyri

There are ninety-two notations of impairments in the *eikones*, though five of these record individuals who appear twice in different texts; hence, eighty-seven individuals. All attestations, along with their gender, age, and their impairment in Greek and English, are listed in tabular format in the Appendix (Table 17.2). The ten attestations recording five individuals have shaded cells. The following subsection is a detailed discussion of the types, frequency, and distribution of these impairments, split into three types: visual, auditory and speech-related, and bodily impairments.

Visual Impairments

The most common impairments were ophthalmological, representing seventy-seven out of ninety-two attestations of an impairment of any kind. Many of these attestations record a form of blindness in one or both eyes, represented by three terms: (1) eyes which are 'shaded' or 'suffused' (ὑποχέω); (2) 'white' eyes (λευκόν); and (3) eyes which are 'impaired' or 'damaged' (βλάπτω). The descriptor 'powerless eyes' – appearing only three times[16] – also likely refers to blindness. However, the term 'hollow-eyed', attested five times for three individuals,[17] is more likely a visible physical characteristic than an impairment.[18]

Of the foregoing terms, the first (ὑποχέω) most likely refers to cataracts, as in Galen.[19] Although cataracts can lead to complete blindness, they are more likely to result in partial blindness – such as the weaver in the first-century CE *P. Oxy.* 1.39, with "shaded eyes" who is still able to see, albeit not much. Cataracts usually result from aging, but the attestations with cataracts have somewhat of a wide age range: the three attestations include a person aged twenty,[19] another aged forty-four,[20] and another aged sixty-five.[21] Age, however, is not the only cause for cataracts, which can occur as a result of extended exposure to sunlight,[22] certainly likely in Egypt.

"White" eyes may also refer to cataracts, but equally to glaucoma.[23] Like cataracts, glaucoma may cause the appearance of a white or clouded iris.[24] There are seventeen attestations of 'white' eyes recording sixteen individuals. Seven of these note a spot in the eye (*leukōma*) associated with traumatic glaucoma.[25] Distribution between eyes is fairly even: three do not specify which eye has been afflicted,[26] seven record the right eye,[27] and five record the left.[28] In two *eikones* of the same man, the earlier *eikōn* specifies the left eye,[29] but the later has his affliction in both eyes.[30]

The final term, βεβλαμμένος, is a derivative of βλάπτω, which carries the general meaning of 'hindered' or 'impaired'. Partial or complete blindness is implied, but not explicitly stated. Much like glaucoma and cataracts, this type of blindness was more likely to appear in one eye rather than both: out of eleven attestations, only one refers to blindness in both eyes.[31]

Poor eyesight appears most commonly as myopia, but also as 'weak' or 'poor' eyes and 'squinting'. Unlike senile cataracts and glaucoma, the age of onset of myopia ranges between six and fourteen years old, stabilizing in the late teens and early twenties.[32] Age is only preserved for eight of the seventeen attestations of myopia, but the range (forty to sixty years old) and average (fifty-three) are oddly high. A squint is attested eleven times,[33] possibly a manifestation of myopia. 'Squinting' may also have referred to cataracts, following description of a man with a squint (*P. Oxy.*1.99) only three years after he is described as having cataracts (*P. Oxy.* 1.39). 'Weak' eyes (ἀσθενῶν, *UPZ* 2.180a, *P. Oxy.* 6.911) and 'bad eyes' (κακόψις, *P. Lips.* 1.1, *P. Grenf.* 2.28) only appear twice each, but the 'bad eyes' are for the same individual.

Other ophthalmological impairments are more rarely noted. Inflamed eyelids (likely trachoma) appear twice (*CPR* 1.218, *P.Mich.* 5.264). The existence of only one eye ('one-eyed', μονόφθαλμόν) is directly attested only once (*P. Brux.* 1.10). Also included in the list of attestations with visual impairments are those individuals described as 'well-marked' (*eusēmos*).[34] This descriptor is often associated with the eyes: attestations record individuals as being *eusēmos* on or with regard to a specific eye, usually the right.[35] Three attestations with the *eusēmos* descriptor are paired with an additional eye affliction: inflamed eyelids,[36] a squint,[37] and cataracts.[38]

Auditory and Speech-related Impairments

The term often translated as 'mute' or 'deaf' (κωφός) is attested in other Greek writings as referring to deafness, muteness, or even mental impairment.[39] The word κωφός could also be a personal name (TM Nam 3805 in the *trismegistos.org* papyrological database), albeit an uncommon one: Κωφός is attested by thirteen individuals from 93 BCE to 417 CE as a personal name. In those cases, it is additionally not entirely clear whether it is in fact a name or a (perhaps derogatory) alias. There is only Roman attestation (c. 250 CE) of a stammer (ψέλλος) though this highly specific attribute may have been a result of its context: a possible parody of a runaway slave notice.[40]

Bodily Impairments

In the *eikones*, bodily impairments are apparent in the notation of a limp (ἐπισκάζω) and partial paralysis (χωλός).[41] Limping appears without any further qualifiers, whereas paralysis can be limited to a certain limb (e.g. leg[42] or arm[43]). One *eikōn* describes a man as 'bent' (σκαμβός),[44] though it is not clear whether this is an indication of bow-leggedness, which is usually referred to as 'bent legs' (σπαμβόπους)[45] or kyphosis more generally.

In two attestations, individuals are described as having one or more fingers which are 'gulped down' (κεκαμμένον),[46] meaning "gulped".[47] The second-century CE date of these descriptors suggests that they may represent an appropriation of the Latin word *capio*, which has a secondary meaning of 'harmed' or 'deprived'.[48] The fingers in these attestations may be read as 'impaired', or alternatively as 'captured' (i.e. missing).

Distribution by Occupation and Gender

There does not appear to be a significant correlation between gender or occupation and type of impairment, with one exception: enslaved persons appear with higher incidence than in the larger corpus of texts, suggesting that impairment played a role in their description, especially when recording a sale transaction.

Gender

Eighteen out of the ninety-two attestations are female, representing roughly 20% of the total attestations with noted impairments. This statistic is only slightly higher than the total corpus of papyrological documents with physical descriptions (17%). All but one of these women evidence ophthalmological impairments; the exception is a woman described as 'limping'.[49]

The high incidence of ophthalmological impairments among women is likely a reflection of the high incidence of such impairments overall in the corpus rather than correlation of gender with eye impairment. Modern research suggests that gender does indeed play a role in the incidence of glaucoma and cataracts,[50] but this data is affected by modern life expectancy discrepancies, which are irrelevant for this data set. Firstly, women did not necessarily live longer in the ancient world, due to the high risk of death in childbirth.[51] Secondly, the age distribution of the women in this corpus range between fifteen and fifty-eight years of age, with an average age of thirty. Therefore, age is not the likely cause for a high rate of eye impairments in women, at least in this data set.

Occupations

Occupations are listed for ten individuals with impairments: three priests,[52] three soldiers,[53] two scribes,[54] one farmer,[55] one weaver,[56] and one choachyte.[57] One individual is also described as "unskilled".[58] Fifteen attestations include the Ptolemaic pseudo-ethnonym "of the epigone", which may have referred to reservist soldiers.[59] There did not seem to be a limitation on what professions in which an impaired person could engage: one priest has 'powerless eyes',[60] two scribes have a white spot in their eyes, and one soldier has a limp.[61]

There is a long-standing Egyptian cultural archetype of the "blind musician": unsighted or partially sighted persons are depicted as playing the harp,[62] and in the Amarna period musicians are depicted wearing a blindfold.[63] However, none of the blind or partially blind persons in this group of papyri are listed as musicians or associated with music. Indeed, it seems that in daily life partially unsighted persons were able to perform a variety of professions, such as land measurers, doorkeepers, cadastral recorders, and herdsmen.[64]

Enslaved Persons

It has previously been assumed that descriptions of enslaved persons were more detailed than descriptions of unenslaved persons.[65] However, this assumption is contradicted by evidence from the *eikones*; descriptions of enslaved persons rarely differed from those of unenslaved persons. That said, the higher incidence of enslaved persons in the impairment attestations (6% of all attestations) compared to their appearances in the total corpus (3%) suggests that impairment may have played a part in the description of enslaved persons.

Four enslaved persons appear with impairments, aged between fourteen and nineteen years old. Three of the four are sales documents and note ophthalmological impairments: inflamed eyelids (*P.Mich.* 5.264), a white spot in the eye (*P. Ant.* 3.187), and squinting (*P. Oxy.* 36.2777). The remaining attestation notes a stammer (*P. Oxy.* 51.3616).

The first three attestations previously listed record a slave sale. It is possible that the notation of an impairment affected the price, though it is difficult to determine with any certainty since prices of this period are not always included or preserved. Even when comparison is possible, price may have been affected by factors other than impairments.[66]

Impairments Absent from the Papyri

There are certain impairments that we might expect to encounter due to their appearance in artistic or paleopathological evidence, such as missing limbs and teeth as well as dwarfism – which are simply not present in the *eikones*. This discrepancy may be a matter of preservation of papyri, but nevertheless the absence of these impairments is worthy of note.

Paleopathological evidence points to both congenitally missing as well as amputated limbs.[67] Notwithstanding the possibly missing fingers, there are no *eikones* with missing limbs. There is also archaeological evidence that people with amputated limbs and digits were given prostheses, which were likely used in life.[68] Nonetheless, assistive aids do not appear in the *eikones*, likely because they were not permanent enough to serve as identifiers.

Dental diseases and treatments were present in Egypt as a result of the coarseness of the diet, which caused extensive wear of tooth enamel.[69] Congenitally missing teeth are also noted in physical remains,[70] along with evidence of dental intervention.[71] Neither missing teeth nor dental work is mentioned in the papyri. There are four attestations of individuals whose identifying mark was on their teeth,[72] which could equally refer to an impairment, dental work, or body modification.

Lastly, dwarfism in any form is not mentioned. In Egyptian artistic and textual traditions, dwarfism is particularly present.[73] Achondroplastic dwarfism is a relatively common genetic disorder,[74] and certainly would have aided in identification. The reason for its absence from the *eikones* is unclear. However, I suggest that unlike the other impairments discussed here (e.g. blindness, partial paralysis), individuals with dwarfism were *disabled*, rather than impaired; in other words, their physical impairment restricted their participation in the financial and social transactions for which *eikones* were recorded.

Comparison with Artistic Depictions and Physical Remains

The data set presented here is particularly useful because evidence from physical remains and artistic depictions are limited in the information they can provide. The contemporary evidence from 'mummy' portraits, usually[75] limited to the head and shoulders, do not show any corporal impairments, and cannot demonstrate deafness in any way. Physical remains do not preserve speech-related impairments, and only rarely preserve ophthalmological or auditory impairments – with few exceptions, discussed below.

Artistic Depictions in the 'Mummy' Portraits

One of the best resources for comparanda are the contemporaneous 'mummy portraits', namely[76] realistic painted depictions of individuals on wooden boards which were attached to Egyptian mummified human remains in the Roman period. The realism of these portraits, including potentially unflattering details such as wrinkles,[77] grey hair,[78] and sunken eyes,[79] was a departure from earlier Egyptian art, which presented an idealized and stylized image of the deceased.[80] Their realistic elements suggest that they are likely to have included impairments such as those listed in the *eikones*.

Considering the high incidence of ophthalmological impairments present in the corpus, the depictions of eye disease in these portraits are particularly relevant. For example, the 2nd century CE portrait of a young man housed at the Metropolitan Museum of Art, now titled *Youth with a Surgical Cut in the Right Eye* (MMA 09.181.4). The boy's right lower lid is discolored and fixed so that the eye is partly closed. The margin of the lower lid is unnaturally straight, hence the assumption for a surgical cut, and the lashes of the lid are missing.

As suggested by Arthur Lehrman[81] and later discussed by Horton Johnson,[82] this portrait reflects a therapeutic treatment for trachoma: a bacterial infection that affects the inner surface of the eyelids. Untreated trachoma leads to corneal abrasion and blindness. The treatment for trachoma in Roman Egypt was almost certainly cautery, which would have treated the painful trichiasis, but would not have saved the boy's vision in that eye: the pupil of the right eye is out of alignment. Trachoma was also very likely the source of the 'inflamed eyelids' (ὑπόστιλλος) in the *eikones*,[83] disproving that "the evidence for ocular disease is purely literary".[84]

A possible depiction of cataracts is in the portrait of an older man, housed at the Galerie Cybèle in Paris. His light grey irises are ill-defined, and the pupils misshapen. It is tempting to consider the 'white' eyes of the *eikones* as representations of light-colored irises, rather than an eye impairment. But although notations of iris color are rare, light-colored irises are indeed attested: in the *eikones* as 'blue-grey'[85] and in the mummy portraits (Pushkin Museum I 1a 5771/429, Petrie Museum UC 36215).

The man portrayed in the Galerie Cybèle portrait is not a light-eyed individual, but rather subject to cataracts or a different form of blindness. The lack of a bright spot of white to indicate reflection could also be an attempt at portraying blindness. In comparison, for instance, a similar light-eyed elderly man (Neues Museum 31161.15) has clear pupils with a bright reflective spot; the eyes of the man in the Galerie Cybèle portrait appear to be unseeing.

Although the evidence for corporal impairment from the 'mummy' portraits is difficult to ascertain, the evidence for ophthalmological impairments, like trachoma and/or glaucoma, supports the evidence from the *eikones*.

Physical Remains

The paleopathological evidence from Egypt is rich. The dry climate of the desert location produces natural preservation of body tissue, and from at least 2600 BCE the process was replicated through artificial means by enhanced ritual mummification.[86]

The limping attested in the *eikones* may be representative of several different conditions evidenced in physical remains: congenital club foot (*talipes equinovarus*),[87] a traumatic or chronic[88] injury, gout, arthritis, cerebral palsy, or poliomyelitis.[89] The partial paralysis from the *eikones,* which can be detailed as occurring in a specific limb, may also point to evidence of polio or cerebral palsy.

The description of 'bent' in the *eikones*[90] may represent scoliosis or angular kyphosis. The latter is often caused by a progression of tuberculosis (Pott's disease), a widespread disease in Egypt; it may also be ankylosing spondylitis, a form of arthritis which causes the fusion of the spine and causes progressive kyphosis.[91] In Greek, this term was also used to describe the bow-leggedness of rickets, a childhood disease primarily caused by a lack of vitamin D but for which there are hereditary variations. Adults with healed rickets will present with bowed femurs or tibias; as of yet, no remains with hereditary or acquired rickets have been identified in Egypt.[92]

Blindness is only diagnosable in remains when the eyes are preserved intact, and they usually are not; Egyptians made no effort to preserve the eyeball in the process of mummification.[93] Even when preserved, cataracts and glaucoma are not readily identifiable in mummified remains.[94] Trachoma, represented in the *eikones* by 'inflamed eyelids', may have been a cause for blindness. However, trachoma is only recognizable in mummified remains if it had been left untreated.[95]

Deafness can only be assessed in physical remains if the condition arose from pathological conditions preserved in mummified and osteological remains such as otitis media (infection of the middle ear) and subsequent perforated eardrum,[96] mastoiditis,[97] or exostoses of the auditory canal.[98] Deafness unrelated to pathology (e.g. senile) would not be evident in physical remains.

Reception of Impairments in the Papyri and Implications

Within the larger context of the *eikones* and their role in biometric identification, we must return to the implication of the use of impairment as a biometric modality. A modality is an identifying marker employed in a biometric system;[99] for instance, a type of fingerprint ridge or a scar on the forehead. The corpus of *eikones* adheres to 'soft' biometrics, in which modalities are not unique to an individual. The term 'soft' is intended as a contrast with 'hard' biometrics, which rely on unique attributes (for example, a retina or fingerprint scanner). In soft biometric systems, a single modality is not enough to identify an individual; rather, several modalities together (multimodal) form an identifying picture.

In the initial phase of this system, in which *eikones* were detailed for all individuals, it is perhaps unsurprising that impairments were included. The impairment played the role of an additional biometric modality, much like from other identifying details such as pierced ears or a mole. But it is notable that the inclusion of impairment persisted into the second phase of this system, in which each person had a single identifying mark (*oulē*); this mark could be anything which identified the person in question, including an impairment. Rather than another modality in a long list, impairment served as an identifying mark.

This does not mean, however, that individuals with impairments in their *eikones* were necessarily treated differently after this shift, only that their impairment could serve as identification. When a man in the fourth century CE[100] was too visually impaired to sign a contract, he had someone sign for him, little different from another individual in the same contract who also had someone sign for him because he was illiterate. Similarly, a man claiming that his identity had been stolen in a second-century CE petition[101] was only able to do so because the fictitious name did not include any of his identifying marks, including his 'disability' (πηρός) and 'impairment' (ἐπισινὴς).

On the other hand, pretence at impairment was poorly received. In a second-century CE petition,[102] a man requested an official to act against the administrator of the village, who had treated him poorly. The man complained that his ill treatment was a result of a non-functioning eye, which "appears to see" but did not. The appearance of able-bodiedness despite the presence of a physical impairment was possibly more disabling or stigmatizing than the impairment itself.

In Egypt of this period, individuals with physical impairments may have been exempted from public service, but this exemption was a matter of practicality. In *P. Oxy*. 1.39 (first century CE), a blind weaver conscripted for public service was exempted because his tasks required eyesight. He was exempted because he could not physically perform the duties required, rather than as a result of alienation.

Impairment did not serve as a justification for exemption or exclusion from full and complete participation in legal and economic transactions as it did in the Athenian and Roman legal systems. In Rome, an individual with physical impairments was legally defined as a minor, unable to sign a contract or testify in court without an appointed guardian.[103] Similarly, women in the Greek courts of the Ptolemaic period necessitated the appearance of a legal guardian for any transaction,[104] rendering them legally incapacitated; individuals with impairments required no such guardian. In other words, returning to the DPI definitions of disability and impairment, impaired individuals were not socially disabled.

Egyptian persons with physical impairments were cared for,[105] following a general tolerant attitude exemplified in teachings towards those needing assistance, for example the elderly, orphaned, and blind.[106] The crucial takeaway from this corpus of documentary texts (which recorded important economic transactions) is that individuals with physical impairments functioned as participatory members of society.

The use of impairments as biometric modalities demonstrates that impairments were noted as a feature that could be used to identify a person in a legal document, not as a marker of social exclusion. In a very real sense, these attestations of impairment were little different from the notation on modern driving licenses which indicate that one needs to wear corrective lenses in order to operate a vehicle. Although the impairment is noted for identification, the fact of its notation does not afford its bearer a manifested stigma. In much the same way, the impairments noted in these documentary papyri certainly aided in identification but did not serve as markers of alienation.

Appendix

Table 17.1 Terminology of Impairment

Type	Subtype	Greek	Number of attestations
Visual	Blindness ('impaired' or 'powerless' eyes)	βεβλαμμένος, ἀδύνατος	14
	Cataracts ('shaded' eyes)	ὑποκεχυμένος	3
	Glaucoma ('white' in the eyes)	λευκόν/λεύκωμα	17
	Myopia	ὑπόσκνιφος	16
	Squinting	ὑπόστραβος	11
	Poor eyesight ('bad eyes', 'weak' eyes)	κάκοψις, ἀσθενῶν	4
	'Well-marked'	εὔσημος	11
	Trachoma	ὑπόπτιλλος	2
	One-eyed	μονόφθαλμος	1
	Total:		**77**
Bodily	Paralysis	χωλαίνων	6
	Limping	ἐπισκάζων	4
	'Gulped' fingers	κεκαμμένος	2
	Bent	σκαμβός	1
	Total:		**13**
Auditory/speech	Deaf/mute	κωφός	2
	Stammer	ψελλόν	1
	Total:		**3**

Table 17.2 Attestations of Impairments

Type	*Subtype*		*Greek*	*Gender*	*Age*	*Text*	*Date*
Visual	'Bad' eyes		κάκοψις	Female	25	P. Lips. 1.1	104 BCE
			κάκοψις	Female	25	P. Grenf. 2.28	103 BCE
	Blind	Both eyes	<β>εβλαμμένος* ὀφθαλμοὺς ἀμφοτέρους	Female	35	P. Grenf. 1.33	103 BCE
		Left eye	τὸν [ὀ]φθαλμὸν ἀριστερὸν βεβλαμμένος	Female	15	P. Köln 4.187	146 BCE
			[βεβλαμμέν]ος τὸν ἀριστερὸν ὀφθαλμόν	Female	28	CPR 18.16	231 BCE
			[βεβλαμμέν]ος τὸν ἀρι[σ]τερ[ὸν ὀφθαλμὸν	Male	60	P. Petrie (2) 1.25	226 BCE
			βεβ[λ(αμμένου)][τὸ(ν) ἀρ(ιστερὸν)][ὀφθ(αλμὸν)]	Male	65	P. Strasb. Gr. 1.52	151 CE
			βεβλ(αμμένου) τὸ(ν) ἀρισ(τερὸν) ὀφθ(αλμὸν)	Male	67	P. Flor. 1.1	153 CE
			τὸν ἀρ[ιστερὸν][ὀφθαλμὸν] [βεβλαμμέ]νος	Male	60	P. Petrie(2) 1.6	238 BCE
		Right eye	[---βεβλαμμέ]ος δεξιὸν βεβλαμμένης	–	–	PSI 14.1402	125 BCE
			βεβλ(αμμένος) τὸν δεξ(ιὸν) ὀφθα(λμὸν)	Male	28	BGU 6.1258A	143 BCE
			ὀφθαλμὸν δεξιὸν βεβλαμμενος*	Male	50	P. Lips. 1.2	99 BCE
			[. . .. . .ὀφθα]λμῷ δεξιῷ	Male	60	BGU 3.896	161 CE
	Weak eyes		ἀσθενῖ* τὰς ὄψις*	Male	69	UPZ 2.180a	113 BCE
			ἀσθενῶν τοῖς ὄμμασιν	Male	–	P. Oxy. 6.911	233 CE
	Inflamed eyelids		ὑπόπτιλλος	Female	17	P.Mich. 5.264	37 CE
			ὑπόπτιλλος	Male	60	CPR 1.218	c. 150 CE
	Near-sighted		σκνιπὸς	Male	–	P. Petrie(2) 1.6	238 BCE
			[ὑπ]όσκνιφο[ς]	Male	–	P. Petrie(2) 1.14	238 BCE
			ὑπόσκνιφος	Male	–	CPR 18.8	231 BCE
			ὑπόσκνιπος	Male	–	P. Petrie(2) 1.27	226 BCE
			ὑποσκιφος*	Male	–	P. Freib. 3.36	179 BCE
			ὑπόσκνιπος	Male	–	P. Heid. Gr. 8.413	179 BCE
			[ὑπόσκν]ιφος	–	–	P. Tebt. 3.972	c. 125 BCE
			ὑπόσκνιφος	Male	–	P.Mich. 3.190	172 BCE
			ὑπόκκινος*	Male	40	P. Grenf. 2.28	103 BCE
			ὑπόσχνιφος	Male	45	P. Tebt. 3.816	192 BCE
			ὑπόσκνιφος	Male	50	P. Grenf. 2.35	98 BCE
			ὑπόσκνιφος	Male	55	P. Grenf. 2.35	98 BCE

(*Continued*)

Table 17.2 (Continued)

Type	*Subtype*		*Greek*	*Gender*	*Age*	*Text*	*Date*
			ὑπόσκνιφος	Female	58	P. Adler Gr. 8	104 BCE
			ὑπ̣ό̣σ̣κνιφ̣ο̣ς	Female	58	P. Adler Gr. 7	104 BCE
			ὑπόσκνειφος*	Male	60	SB 12.10859	220 BCE
			[ὑπ]όσκνειφος*	Male	60	PSI 9.1057	32 CE
			ὑποσκνίφο[υ]	Male	–	SB 1.428	99 BCE
	One-eyed		μονόφθ(αλμος)	Male	11	P. Brux. Gr. 1.10	174 CE
	Powerless eyes		ἀδύνα(τος) τοῖς ὄμμασ(ιν)	Female	35	P. Strasb. Gr. 2.81	115 BCE
			[ἀ]δύνατ[ος] [ὄμμ]ασι	Male	54	P. Lond. 3.678	99 BCE
			ἀδύνατος τοῖς ὄμμασι	Male	72	P. Adler Gr. 17	99 BCE
	Shaded eyes		ὑποχυμένος(*)	Male	–	P. Oxy. 1.39	52 CE
			ὑποκεχυμένη τὰς ὄψεις	Female	20	P. Coll. Yout. 1.19	44 CE
		Left eye	ὑποκεχυμένος τὸν ἀριστερὸν ὀφθαλμὸν	Male	65	P.Mich. 5.321	42 CE
	Squinting		στραβίζ[οντος]	–	–	PSI 14.1402	125 BCE
			σ̣τ̣ρα(βὸς)	–	–	P. Tebt. 3.972	c. 125 BCE
			ὑπόστραβος	Male	–	P. Oxy. 2.256	34 CE
			παράστραβον	Male	19	P. Oxy. 36.2777	212 CE
			ὑ̣π̣ό̣σ̣τρα̣(βος)	Male	21	BGU 6.1258A	143 BCE
			ὑπόστραβος	Female	23	P. Hamb. 1.15	209 CE
			ὑποστρα(βος)	Male	30	P. Grenf. 1.33	103 BCE
			παραστραβω*	Female	30	P. Aberdeen 56	176 CE
			παραστραβος*	Female	37	PSI 9.1028	15 CE
			ὑπόστραβος	Male	47	P. Oxy. 1.99	55 CE
			ὑπόστρ[α]β(ος)	Female	23	BASP 50 p. 89	88 CE
	Well-marked		εὔσ(ημος)	Male	14	P. Oxy. 18.2186	260 CE
			εὔση(μος)	Female	23	BASP 50 p. 89	88 CE
		On eye	[ε]ὔσημος ὀφθαλμὸν ἀριστερὸν	Male	–	P. Flor. 1.51	138 CE
			εὔσημον ὀφθαλ̣(μὸν) δεξιὸν	Male	8	P. Amh. Gr. 2.74	147 CE
			εὔσ(ημος) τὸν ὀφθαλμ(ὸν) δεξιὸν	Male	26	PSI 8.922	180 CE
			εὔσημος ὀφθαλμὸν δεξιὸν	Female	35	P. Amh. Gr. 2.102	180 CE

(*Continued*)

Table 17.2 (Continued)

Type	*Subtype*		*Greek*	*Gender*	*Age*	*Text*	*Date*
			εὐσή[μ]ο̣υ τὸ̣[ν δ̣εξιὸ̣ν ὀφθ(αλμὸν)]	Male	35	P. Flor. 3.383	234 CE
			εὐσημος* τὸν δεξιὸν ὀπθαλμὸν*	Male	38	PSI 9.1028	15 CE
			εὐσήμωι ὀ[φθαλ]μῷ δεξιῷ	Male	50	P. Flor. 3.316	c. 150 CE
			εὔσημος ὀφθαλμῶι δεξ[ιῶι]	Male	65	P.Mich. 5.321	42 CE
	White in eye		λευκῷ ὀφθαλμῷ	Male	19	P. Ant. 3.187a	198 CE
			λεύκωμα ὀφθαλμόν	Female	37	P. Grenf. 1.33	103 BCE
			λευκὸν ἐν ὀφθαλμῷ	Male	62	P. Hamb. 1.38	182 CE
		Both eyes	[λευ]κὸ̣ν ὀφ̣θαλμοῖς ἀμφοτέρωις*	Male	36	SB 10.10571	194 CE
		Left eye	λευκῷ ὀφθαλμῷ ἀριστερῷ	Male	–	SB 24.15987	208 CE
			λευκον* ὀφθαλμὸν ἀριστερὸν	Male	25	Stud. Pal. 22.42	185 CE
			λευκὸν ὀφθαλμῷ ἀριστερῷ	Male	30	PSI 13.1324	173 CE
			λ̣εύκωμα ὀφθαλμῷ ἀριστερῷ	Male	35	P. Grenf. 2.51	143 CE
			λευκὸν ὀφθαλμῷ ἀριστερῷ	Male	50	P. Tebt. 2.397	198 CE
			λευκῷ ὀφθαλμῶι ἀριστερῶι	Male	55	P. Adler Gr. 5	108 BCE
		Right eye	λευκὸν ὀφθαλμοῦ δ̣ε[ξιοῦ –]	Female	22	P. Coll. You. 1.19	44 CE
			λεύκωμα ὀφθαλμῷ δεξιῷ	Male	23	SB 1.4414	143 CE
			λ̣εύκω(μα) ὀφθαλ(μῷ) δε(ξιῷ)	Male	25	SB 20.14481	158 BCE
			λευκ(ὸν) ὀφθ(αλμῷ) δεξι(ῷ)	Male	25	P.Mich. 5.285	1–56 CE
			λεύκωμα ὀφθαλμὸν δεξιὸν	Male	30	BGU 3.834	125 CE
			λεύκ(ωμα) ὀφθ(αλμῷ) δεξιῷ	Male	45	P. Berl. Frisk. 1	155 CE
			λεύκω(μα) ὀφθαλ(μῷ) δεξ(ιῷ)	Male	60	SB 20.14471	160 BCE
Bodily	Paralysis		χωλ[οῦ]	Male	–	SB 1.428	99 BCE
			κυλλώς*	Male	17	P. Bingen 31	c. 275 CE
			χωλαινω(ντος)*	Male	52	P. Brooklyn Gr. 8	177 CE
		Arm	κυλλὸ[ς] χῖρα(*) δ̣εξιὰ[ν	Male	5	P. Cair. Mich. 3.21	188 CE
		Limb	χωλένων* ἐν δ[εξιῶι –]	Male	–	P. Freib. 4.55	71 CE
		Leg	χωλαίνων τὸ δεξιὸν σκέλος	Male	40	CPR 18.24	232 BCE
	Limping	Right foot	ἐπισχάζων* τὸν πόδα δεξιὸν	Male	40	BGU 3.997	103 BCE

(*Continued*)

Table 17.2 (Continued)

Type	*Subtype*	*Greek*	*Gender*	*Age*	*Text*	*Date*
		ἐπισ[κάζω]ν τὸν πόδα δεξιὸν	Male	55	BGU 3.998	101 BCE
		ἐ̣[π]ι̣ς̣κάζων	Male	–	CPR 18.19	231 BCE
		[ἐπισκα]ζούσηι	Female	20	SB 20.14771	260 BCE
	Bent	σκαμβοῦ	Male	45	P. Tebt. 3.814	227 BCE
	Bent fingers	κεκαμμένου δακ[τύλ]ους τρεῖς χειρὸς δε[ξιᾶς]	Male	–	CPR 1.170	103 CE
		κεκαμμένον δάκτυλον μικρὸν χειρὸς ἀριστερᾶς	Male	55	P. Tebt. 2.397	198 CE
Auditory/ Speech	Deaf/mute	κ̣ω̣φός	Male	–	BGU 4.1196	29 CE
		κωφὸς	Male	–	Stud. Pal. 22.67	208 CE
	Stammer	ψελλόν	Male	14	P. Oxy. 51.3616	c. 250 CE

Notes

1 References to papyrological sources follow the conventions set forth in John Oates and William Willis, "Checklist of Greek, Latin, Demotic and Coptic Papyri, Ostraca and Tablets," https://papyri.info/docs/checklist.
2 Alphonse Bertillon (1853–1914) is often credited with inventing standardized biometrics for identifying criminals; Kaluszynski (2001, 123–38), Karev (2024, 18–21).
3 A similar method of identification in China's Han Dynasty (202 BCE–220 CE); see Barbieri-Low and Yates (2015, 1115–17).
4 The first attested description dates to 299 BCE (*P. Cair. Preis*. 2.37).
5 The classification of "documentary texts" is generally understood to mean "non-literary"; on this classification for Demotic documentary texts and examples of types of documentary texts, see Depauw (1997, 84).
6 On the significance of *eikones* as documents of identification, see Karev (2024, 34–35).
7 *UPZ* 1.121 (180 BCE); *BGU* 6.1258 (143 BCE).
8 *CPR* 18.24 (232 BCE); *P. Lond.* 2.219 (199 BCE); *BGU* 10.1971 (150 BCE); *P. Grenf.* 2.15 (139 BCE); *SB* 18.13168 (123 BCE); *P. Ryl. Gr.* 4.581 (121 BCE); *P. Strass*. 2.87 (107 BCE); *P. Adl. Gr.* 12 (101 BCE); *P. Lond.* 3.882 (101 BCE); *P. Adl. Gr.* 15 (100 BCE); *P. Adl. Gr.* 17 (99 BCE); *P. Lond.* 3.883 (88 BCE).
9 *P. Trier* 1.3 (183 BCE); *P. Köln* 4.187 (146 BCE).
10 "Greek-speaking" does not necessarily indicate ethnic origin. Greek was the administrative language of Graeco-Roman period in Egypt. The overwhelming majority of the *eikones* are written in Greek, except for eight in Latin and twelve in Demotic.
11 Karev (2024). For earlier – though less comprehensive – collections of these data, see: Smolka (1924), Hasebroek (1921), Hübsch (1968).
12 The descriptors used in the *eikones* were used for identification throughout a person's lifetime, and therefore would need to be permanent or (as in, e.g., "balding") semipermanent. Excepting "inflamed eyelids", the impairments discussed here are permanent.
13 There is one possible exception: a runaway slave and thief is described in. *P. Paris* 10 (156 BCE) as "well-legged (εὔκνημος)". But whether this description is meant to highlight his abled body or simply included in his unusually detailed description is unclear, since the term does not reappear in the *eikones.*
14 As quoted in Goodley (2011, 6).
15 There are ninety-two *eikones* with impairments, but ten of those refer to five individuals: Eudaimonos son of Sarapion (*P. Strasb. Gr.* 1.52, *P. Flor.* 1.1); Thaibis daughter of Phibis (*P. Adler Gr.* 7 and 8); Sennesis daughter of Psenthotos (*P. Grenf.* 2.28, *P. Lips*. 1.1); Tryphon son of Dionysius (*P. Oxy.* 1.99 and 1.39); and Psenmenches son of Panechatos (*BGU* 3.997 and 998).
16 *P. Strasb. Gr.* 2.81 (115 BCE); *P. Adler Gr*. 17 (99 BCE); *P. Lond.* 3.678 (99 BCE).
17 *CPR* 18.11 (231 BCE) and 18.9 (231 BCE), *UPZ* 2.175a (145 BCE); in Demotic, *P. BN.* 218 (146 BCE), *P. Berl.* 3119 (146 BCE).
18 Cf. the same term regarding horses (*Xen. Eq.* 1.19), in contrast with a "prominent eye".
19 *P. Coll. Youtie* 1.19 (44 CE).
20 The age of Tryphon in *P. Oxy.* 1.39 (52 CE) is not preserved, but he re-appears at forty-seven years old and "squinting" in *P. Oxy.* 1.99 (55 CE).
21 *P.Mich.* 5.321 (42 CE).
22 Asbell et al. (2005, 602).
23 "Glaucoma" is an umbrella term for a group of eye diseases; see Gross (2018, 1261–63). The term itself originates from γλαυκὸς ("bright, gleaming"), which in the *eikones* referred to light-colored irises, as in *P. Petrie* 2.6 (238 BCE).
24 Sihota, Sood, and Agrawal (1995, 252–54).
25 "Leucoma" also in modern medical literature, ibid.
26 *P. Grenf.* 1.33 (103 BCE), *P. Hamb.* 1.38 (182 CE), *P. Ant.* 3.187a (198 CE).
27 *SB* 20.14471 (160 BCE), *SB* 20.14481 (158 BCE), *P.Mich.* 5.285 (1–56 CE), *P. Coll. Youtie* 1.19 (44 CE), *BGU* 3.834 (125 CE), *SB* 1.4414 (143 CE), *P. Berl. Frisk.* 1 (155 CE).

28 *P. Adler Gr.* 5 (108 BCE), *P. Grenf.* 2.51 (143 CE), *PSI* 13.1324 (173 CE), *P. Tebt.* 2.397 (198 CE), *SB* 24.15987 (208 CE).
29 *Stud. Pal.* 22.42 (185 CE).
30 *SB* 10.10571 (194 CE).
31 *P. Grenf. 1.33* (103 BCE).
32 Saw et al. (1996, 175–87).
33 As ὑπόστραβος: *BGU* 6.1258a (143 BCE), *P. Grenf.* 1.33 (103 BCE), *P. Oxy.* 2.256 (34 CE), *P. Oxy.* 1.99 (55 CE), *BASP* 50, 89 (88–96 CE), *P. Hamb.* 1.15 (209 CE); as παράστραβος: *PSI* 9.1028 (15 CE), *P. Aberdeen* 56 (176 CE), *P. Oxy.* 36.2777 (212 CE); στραβός: *P. Tebt.* 3.972 (125–100 BCE); στραβίζοντος: *PSI* 14.1402 (125 BCE).
34 See Karev (forthcoming).
35 Right eye: *PSI* 9.1028 (15 CE), *P. Flor.* 3.316 (100–199 CE), *P. Amh. Gr.* 2.74 (147 CE), *P. Amh. Gr.* 2.102 (180 CE), *PSI* 8.922 (180–192 CE), *P. Flor.* 3.383 (234 CE): Left eye: *P. Flor.* 1.51 (138–161 CE); not preserved: *CPR* 1.218 (100–199 CE); not specified: *P. Oxy.* 18.2186 (260 CE).
36 *CPR* 1.218 (100–199 CE).
37 *BASP* 50, 89 (88–96 CE).
38 *P.Mich.* 5.321 (42 CE).
39 Mute or noiseless: Il. 14.16 and 24.54, Hdt. 4.200, Xen. HG 2.5.31, Aen. Taxt. 19, Plu. 2.721, Ph. 2.520; Dumb (men or animals): Parm. 6.7, Cratin. 6; Deaf: Herclit. 34, Hdt. 1.34, Dialex. 6.12, Plu. 2.1108d.
40 On detailed runaway notices as a literary trope, see Karev (2024, 154–155).
41 The dictionary definition of χωλός (Liddell, Scott, and Jones [1940, *s.v.* χωλός]) is usually "lame", but this is an outdated and negative term; hence, I have opted for the translation "partial paralysis" implied by the secondary meaning of "halting".
42 *CPR* 18.24 (232 BCE).
43 *P.Cair. Mich.* 3.21 (188 CE).
44 *P. Tebt.* 3.814 (227 BCE).
45 As in *Ps. -Archyt.* quoted in *Cat.* 396.1.
46 *CPR* 1.170 (103 CE); *P. Tebt.* 2.397 (198 CE).
47 Usually of liquids; see Liddell, Scott, and Jones (1940, *s.v.* κάπτω).
48 Lewis and Short (1975, *s.v.* capio); cf. Cic. *Rab. Perd.* 7.21.
49 *SB* 20.14771 (160 BCE).
50 Vajaranant et al. (2010, 91–99).
51 On the challenges of life expectancy calculation, see Bagnall and Frier (1994, 75–110).
52 *P. Grenf.* 2.35 (98 BCE); *P. Lond.* 3.678 (99 BCE); *Stud. Pal.* 22.42 (185 CE).
53 Two in *P. Petrie* 2.6 (238 BCE); one in *CPR* 18.19 (231 BCE).
54 *BGU* 3.834 (125 CE); *SB* 24.15987 (208 CE).
55 *SB* 1.4414 (143 CE).
56 Same individual in *P. Oxy.* 1.39 (52 CE); *P. Oxy.* 1.99 (55 CE).
57 *UPZ* 2.180b (113 BCE).
58 "ἄτεχνος," *P. Oxy.* 2.256 (34 CE).
59 Vandorpe (2008).
60 *P. Lond.* 3.678 (99 BCE).
61 *CPR* 18.19 (231 BCE).
62 David (2017, 75–89), Jefreys and Tait (2000, 91).
63 Anderson (2009, 343).
64 David (2017, 83).
65 Notably Montserrat (1998); extensive discussion in Karev (2024, 151–156).
66 On the difficulty in determination of slave prices: Scheidel (2005), Harper (2010). Notably, Roman-period slave sales included a standardized clause declaring the enslaved person to be free of epilepsy, which warrants an impairment-aware discussion in its own right. On the clause, see Urbanik (2010).
67 Dupras et al. (2008), Nerlich et al. (2000), Finch et al. (2012), David (1979, 83–89).

68 Finch et al. (2012), Gray (1966, 138).
69 Harris, Ponitz, and Ingalls (1998, 60).
70 Ibid., 62–63.
71 Harris, Iskander, and Farid (1975, 401–4), Massingham and Power (2022, 64–75).
72 *BGU* 3.999; *P. Grenf.* 2.32; *P. Lips.* 1.1; *SB* 20.14393.
73 Nunn (1996, 198). On dwarfism in Egypt in general el-Aguizy (1987, 53–60), Dasen (1993), Jefreys and Tait (2000, 88–90), David (2017, 83).
74 Harer (1993, 19).
75 Full-body mummy paintings are attested (e.g. Getty Museum 81.AP.42; Louvre N3076; British Museum EA6709; British Museum EA 68509; British Museum EA 6715) but bust-length portraits are far more common.
76 Bagnall (1997, 17–20).
77 E.g. British Museum GRA 1890.9–20.1 (Painting 87).
78 E.g. Altes Museum 31161.10.
79 E.g. Altes Museum 3116.9.
80 Jefreys and Tait (200, 88).
81 Lehrman (1993, 378).
82 Johnson (2005, 31).
83 *P.Mich.* 5.264 (37 CE); *CPR* 1.218 (100–199 CE).
84 As stated in Sandison and Tapp (1998, 44). On trachoma as the likely cause of blindness in Egypt, see Sandison (1967, 457–58).
85 As in, e.g., *P. Oxy.* 51.3167 (200 BCE); *P. Tebt.* 3.817 (182 BCE).
86 Aufderheide (2003, 212, 248–49).
87 David (2017, 79).
88 E.g. periostitis, as in PUM II; Sandison and Tapp (1998, 81).
89 David (2017, 80).
90 *P. Tebt.* 3.814 (227 BCE).
91 On ankylosing spondylitis in Egypt: Aufderheide and Rodriguez-Martin (1988, 102–4), Feldtkeller, Lemmel, and Russell (2003, 1–5); *contra* Saleem and Hawass (2014, 3311–16).
92 Waldron (2009, 127).
93 Sandison (1957, 336).
94 Aufderheide (2003, 424).
95 Ibid., 423.
96 Evidenced in the mummy PUM II. See Benitez (1988, 485–90).
97 Smith and Jones (1910, 284), Leek (1986, 191).
98 Aufderheide (2003, 428), for Egyptian examples, Hrdlička (1935, 92).
99 Dantcheva, Elia, and Ross (2015, 441–67), and citations *indem.*
100 *P. Oxy.* 41.2993 (323 CE).
101 *P.Mich.* 6.426 (199 CE).
102 *P. Brux.* 1.10 (174 CE).
103 Vlahogiannis (1998, 18).
104 In Egyptian courts, women needed no such oversight; see Pestman (1961, 184), Depauw (2017, 45–56).
105 Jefreys and Tait (2000, 94).
106 David (2017, 82–83).

Bibliography

Anderson, S. R. "The Eye and Its Diseases in Ancient Egypt." *Acta Ophthalmologica Scandinavica* 75, no. 3 (2009): 343.

Asbell, P., J. Dualan, D. Mindel, D. Brocks, M. Ahmad, and S. Epstein. "Age-Related Cataracts." *The Lancet* 365 (2005): 599–609.

Aufderheide, Arthur. *The Scientific Study of Mummies.* Cambridge: Cambridge University Press, 2003.

Aufderheide, Arthur, and Conrado Rodriguez-Martin. *The Cambridge Encyclopaedia of Human Palaeopathology.* Cambridge: Cambridge University Press, 1988.

Bagnall, Roger. "The Faiyum and Its People." In *Ancient Faces: Mummy Portraits from Roman Egypt,* edited by S. Walker and M. Bierbrier, 17–20. London: British Museum Press, 1997.

Bagnall, Roger, and Bruce Frier. *The Demography of Roman Egypt.* Cambridge: Cambridge University Press, 1994.

Barbieri-Low, Anthony, and Robin D. S. Yates. *Law, State, and Society in Early Imperial China. Vol. 2: A Study with Critical Edition and Translation of the Legal Texts from Zangjiashan Tomb No. 247.* Leiden: Brill, 2015.

Benitez, Jaime. "Otopathology of Egyptian Mummy PUM II: Final Report." *Journal of Laryngology and Otology* 102 (1988): 485–90.

Bierbrier, M. "The Discovery of the Mummy Portraits." In *Ancient Faces: Mummy Portraits from Roman Egypt,* edited by S. Walker and M. L. Bierbrier, 23–24. London: British Museum Press, 1997.

Collomp, Paul. "L'ethnographie égyptienne d'après les signalements contenus dans les papyrus." *Bulletin de l'Association G. Budé*, no. 49 (1935): 2–8.

Dantcheva, Antitza, Petros Elia, and Arun Ross. "What Else Does Your Biometric Data Reveal? A Survey on Soft Biometrics." *IEEE Transactions on Information Forensics and Security* 11, no. 3 (2015): 441–67.

Dasen, Veronique. *Dwarfs in Ancient Egypt and Greece.* Oxford: Clarendon Press, 1993.

David, Rosalie. *The Manchester Mummy Museum Project.* Manchester: Manchester University Press, 1979.

David, Rosalie. "Egyptian Medicine and Disabilities from Pharaonic to Greco-Roman Egypt." In *Disabilities in Antiquity*, edited by C. Laes, 75–89. London: Routledge, 2017.

Depauw, Mark. *A Companion to Demotic Studies.* Bruxelles: Fondation Égyptologique, 1997.

Depauw, Mark. "Legal Incapacity in Ancient Egypt." In *Ancient Guardianship: Legal Incapacities in the Ancient World,* edited by U. Yiftach and M. Faraguna, 45–56. Trieste: Edizioni Università di Trieste, 2017.

Doxiadis, Euphrosyne. *The Mysterious Fayum Portraits: Faces from Ancient Egypt.* New York: Harry N. Abrams, 1995.

Dupras, Tosha, Stevie Mathews, Marleen De Meyer, Christoph Peeters, and Bart Vanthyune. "Just Cut It Off: Amputation in Ancient Egypt." *Palaeopathological Association 35*th *Meeting, Abstracts* (2008): 6–8.

El-Aguizy, Ola. "Dwarfs and Pygmies in Ancient Egypt." *Annales du Service des Antiquités de l'Égypte* 71 (1987): 53–60.

Feldtkeller, Ernst, Ernst-Martin Lemmel, and Anthony S. Russell. "Ankylosing Spondylitis in the Pharaohs of Ancient Egypt." *Rheumatology International* 23 (2003): 1–5.

Finch, Jacqueline, Glyn Heath, Ann David, and Jai Kulkari. "Biomechnical Assessment of Two Artificial Big Toe Restorations from Ancient Egypt and their Significance to the History of Prosthetics." *Journal of Prosthetics and Orthotics* 24 (2012): 181–91.

Goodley, Dan. *Disability Studies: An Interdisciplinary Introduction.* London: Sage, 2011.

Gray, P. H. K. "Embalmers' 'Restorations'." *Journal of Egyptian Archaeology* 52 (1966): 138–40.

Gross, Ronald. "Open Angle Glacuomas." In *The Encyclopedia of Ophthalmology,* edited by U. Schmidt-Erfurth and T. Kohnen. Berlin: Springer, 2018.

Harer, W. Benson. "Health in Pharaonic Egypt." In *Biological Anthropology and the Study of Ancient Egypt,* edited by W. V. Davies and R. Walker. London: British Museum Press, 1993.

Harper, Kyle. *"Slave* Prices in Late Antiquity (and in the Very Long Term)." *Historia: Zeitschrift für alte Geschichte* 2 (2010): 206–38.
Harris, James, Z. Iskander, and S. Farid. "Restorative Dentistry in Ancient Egypt: An Archaeological Fact." *Journal of the Michigan Dental Association* 57 (1975): 401–4.
Harris, James, Paul Ponitz, and Brian Ingalls. "Dental Health in Ancient Egypt." In *Mummies, Disease, & Ancient Culture,* edited by A. Cockburn, E. Cockburn, and T. Reyman. Cambridge: Cambridge University Press, 1998.
Hasebroek, Johannes. *Das Signalement in Den Papyrusurkunden.* Berlin: De Gruyter, 1921.
Hrdlička, Aleš. "Ear Exotoses." *Smithsonian Miscellaneous Collections* 93 (1935): 1–99.
Hübsch, Gerbert. *Die Personalangaben als Identifizierungsvermerke im Recht der gräko-ägyptischen Papyri.* Berlin: Duncker & Humblot, 1968.
Jefreys, David, and John Tait. "Disability, Madness, and Social Exclusion in Dynastic Egypt." In *Madness, Disability, and Social Exclusion: The Archaeology and Anthropology of "Difference"*, edited by J. Hubert. London: Routledge, 2000.
Johnson, Horton. "Fish Bile and Cautery: Trachoma Treatment in Art." *Journal of the Royal Society of Medicine* 98 (2005): 31.
Kaluszynski, Martine. "Republican Identity: Bertillonage as Government Technique." In *Documenting Individual Identity,* edited by J. Caplan and J. Torpey. Princeton: Princeton University Press, 2001.
Karev, Ella. *Physical Descriptions, Biometrics, and Eikonographia in Graeco-Roman Papyri from Egypt.* Leiden: Brill, 2024.
Leek, Frank. "Cheops' Courtiers: Their Skeletal Remains." In *Science in Egyptology*, edited by R. David. Manchester: Manchester University Press, 1986.
Lehrman, Arthur. "The Fayyum Portraits." *Plastic and Reconstructive Surgery* 92 (1993): 378.
Lewis, Charlton, and Charles Short. *A Latin Dictionary: Founded on Andrews' Edition of Freund's Latin Dictionary Revised, Enlarged and in Great Part Rewritten.* London: Clarendon Press, 1975.
Liddell, Henry George, Robert Scott, and Henry Stuart Jones. *A Greek-English Lexicon.* 9th ed. Oxford: Oxford University Press, 1940.
Massingham, S., and R. Power. "Interventive Dental Therapy in Ancient Egypt (*c.* 2686 BC–323 AD): A Critical Review." *International Journal of Palaeopathology* 38 (2022): 64–75.
Montserrat, Dominic. "Experiencing the Male Body in Roman Egypt." In *When Men Were Men: Masculinity, Power and Identity in Classical Antiquity,* edited by L. Foxhall and J. Salmon. London: Routledge, 1998.
Nerlich, Andreas, Albert Zink, Ulrike Szeimies, and Hjalmar Hagedorn. "Ancient Egyptian Prosthesis of the Big Toe." *The Lancet* 356 (2000): 2176–79.
Nunn, J. F. *Ancient Egyptian Medicine.* Norman: University of Oklahoma Press, 1996.
Pestman, P. W. *Marriage and Matrimonial Property in Ancient Egypt.* Leiden: Brill, 1961.
Saleem, Sahar, and Zahi Hawass. "Ankylosing Spondylitis or Diffuse Idiopathic Skeletal Hyperostosis in Royal Egyptian Mummies of the 18th–20th Dynasties? Computed Tomography and Archaeology Studies." *Arthritis & Rheumatology* 66 (2014): 3311–16.
Sandison, Andrew. "The Eye in the Egyptian Mummy." *Medical History* 1 (1957): 336.
Sandison, Andrew. "Diseases of the Eyes." In *Diseases in Antiquity,* edited by A. Sandison and D. Brothwell, 457–58. Springfield, IL: Charles Thomas, 1967.
Sandison, Andrew, and Edmund Tapp. "Disease in Ancient Egypt." In *Mummies, Disease, & Ancient Culture,* edited by A. Cockburn, E. Cockburn, and T. Reyman. Cambridge: Cambridge University Press, 1998.
Saw, Seang-Mei, J. Katz, O. Schein, S. Chew, and T. Chan. "Epidemiology of Myopia." *Epidemiologic Reviews* 18, no. 2 (1996): 175–87.
Scheidel, Walter. "Real Slave Prices and the Relative Cost of Slave Labor in the Greco-Roman World." *Ancient Society* (2005): 1–17.

Sihota, R., N. Sood, and H. C. Agrawal. "Traumatic Glaucoma." *Acta Ophthalmologica Scandinavica* 73, no. 3 (1995): 252–54.

Smith, Grafton, and Frederick Jones. *The Archaeological Survey of Nubia: Report for 1907–1908.* Cairo: National Printing Press, 1910.

Smolka, F. "De ratione personarum describendarum in papyrorum actis adhibitis." *Eos* 27 (1924): 75–88.

Urbanik, Jakub. "P. Cairo Masp. I 67120 Recto and the Liability for Latent Defects in the Late Antique Slave Sales, or Back to *Epaphe*." *Journal of Juristic Papyrology* 40 (2010): 219–47.

Vajaranant, Thasarat, Sushma Nayak, Jacob Wilensky, and Charlotte Joslin. "Gender and Glaucoma: What We Know and Need to Know." *Current Opinions in Ophthalmology* 21 (2010): 91–99.

Vandorpe, Katelijn. "Persian Soldiers and Persians of the Epigone: Social Mobility of Soldiers-Herdsmen in Upper Egypt." *Archiv für Papyrusforschung* 54 (2008): 87–108.

Vlahogiannis, Nicholas. "Disabling Bodies." In *Changing Bodies, Changing Meanings: Studies on the Human Body in Antiquity,* edited by D. Montserrat, 13–36. London: Routledge, 1998.

Waldron, Tony. *Palaeopathology.* Cambridge: Cambridge University Press, 2009.

18 Disability in the Greek Papyri from Roman Egypt

A Public Concern

Nicola Reggiani

Introduction

The study of physical disability in the Graeco-Roman world has gained significant attention in recent years.[1] Scholars have analysed various literary and material sources to reconstruct the experiences of disabled people in classical societies.[2] By exploring the ways in which disability was understood and accommodated in the past, scholars can help to shed light on the broader issues of difference, diversity, and social inclusion in human history.

The present contribution aims to explore a category of sources that has been understudied: Greek documentary papyri from Hellenistic, Roman, and Byzantine Egypt. These documents offer glimpses into everyday life, thus providing a direct way to approach the topic of disability without the potential distortions imposed by literary or artistic sources. The chapter first outlines key terms[3] related to disability in the papyrological corpus in terms of meaning and context. A particular focus is on Roman-age documents of a public nature, in which some of these terms are used to indicate specific categories of people. From the viewpoint of state administration, it was crucial to determine whether an individual was able to work or not, essentially to establish their liability to pay certain taxes. Physical impairments were considered valid reasons for tax exemptions, especially concerning the capitation tax.[4] In official terminology, the exemption for physical 'weakness' was indicated by the general term ἀπολελυμ(μ)ένος (i.e., τῆϲ λαογραφίαϲ) "having been released (from the capitation tax)".[5] It was used as a personal identifier in census registers and tax reports, alone or in combination with other terms related to physical 'weakness', namely, ὑπερετήϲ "overage", ἀϲθενήϲ "sick, weak", and ἐπιϲινήϲ "disabled, impaired".[6]

ἐπιϲινήϲ (*episines*) and πηρόϲ (*peros*)

The term ἐπιϲινήϲ, derived from ϲίνομαι ("to harm, injure, damage").[7] It is a general word indicating a physical impediment without specification of the actual injury.[8] The official application of such terminology as introduced earlier is immediately clear from the census register P. Oxy. VI 984 (=P.Oxy.Census, Ox., 91/2 CE), which records a person, whose name is now lost, defined as ἐπιϲινὴ(ϲ) ἀπολελυμμένο(ϲ) "disabled released" (l. 220). Another entry of the same text, related to a young man,

DOI: 10.4324/9781003440369-21

runs Τιθοῆϲ [υἱὸ(ϲ)] μητρὸ(ϲ) Cενύριο(ϲ) ὃϲ ὕϲτερο(ν) ἐν ἐπιϲινέ(ϲιν) ἀπελ(ύθη) (ἐτῶν) ιζ (l. 346) "Tithoes, son (i.e., of the preceding person), whose mother is Senuris, who eventually was released among the disabled, 17 years old."

The information stored in these general population registers that were used by authorities to manage tax collection was taken by the public offices from house-by-house census declarations (κατ' οἰκίαν ἀπογραφαί), which were personal reports concerning the inhabitants of single dwellings.[9] There are several papyrological examples of this procedure, among which SB VIII 9870 (Hermopolites, 2nd CE) contains a fragmentary reference to a "disabled" person: Cτοτ⟨ο⟩ῆτι⟨ϲ⟩ [Cτοτοή]τιοϲ | τοῦ Φα[... μ]ητρὸϲ Θερ[......] ἐπι|ϲινήϲ (ll. 8–10) "Stotoetis, son of Stotoetis, grandson of Pha . . ., whose mother is Ther . . ., disabled."

The second reference in the aforementioned Oxyrhynchus census register (ὕϲτερον ἐν ἐπιϲινέϲιν ἀπελύθη) suggests that there was some official procedure to declare a person as ἐπιϲινήϲ, i.e., belonging to the category of the ἐπιϲιναί, but we do not know exactly how this worked. Official certificates for the status of ἀϲθενήϲ existed (see the following), and the same must have existed for ἐπιϲινήϲ as well. A most interesting papyrus, P. Oxy. XXXVI 2754 (Ox., 111 CE), contains the text of an edict of the prefect of Egypt concerning the legal procedure in the production of such certifications:

> The village secretaries are to present under oath the names of those who are disabled or who wish to be released (i.e., from the capitation tax) on other grounds (τῶν ἐπιϲινῶν ἢ ἄλλαιϲ αἰτίαιϲ ἀπολυθῆναι βουλομένων), with the strategus supervising. It will be no monetary penalty that those will suffer who assume feigned names, abusing the clemency of the most manifest of gods, the Emperor Caesar Nerva Trajan Augustus Germanicus Dacicus. Those concerned in the petitions and wishing to defer the case will have no excuse, having known long ago the time fixed for the *conventus* (i.e., the periodical visit of the prefect in the countryside to administer justice). I absolutely prohibit the receiving of bribes, not now for the first time forbidding this evil. . . . If anyone of those whose names have been posted at the termination of the *conventus* has not already obtained a hearing, he will be able to be judged before the strategus of the nome. But should the judges be responsible for the delay, I will detain them until they settle the cases. Let this be publicly displayed. The 14th year, Pharmouthi 1.[10]

Once the exempted status was obtained, it was recorded not only in the census declarations, but also in other documents related to the public life of the disabled individuals. For example, in a fragment from a register of people cultivating different types of land (γεωργοῦντεϲ), we find a final total account of the workers and also of those who were not able to work: ὑπερ(ετεῖϲ) ιγ ἐνϲινὴϲ α "overage: 13; disabled: 1" (BGU II 560, Ars., 2nd CE).[11] In a dossier concerning obligations and exemptions of the weavers (P.Phil. 1, Ars., after 119 CE), the second document (an extract of an edict of the prefect C. Vibius Maximus, 103–107 CE) contains a list of persons exempted from public duties (εἰϲὶ δὲ οἱ ἀπ[ολ]υόμενοι δημο[ϲίων κτλ.), among which were ὑπερετεῖϲ ἐπιϲινεῖϲ ἐπικριθέντε[ϲ (col. i, l. 29) "over-age, disabled, those who passed the *epikrisis*".[12] In one of the *libelli* imposed by Emperor Decius to prove that individuals had offered sacrifices to the Roman gods, the involved person is recorded as Ἀϲῆϲιϲ ὡϲ (ἐτῶν) λβ ἐπιϲινήϲ "Asesis, 32 years old, disabled" (SB I 4435, Theadelphia, 250 CE).

However, a problem is raised by the precise extent of the 'damage' denoted by the term ἐπιϲινήϲ. Was it a temporary or a chronic impediment? Was it a physical injury or a disease? Some documents may shed light on this issue. The tax rolls from Karanis, a collection of extensive and detailed registers of payments for various types of taxes, contain recurring entries for the same individuals identified as ἐπιϲινήϲ over different years. "Ptolemaios son of Onnophris, grandson of Petheus, whose mother is Tapetheus" is recorded as ἐπιϲινήϲ in 171/2 CE (P.Mich. IV 223, 1781–82) and again in 173/4 (P.Mich. IV 225, 1493). Similarly, "Apollonios s. Petronius, g. Apollonios, m. Ptolemais" is listed as ἐπιϲινήϲ in 172/3 (P.Mich. IV 224, 313–4), 173/4 (P.Mich. IV 225, 1241–42) and twice in 175 (P.Cair. Mich. I 359, 635 and 1696). "Onnophris s. Onnophris" is identified as ἐπιϲινήϲ in 172/3 (P.Mich. 224, 2101) and twice in 173/4 (P.Mich. IV 225, 1671 and 2509).[13] Finally, "Ptolemaios s. Petermouthis, g. Apunchis, m. Thermouthis" appears as ἐπιϲινήϲ twice in 173/4 (P.Mich. IV 225, 2780 and 3136–37) and again in 175 (P.Cair. Mich. I 359, 1702). These instances suggest that the status of ἐπιϲινήϲ could persist over time. However, there are instances where the same individuals who are identified as ἐπιϲινήϲ in some years are not labelled as such in other years. Thus, Ptolemaios s. Onnophris is listed without the attribute in P.Mich. IV 224, 2131 and 4754–55 (172/3 CE); Ptolemaios s. Petronius is also registered without the attribute in another moment of 172/3 CE (P.Mich. IV 224, 4717); Ptolemaios s. Petermouthis is recorded throughout P.Mich. 223, 224, 225 without the attribute. A new instance, "Heron s. Heron alias Heras, g. Sisois, m. Segathis", is identified as ἐπ⟨ι⟩ϲινῆϲ in 173/4 (P.Mich. IV 358d, 8) but not elsewhere (P.Mich. IV 224, 4726–27 and 3671).[14] This suggests that in some cases, ἐπιϲινήϲ may not have referred to a permanent disability, unless its omission was due to a careless scribe.

The only instances that provide information on what ἐπιϲινήϲ could refer to are some petitions related to mistreatments experienced by disabled people. In addition to the terminological interest, these documents are very important to understand the general attitude towards disability. The idea conveyed by these texts is that an ἐπιϲινήϲ is vulnerable due to their impairment, and is subject to discrimination and abuse, not unlike fatherless or widowed women in comparable cases.

P.Mich. VI 425 (Karanis, 198 CE) is a petition addressed to the epistrategus (chief judicial official) by a certain Gemellus alias Horion,[15] who denounces violence and attempted extortion committed against him and his mother by a tax collector's assistant. The violence is stressed by the petitioner as even more deplorable because he was blind:

> ὅδε̣ καταφρονήϲαϲ μου ὡϲ ἐπιϲουνοῦϲ (=ἐπιϲινοῦϲ), | μονόφθαλμοϲ γὰρ ὢν τῷ δοκοῦντι ὁρᾶν οὐ βλέπω ὡϲ ἐν ἀνφοτέροιϲ (=ἀμφοτέροιϲ) | πονηρὸν εἶναι ἄντικροιϲ (=ἄντικρυϲ), ἠργολ[ά]βηϲέν με κ̣α̣ὶ πρότερον ἐμὲ ἐξυβρ{ε}

ίcαc | δημοcίᾳ καὶ τὴν μητέρα{ν} μου, μετὰ τ̣ὸ π̣λ̣⟨ε⟩ί̣cταιc αὐτὴν πληγαῖc αἰκίcαcθαι | καὶ πέλυκι ὅλαc μου τέccαρεc (=τέccαραc) θύραc καταcχ{ε}ίcαι ὥcτε ὅλην ἡμῶν τὴν | οἰκίαν ἀν⟨απ⟩επταμένην γενέcθαι καὶ εὐεπ{ε}ίβατον παντὶ κακού[ργῳ (ll. 11–16) This person, who held me in contempt because of my infirmity – for I have only one eye and I do not see with it although it appears to have sight, so that I am utterly worthless in both – victimised me, having first publicly abused me and my mother, after maltreating her with numerous blows and demolishing all four doors of mine with an ax so that our entire house is wide open and accessible to every malefactor.[16]

One year later, the same Gemellus submitted another petition to the epistrategus (P.Mich. VI 426, Karanis, 199/200 CE), requesting confirmation of his right to exemption from compulsory public service as a village elder, also in accordance with his privileges as an inhabitant of Antinoupolis. Throughout the text, he repeatedly refers to his impairment, providing further details about that (such as the cause for his blindness), citing it as the reason for both the abuse and the privileges he is requesting:

Ἀρρίῳ Οὐί{ο}κτορι τῷ κρα(τίcτῳ) ἐπιcτρατήγωι | παρὰ Γεμέλλου τοῦ καὶ Ὡρίωνοc Γαίου Ἀπολι|ναρίου Νίγεροc ἀcθενοῦc τὴν ὄψιν γεου|χοῦντοc ἐν κώμῃ Καρανίδι τῆc Ἡρακλείδου μερίδο(c). | τῆc εἰc πάνταc ἀνθρώπουc φθανούcηc δικαιοκρι|cίαc, ἐπιτρόπ̣ων μέγιcτε, καὶ αὐτὸc βίαν πάcχων | δέομαι τῶν ἀπὸ c̣ο̣ῦ δικαίων τυχεῖν. ἔχει δὲ οὕτωc· | οἱ κώμηc Καραν̣ίδοc τῆc αὐτῆc Ἡρακλείδου μερίδοc | πρεcβύτεροι ἀδεέcτατοι τυγχάνοντεc, τῇ ἑαυ|τῶν βίᾳ καὶ αὐθαδ⟨ε⟩ίᾳ χρηcάμενοι, ὡc κοινωνω (=κοινωνὸν) αὐ|τῶν ἀναδοθέντα ὡc Ὧρον Ἀπολιναρίου ἀνύπαρ|κτον ὄνομα ὃ καὶ ἀγνοῶ οὕτωc ἀγνοῶ, οὔτε γὰρ | ἐδήλωcεν ὅτι πηρὸc ἢ ἐπιcινὴc ἢ ἄλλο τι τῶν | ἐμῶν cημείων, οὐδὲ μὴν ἐξόν μοι ἄλλωc χρημα|τίζ⟨ε⟩ιν μοι Ἀντινοεῖ ὄντι, οὐδὲ μὴν πάλιν λ⟨ε⟩ιτουρ|γεῖν εἰ μὴ ἐν μόνῃ τῇ Ἀντινόου πόλει. ἔτι δὲ καὶ | ὑπὸ τῶν τῆc πόλεωc βουλῆc γενομένηc cυνε|χωρήθην χλαμυδοφ[ορεῖ]ν. διὰ τὸ ὡc οὐ μόνον | μονόφ̣θαλμόν μ[ε] εἶναι [ἀλ]λὰ καὶ τῷ νομιζομένῳ | ὑπάρχειν ἑτέρῳ ὀφθαλ[μ]ῷ οὐ βλέπω, λευκώμα|τοc ἐκ τῆc κόρη[c] αὐτο[ῦ] διαφανέντοc καὶ τῷ πλέ|πιν (=βλέπειν) ἐπιcινοῦ[c μου ὄντοc, δι]ὰ τοῦτο ἐνέτυχον | καὶ τῷ κρα[τίcτῳ ἡγεμόνι ἡμ]ῷν καὶ ἔcχον αὐτοῦ ἱερὰν | ἐπιcτο[λήν, ἧc ἀντίγραφ]ο̣ν̣ (ll. 1–24) To his excellency Arrius Victor, epistrategus, from Gemellus also called Horion, son of Gaius Apolinarius Niger, who is afflicted with weak vision, landholder at the village of Karanis in the division of Herakleides. Since your righteous judgment extends to all men, mightiest of overseers, I also, a victim of violence, beg to partake of your justice. The situation is as follows: the elders of the village of Karanis of the same division of Herakleides, men without the least scruple, with their habitual violence and arrogance < – – – > me whom they nominated as their colleague under the name "Horos, son of Apolinarius," a fictitious name which I do not know. For this reason, I do not know it, for neither did it set forth "disabled" or "infirm" or any other of my distinguishing marks, nor is it indeed permissible for me, since I am an Antinoite, to be styled otherwise, nor indeed to perform a liturgy again except in Antinoupolis alone. Furthermore, I was granted the right to wear the chlamys by the citizens at a meeting of the senate. Since not only am I one-eyed, but also, I do not see with the eye that supposedly remains, because a leucoma has appeared in its pupil and my sight is impaired, on this account I addressed a petition also to his excellency the prefect, and I received the sacred rescript, of which a copy follows (the rest is very fragmentary).[17]

In the same time span, another petition was addressed to a police officer of Theadelphia by a woman denouncing an extortion undergone by an unfortunate lame man (SB VI 9105, 198 CE):

Φιλίπ[π]ῳ ἐξ εὐ[cχ]ημ⟨όν⟩ων γ | αἱρεθέντι εἰρηνοφύλ(ακι) Θεαδ|ελφείας | παρὰ Οὐλπίας Ἡρωείδος |μετὰ κυρίου τοῦ δεδ[ο]μέ|νου μοι κατὰ τὰ Ῥωμαίων | ἔθη Γαίου Λουκρητίου | Παπιριανοῦ. οὐκ ἀγνοεῖς | τὰς ἀναιδείας καὶ τὰς πει|ράσεις τὰς περὶ Ἀβαβῖ|κειν, ᾧ καὶ ἄλλοτε πλη|γὰς ἐπέθηκας ἀναιδειῶν | ἕνεκεν· καὶ νῦν αὐτὸς | τὴν τυραννίαν ἐπιδεί|ξαςθαι ἠθέληςεν· τὸν | γὰρ ἐν τῷ πωμαρίῳ | μου τρεφόμενον ἐπι|ςινῆ χωλὸν ἀπολελυ|μένον ἁπάςης ὀχλή|ςεως καὶ λαογραφίας | κατὰ τὴν τοῦ ἡγεμόνος | δικαιοδοςίαν ἀπ⟦α⟧\ή/ ιτη|ςεν (=ἀπῄτηςεν) ⟦αὐτὸν⟧ ἀργυρ{ε}ίδιον | προφάςει τοῖς πρεςβυ|[τέ] ρο[ι]ς χ̣ωρεῖν. ἐπεὶ | οὖν τὰ τοια̣ῦ̣τ̣α̣ δεῖται | ἐγδικίας μεγάλης, ἢ μά|λιςτα ἀπολυτέον ἄν|θρωπον διαςείεςθαι, | ἐπιδίδωμί ςοι τόδε τὸ βι|βλίδιον ὅπως μετ' ἀςφα|λείας αὐτὸν εἰς τὴν μη|τρόπολιν ἀγάγῃς ςὺν τῷ | χωλῷ· φάςκει γὰρ καὶ δε|δωκέναι τοῖς ἐπὶ τοῦ | θηςαυροῦ δημοςίοις | τὰ ἴςα. ⟦ι⟧ \ᾧ/καὶ μάρτυρας | ἐπέςτηςα (ll. 1–38) To Philip, chosen *eirenophulax* of Theadelphia out of 3 *euschemones,*[18] from Ulpia Herois with the guardian granted me according to Roman usage, Gaius Lucretius Papirianus. You are not unaware of the shameless enterprises connected with Ababikis, whom you have at other times chastised for shameless extortion: now this same man has elected to give an exhibition of his tyranny; for he has demanded a sum of money from the man who is being cared for in my orchard, a diseased cripple, who had been exempted from all liability for poll-tax according to the ruling of the prefect; this on the pretext that he was deferring to the elders. Since therefore such conduct demands severe punishment, or certainly (?) the man must be delivered from extortion, I tender this petition, that you may take him under guard to the metropolis together with the cripple; for he further alleges that he has given the copies to the public officials in charge of the storehouse; and I have produced witnesses to this.[19]

Gemellus' second petition demonstrates a close equivalence between the terms ἐπιςινής and πηρός, with the latter being a less common and less official synonym.[20] In addition to the petition mentioned earlier, only two attestations of πηρός are found. In a second-century private letter (BGU III 846, Ars.), a son complains to his mother about his poverty, ending his lament with a meaningful exclamation: οὐκ οἶδες, ὅτι θέλω πηρ̣ὸς γενέσται (=γενέσθαι) | εἶ (=ἢ) γνοῦναι (=γνῶναι) ὅπως ἀνθρόπωι (=ἀνθρώπωι), [ἔ]τ[ι] ὀφείλω ὄβολον (ll. 15–16) "Don't you know that I would rather be a disabled person than be conscious that I am still owing anyone an obol?"[21] While in the official context of the petitions impairment was evoked as a way of stressing the cry for help and justice, in the colloquial context of this letter this condition is presented as an inferior state, though better than misery. A flaw is also intended in a contract of sale of a donkey (P.Lond. II 203, Herakleia, Ars., 142 CE), which describes the animal as ὄνον ἄρρενα | τέλει[ο]ν λευκομυόχρουν τοῦτον | τοιοῦτον ἀναπό⟨ρ⟩ριφον χωρὶς πηροῦ (ll. 15–17) "a donkey, male, adult, white-coloured, not liable to be rejected except if blemished".

χωλός (*cholos*) and τυφλός (*tuphlos*)

While ἐπισινής was mainly used to refer to a tax- and duty-exempted category, πηρός was an ordinary word with a more negative connotation, though the cited petition P.Mich. 426 seems to equate them on an official level. There were also more specific terms used to indicate particular cases of physical disability, which appear to have been used as bodily distinctive features in official identifications, just like other common characteristics such as skin colour, size and shape of body parts, and scars.[22] As Ulpia Herois' petition makes clear, a case of ἐπισινής could be represented by χωλός "limping". χωλός is indeed among the most frequently used terms and was continuously employed from the Ptolemaic to the Byzantine age to identify a personal peculiarity that became a distinctive identity characteristic, even when the use of personal identifiers declined in the Roman administrative practice.[23] The most relevant document is a petition addressed by a royal cultivator to the strategos (UPZ I 122, Memphis, 157 BCE), which denounces a crime that caused the petitioner to develop a limp, and stresses the precariousness of such a condition:

> Π[οσ]ειδωνίωι [ἀρ]χισωμα[τ]οφύλακι | καὶ στρατηγῶι παρ' Ἁρμάιος | βασιλικοῦ γεωργοῦ τοῦ (=τῶν) ἐκ Παανάμεὺς | τοῦ Ἡρακλεοπολίτου. εἰθισμένος | ἔρχεσθαι εἰς τὸ πρὸς Μέμφει μέγα | Σαραπιεῖον κατ' ἐνιαυτόν, ὅπως θυσιάσω, | τοῦ δὲ κε (ἔτους) Ἀθὺρ κη θυσιάσαντός μου | κατέλυσα ἐν τῶι Ἀνουβιείωι. τῆι δὲ κθ | ἀναβάντος σου εἰς τὸ Ἀνουβιεῖον ἐπὶ | τοὺς λῃστὰς καὶ εὐλαβῶς μου σχόντος | καὶ βουλομένου ἀναχωρῆσαι εἰς τὸ | Σαραπιεῖον, τῶν μετὰ σοῦ τις ἐν τῶι | θορύβωι βουλόμενός μου περιελέσθαι | τὸ ἱμάτιον καὶ ἐμοῦ ἀντιποιουμένου | σπασάμενος λέπει με τῆι μαχαίραι | εἰς τὸ σκέλο[ς], ὥστε χωλὸν ἕως τοῦ νῦν | μ' εἶναι. διὸ ἀξιῶ, ἐπεὶ σὺν τοῖς θεοῖς | καὶ τῆι σῆι τύχηι ἐκ θανάτου σέσωμαι, | ἐὰν φαίνηται, συντάξαι τοῖς παρά σου | μὴ κωλύειν με, ἐὰν βούλωμαι ἐπανάγειν | εἰς τὴν κώμην διὰ τὸ χωλὸν ὄντα τοῖς | ἀναγκαίοις θλίβεσθαι, ὅπως μὴ ὑπὸ τῆς | λιμοῦ διαλ[υ]θῶ
> To Poseidonios, chief bodyguard and strategos, from Harmaios, royal farmer from Paanameus in the Herakleopolites. It is customary for me to come to the great Sarapieion near Memphis every year to make a sacrifice. On the 28

> Hathyr of the 25th year, while I was sacrificing, I stayed at the Anubieion. On the 29th, when you went up to the Anubieion against the robbers and I was with you, being cautious and wanting to retreat to the Sarapieion, someone who was with you in the confusion wanted to grab my cloak, and when I tried to resist, he stabbed me in the leg with the sword, leaving me lame until now. Therefore, I ask, since with the help of the gods and your good fortune I have been saved from death, that you order your men not to hinder me, if I wish to return to the village because my lameness makes it difficult for me to endure the necessary things, so that I will not be destroyed by hunger.

Variant ways to indicate lower limb impairment (that causes a limp) as a personal identifier were the rare compound χωλόπους "limping at the foot"[24] and the present participle of the verb χωλαίνω "to be lame", often followed by the indication of the affected leg.[25] Similarly, the participle of the verb ἐπισκάζω "to limp" was used, with the indication of the affected foot.[26] This may suggest a distinction between the two terms (impairment at the leg vs at the foot), but it must be noted that the latter is so far attested only in Ptolemaic texts.

Gemellus' petitions, on the other hand, show that blindness was considered another type of ἐπισινής. He first describes himself as μονόφθαλμος "one-eyed," a term which was used elsewhere as a personal identifier.[27] Gemellus then emphasises that his only eye is unable to see due to a leucoma,[28] a technical medical term that was widely used in the everyday language, since we find it in official identifications[29] as well as in private writings.[30] He describes his condition using the phrases οὐ βλέπω "I do not see" and ἀσθενὴς τὴν ὄψιν "sight impaired". The former phrase is not found elsewhere,[31] but the latter appears in two earlier petitions by Gemellus, who again mentions his impairment to stress his weakness in front of an abuse. In these texts (P.Mich. VI 422 and 423, Karanis, 197 CE; duplicates: SB XXII 15774 and P.Mich. VI 424), Gemellus complains to the prefect and to the strategos that people had entered his fields and stolen his crops using violence, and they did so καταφρονήσαντος τῆς περὶ τὴν ὄψιν μου ἀσ|θενείας (422, 4–5) ≙ καταφρονούντω\ν/ | τὴ⟨ν⟩ περὶ τὴν ὄψιν μου | ἀσθέν⟨ε⟩ιαν (423, 29–31) "despising my impaired vision". Comparable phrases are ἀσθενὴς τοῖς ὄμμασι[32]/ ὀφθαλμοῖς,[33] ἀδύνατος τοῖς ὄμμασι[34]/ὀφθαλμοῖς (both meaning "weak in the eyes"),[35] τοῖς ὀφθαλμοῖς ἀμβλυωπῶν/ἀμβλυωπήσας[36] (with participle forms of the verb αμβλυωπέω "to be dim-sighted"), ὑποκεχυμένος τὰς ὄψεις/τὸν ὀφθαλμὸν[37] ("afflicted with cataracts at the eye(s)"). They appear in contracts or other legal documents, in which they act as personal identifiers, and in petitions, in which they are used to stress the petitioner's weakness. The phrase ὑποκεχυμένος ὀλίγον βλέπων[38] ("afflicted with cataracts and seeing little") is of particular interest because it is used in a certificate of release from military service to stress the physical impossibility to serve as a soldier. The lack of a standard terminology appears to indicate that no official categorisation was developed.

The term ἀσθενής in relation to physical impairment will be discussed later. Blindness in the papyri is expressed elsewhere with the attribute τυφλός "blind," which was similarly used as a personal identifier as χωλός.[39] The idea that such a physical impairment implies particular weakness and defencelessness is echoed in a late request for clemency to an unnamed supreme authority (P.Cair. Masp. I 67020, Aphrodito, c. 566–573 CE), where the addressees are praised for being πενήτων θρεπτητορες (=θρεπτῆρες) καὶ τυφλῶν καὶ εὔϲφλαγχνοι (=εὔϲπλαγχνοι) δοτῆρες "nurturers of the poor and compassionate givers to the blind". See also the following passage from a late legal protocol (P.Lond. V 1708, Antinoupolis, 567/8 CE), in which blindness is presented as a cause of general weakness: ὁ πάτηρ ἡμῶν Ἀπολλῶϲ ἀπεβιώϲατο, ἐτυφλώθη δὲ | ὁ αὐτὸϲ ἤτοι τῆϲ ὁράϲεωϲ ὑϲτερηθεὶϲ ἐξηϲθενηκὼϲ | διόλου καὶ ἄπρακτοϲ γέγονεν (ll. 84–86) "our father Apollo passed away: he became blind, or rather was deprived of sight and became completely weakened and inactive". Other personal identifiers related to sight issues were ὑπόϲκνιφοϲ "shortsighted"[40] and ϲτραβόϲ "cross-eyed".[41]

ἀϲθενήϲ (*asthenes*)

The term ἀϲθένεια etymologically derives from a negative form of ϲθένοϲ "physical force"[42] and therefore bears the general meaning of "weakness". The frequent occurrence of this word, along with its adjective ἀϲθενήϲ and the adverb ἀϲθενῶϲ, in the papyri (205 attestations according to the *Papyri.info* database) raises some interpretive issues regarding its actual meaning. ἀϲθενήϲ could sometimes imply the concept of "disabled, impaired", as seen in Gemellus' petitions mentioned earlier. The problem lies in distinguishing this special meaning from the other two that are attested in our reference corpus: "weak" and "sick, ill". The boundary between these meanings is, of course, blurred since disability can be caused by illness, and both impairment and disease produce weakness, so the three concepts are intertwined.[43]

A systematic analysis of all occurrences of ἀϲθενήϲ and similar words in the papyri is beyond the scope of this contribution. In contexts in which a cure is sought, ἀϲθένεια is more likely intended to mean illness: for example, in two copies of an oracular ticket asking the crocodile-gods of Soknopaiou Nesos whether ϲοθῆϲωι (=ϲωθήϲομαι) ταύτηϲ ἧϲ ἐν ἐμοὶ ἀϲθενία⟨ϲ⟩ "if I will be saved from this disease which is in me". A disease is also likely intended when people say they are lying in a state of weakness that temporarily prevents them from doing something. An ἀϲθένεια that was certainly a disease damaged the breast milk of a woman in BGU IV 1109, 10–12 διὰ τὸ τῆϲ | Καλλιτύχηϲ ἐν ἀϲθενείᾳ διατεθείϲηϲ διεφθάρθαι τὸ ταύτηϲ | γάλα (nursing contract, Alexandria, 5 BCE). A very prolonged weakness may refer to something more serious, as in a private letter from Herakleopolis (BGU III 948, 4th/5th CE), in which the writer states that the recipient's mother has been weak (ill) for 13 months (ll. 5–6 ἡ μήτηρ ϲου Κοφαήνα | ἀϲθεν⟨ε⟩ῖ, {ε} ἰδοῦ, δέκα τρ⟨ε⟩ῖϲ μῆνεϲ). In other cases, ἀϲθένεια can be a reference to economic weakness, like that affecting the cultivators petitioning in BGU VIII 1815, 6–7 τῶν ἀϲθενῶϲ διακει|μένων γεωργῶν (Her., 60 BCE), or metaphorical weakness, like that ascribed to women as a gender in P.Lond. III 971, 4 ἀδύνατοϲ γάρ ἐϲτιν ἡ γυνὴ διὰ ἀϲθέν⟨ε⟩ιαν τῆϲ φύϲε[ωϲ "The woman is indeed unable because of the weakness of her nature" (negotiations about a female bailiff, u.p., 4th CE) and in CPR VII

15, 4 γυναῖκας διὰ τὸ τ]ῆς φύσεως ἀσθενές "women (who are) weak by nature" and 12–13 κ̣α̣τ[α]φρο|[νοῦντες τῆ]ς̣ ἀσθενοῦς̣ μου γυναικ[είας φ]ύ̣σ̣ε̣ω̣ς "despising my weak feminine nature" (petition, Hermopolis, c. 330 CE). Perhaps a special meaning is to be intended in BGU VIII 1773, 13 σωματικῆι ἀσθενείαι κατεχομέν[ου] "impeded by a physical weakness" (trial proceedings, Herakleopolis, 58 BCE); the text deals with a person who has been mistreated because someone illegally took possession of his field, harvested the crops, and did not pay the due taxes. The victim is said to have written to the chief guard because of his physical impairment. ἀσθενοῦντες are certainly people who cannot work temporarily in the quarries of Mons Claudianus (1st to 2nd CE) and for this reason they are listed (O. Claud I 118, 122) or individually recorded as such in personnel lists (O. Claud. IV 696, 709, 754). However, other *ostraka* of the same type record ἄρρωστοι, meaning "sick people" (O. Claud. I 83–94, 96, 117, IV 708, 714, 717). According to Hélène Cuvigny, who analysed these texts, the two terms are "parfaitement synonymes".[44]

The clearest example of ἀσθενής as an official category of population is the "list of overage and weak people" filed by the amphodarch (mayor) of the quarter Apolloniou Parembole in Ptolemais Euergetis in 72/3 CE (SPP IV pp. 58–83, xiv 489–92 π]α[ρ]ὰ Ἡρακλείδου ἀμφοδ[άρχ]ου Ἀ[πολλω(νίου) Παρε(μβολῆς)] | γραφὴ {ι} ὑπερετῶν καὶ ἀσθενῶν [ἀναγραφομένων] | ἐπὶ τοῦ προκειμένου ἀμφόδου τῷ [ε (ἔτει)] | Αὐτοκράτορος Καίσαρος Οὐεσπα̣σ̣ι[ανοῦ Σεβαστοῦ]). At first glance, it seems that ἀσθενής may have had a different meaning than ἐπισινής, with the former referring to illness and the latter to physical impairment. However, things are never simple when dealing with partially unknown contexts. For example, the status of ἀσθενής was certainly certified by means of documents such as SB V 8025 (Ars.?, 91/2 CE):

> ἀσθενὴς ἀπο|λελυμένος τῆς | λαογραφίας τῶι .[] (ἔτει) | Δομιτιανοῦ ὑπ[ὸ] | Μεττίου Ῥούφου | τοῦ ἡγεμονεύσαντ(ος) | Σαταβοῦς Ακ̣.. |.. τοῦ Ἀκεί̣ους, | μη(τρὸς) Θενπατύνιος | [τ]ῆς Ἥρωνο[ς] |.[].. (ἔτους) ια Sick released from the capitation tax of the x year of Domitian by Mettius Rufus the former prefect: Satabus son of Ak . . ., grandson of Akes, whose mother is Thenpatunis daughter of Heron,. . .11 years old.

However, what is striking about this document is the young age of the person released from the tax, since children under 14 were not liable to pay it. So why was a certificate of ἀσθένεια necessary in this case? Perhaps was it intended to attest a physical impairment that would have lasted for this person's entire life?

Another case of ἀσθενής related to public exemptions is a petition from Ptolemais Euergetis dated to 192–194 CE (PSI X 1103):

> Ῥουτιλλίωι Ἀχιλλεῖ τῷ κρατίστῳ ἐπ[ι]στρατήγωι | παρὰ Πα̣[.]νος {ηρα} Ἡρακλείδου τοῦ Διδύμου ἀπὸ τῆς | μητροπόλεως τοῦ Ἀρσινοείτου. μηκέτι ἄλλο π̣[ρ]ᾶγμα δέετε (=δέεται) | τῆς σῆς τοῦ κυρίου μισοπονηρίας ⟨ἢ⟩ καὶ τὸ ἡμ̣έ̣τ̣ερον. ἔχει δὲ | οὕτως. ἐκ νέας ἡλικίας λ⟨ε⟩ιτουργήσας ἀλλεπαλλήλους χρεί|ας βαρυτάτας κατὰ δὲ τὴν τῆς ἡλικίας δύναμιν καὶ τὴν τοῦ | σώματος

ὑπηρεcίαν, ἔτι δὲ καὶ ἄπορος παντελῶς τυγχά|ν̣ων, κατ' ἐπήρ[εια]ν̣ ὑπογυίως ἀνεδόθεν ὑπὸ τῶν τῆς πό|λεως γραμματέων εἰς δ̣ιαραματίαν (=διεραματίαν) τῆ[ς] Ἡρακλείδου | μερίδος ἄνθρω[π]ος τῇ ἡλικίᾳ προβεβηκώς· εἰμὶ γὰρ ὑπὲρ | τὰ ἑβδομήκοντα ἔτη· τῶν κατὰ καιρὸν ἡγεμ[ό]νων καὶ ἐπι|τρόπων ἀπολελυκότων λ⟨ε⟩ιτουργιῶν τοὺς ὑπὲρ τὰ | ἑξήκοντα καὶ [π]ε̣ντε ἔτη, [ἐγ]ὼ δὲ οὐ μόνον τῇ ἡλικίᾳ, | ἀλλὰ καὶ τῷ σώ[μ]ατι ἀσθε[ν]ῆ̣ς καὶ τοῖς ὀφθαλμοῖς ἀβλοιοπῶν (=ἀμβλυωπῶν) | [ἐ]πὶ τοσοῦτον ὥ[ς]τε καὶ ἀ̣π̣ρ̣[ ]ε̣ι̣τον εἶναι (ll. 1–15) To Rutillius Achilles, the most excellent epistrategos, from Pa . . . nos son of Herakleides, grandson of Didymos, from the metropolis the Arsinoites. No other fact needs your lordship's hatred of evil than ours. This is how it is: having served various public duties from a young age and according to the strength of the age and the service of the body, yet now being completely destitute, I was deceitfully charged by the scribes of the city of the grain shipment of the division of Herakleides, (though being) a man who have surpassed the age; for I am beyond the seventy years. Among the officials and stewards who were released from the public duties at the appropriate time, those beyond the sixty-five years, I am not only weak in age, but also weak in body and nearsighted in both eyes, to such an extent that I am almost (blind?).

Here ἀσθενής is not intended as a proper official category but hints to something very similar to Gemellus' impaired vision, in this case due to old age. The same connection between physical weakness and old age is evident in two additional documents. One is a petition submitted by an elderly weaver from Karanis seeking exemption from the weavers' tax (P.Oslo III 124, 1st CE). He presents himself as ὑπερετοῦς | ἀρχαίου (ll. 7–8) "overage advanced in years" and asks οὐκέτι | εὐτονῶ{ι} τὴν γερδια|κὴν τ̣έχνη(ν) ποιεῖν | [δ]ι̣ὰ τὸ ἀσθενῆ με εἶ̣ν̣α̣ι | ̣τῇ ὁράσει καὶ ὑπὸ | γήρους̣ σ̣υ̣ν̣εχόμε̣ν[ον] | εἶ̣ναι [ὡς] ἐ̣τῶν π̣ , | διὸ ἀξιῶ σε τὸ̣ν | κύριον ἀπολυθῆ|ναί με τοῦ γερδ̣ι̣α̣|[κοῦ τ]έ̣λους (ll. 8–18) "since I am no longer able to practice the weaving art, due to weak eyesight and old age, being about eighty-x years old, therefore I ask you the lord to exempt me from the weavers' tax". The second document is a public notice (*programma*) by the strategos from Ptolemais Euergetis in 136 CE (SB XVI 12504):

ἀντί]γ̣ρα̣(φον) π̣ρογράμματος̣ ̣[.] () ο̣μ̣. [-ca.?-] | [Ἡ]ρακλείδης στρατη[γὸ]ς Ἀρσινοίτου Θεμίστ[ου μ]ε̣ρίδος. | [Γ]ελλίου Βάσσου τοῦ κρατίστου ἐπι[σ]τρατήγου | γράψαντός μοι ἀντὶ Γαίου Ἀντωνίου Γαλλικοῦ | διὰ γῆρα[ς] ἀσθενοῦς τῷ σώματι καταστῆσαι | ἕτερον εἰς τὴν ἐπιτήρησιν ἐν ᾗ ἐδήλωσεν | ὁ̣ Γαλ̣λ̣ι̣κ̣ὸ̣ς̣ εἶναι, ἀνεδόθη ὑπὸ τῶν τῆς μερίδος | κωμογραμματέων ὧν δὲ κωμῶν μή εἰσι̣ν̣ | κωμογραμματε[ῖ]ς πρεσβυτέρων διαδεχομένων | τὰ κατὰ τὰς κωμογραμματείας | Ἀπίων Ἀμμωνίου τοῦ Μύσθου ἀπὸ Χηνοβοσκ(ῶν) | εἰς τὴν ἐ[πι]τήρησιν ὠνῆς ζυτηρᾶς κώμης | Θ̣ε̣α̣δ̣ε̣λ̣φία[ς.] (col. ii, ll. 25–37) [Copy] of a public notice, (excerpted from the public archives?). Herakleides, strategos of the division of Themistes in the Arsinoites. After his excellency Gellius Bassus, the epistrategos, had written to me to appoint, instead of

> Gaius Antonius Gallicus, who is physically weak owing to old age, another person to the superintendency in which Gallicus (in his petition) stated himself to be, there was nominated by the village scribes of the division and – in villages where there are no scribes – by the elders performing the duties of the office of village scribe: Apion son of Ammonios, grandson of Musthes, of the quarter of the Chenoboskoi, for the superintendency over the farming of the beer-tax of the village of Theadelphia.[45]

In conclusion, both ἐπιcινής and ἀcθενής are associated with bodily weakness. The former seems to be specific to physical impairment or disability without any connection to old age, while the latter looks like a more general term indicating physical limitations, which in some cases could be disability or old age. On the other hand, ἀcθενής was used as a proper official term denoting a population category. The fact that ἀcθενής and ἐπιcινής never appear together, although both appear in combination with ὑπερετής, suggests that they could be interchangeable with each other to officially refer to physical weaknesses, not related to age.

Conclusions

Although it is not always easy to understand the exact meanings of the words, it is possible to conclude that the overall concept underlying the vocabulary of physical disability in the Greek papyri reflects the idea of weakness. On one hand, this attracted particular attention from public administration to establish who was unable to work and, above all, pay taxes, resulting in a somewhat 'privileged' category in population surveys.[46] On the other hand, the same idea of weakness was evoked by those who were impaired in official contexts to seek help, justice, and relief from public burdens. In the end, the everyday aspect of disability is reflected in the system of personal identifiers, wherein several physical impairments were objectively used to check individual identities.

Summary Table of the Discussed Terms

Greek term	*Translation*	*Context*
ἐπιcινής	Harmed/injured/ damaged	Official personal applications, declarations, and records (tax- and duty-exempted status)
ἀcθενής	Weak/ill/sick	Personal communications but also official contexts as previous (tax- and duty-exempted status)
πηρόc	Blemished	Less official context, perhaps not an officially established status
χωλόc χωλόπουc χωλαίνων ἐπιcκάζων	Limping	Personal identification

Greek term	*Translation*	*Context*
μονόφθαλμος	One-eyed	Personal identification
ἀcθενὴc τὴν ὄψιν ἀcθενὴc τοῖc ὄμμαcι ἀcθενὴc τοῖc ὀφθαλμοῖc ἀδύνατοc τοῖc ὄμμαcι ἀδύνατοc τοῖc ὀφθαλμοῖc ἀμβλυωπῶν τοῖc ὀφθαλμοῖc ἀμβλυωπήcαc τοῖc ὀφθαλμοῖc	Dim-sighted/weak in the eyes	Personal identification
ὑπόcκνιφοc	Short-sighted	Personal identification
cτραβόc	Cross-eyed	Personal identification
ὑποκεχυμένοc τὰc ὄψειc ὑποκεχυμένοc τὸν ὀφθαλμὸν	Affected with cataracts at the eye(s)	Personal identification
τυφλόc	Blind	Personal identification

Notes

1 This paper stems from the PRIN 2017 National Project "Greek and Latin Literary Papyri from Graeco-Roman and Late Antique Fayum: Texts, Contexts, Readers" (P.I. Lucio Del Corso, University of Salerno), Research Unit at the University of Parma (coordinator Nicola Reggiani). The papyrological sources are cited according to the official abbreviations of the *Checklist of Editions*, online at https://papyri.info/docs/checklist. Unless differently noted, translations are mine. For the sake of conciseness, the following abbreviations are used throughout: Ars. = Arsinoites; Her. = Herakleopolites; Ox. = Oxyrhynchus; Oxy. = Oxyrhynchites; u.p. = unknown provenance. The indication 'century' is omitted.

2 Some of the most notable works in this area include Dasen (1993), Garland (1995), Ogden (1997), Rose (2003), Breitwieser (2012), Southwell-Wright (2013), Laes, Goodey, and Rose (2013), Laes (2017), Sneed (2018), Laes (2020a), Adams (2021).

3 Critical catalogues of words related to disability have been provided by Caldara (1924), Samama (2017), Laes (2020b).

4 See P.Oxy.Census, p. 39, note to l. 220; Hombert and Préaux (1937, 262), Jördens (2009, 349–50).

5 "Der befreit worden ist von der Kopfsteuer," Wilcken (1893, 249).

6 See Reggiani (2020, 200).

7 Chantraine (1999, 1005), *s.v.* cίνομαι; see also Hdn. *Orth.* III.2, p. 580, 25 καὶ τὰ παρὰ τὸ cίνομαι δὲ διὰ τοῦ ι γράφεται οἷον ἐπιcινήc.

8 The only exceptions are represented by P.Oxy. L 3595, 3596, 3597 (Senepta, 243 CE), lease contracts of a pottery, where the word ἐπιcινήc is used to refer literally to "blemished" pottery. In literature, the term frequently also bears a transitive meaning of "harmful". As such,it is used several times in scientific (Theophrastus' *History of Plants*) and astrological treatises (Claudius Ptolemy, Vettius Valens, etc.).

9 See Hombert and Préaux (1952), Bagnall and Frier (1994, 1–30), Jördens (2009, 62 ff.), Claytor and Bagnall (2015).

10 Translation adapted from the edition.

11 The rare form ἐνcινήc could be a remainder of Ptolemaic terminology, in which the word was used in public documents (contracts, tax accounts) as a personal identifier. The only two extant instances are P.Genova IV 150 (account of payments in kind, Ars., mid-3rd BCE), 23 Εὐάρχῳ ἐνcιν(εῖ) and P.Strasb. VIII 761v (contract, 2nd BCE), 11 ἐ̣νcίνου. The term is not unproblematic (see short discussion in P.Genova IV 150, 23 n.) but seems certain.

12 *Epikrisis* was a legal procedure aimed at establishing other categories of privileged people: those possessing the gymnasial status, the metropolitans, the Arsinoitic *katoikoi*; see Nelson (1979), Jördens (2009, 331–54).

13 P.Mich. IV 225, 3316 Ὀ]ννῷφρ[ε]ῳϲ ἐ̣π̣ι̣ϲ̣ι̣ν[ή]ϲ̣ may refer either to Onnophris s. Onnophris or to Ptolemaios s. Onnophris; however, since the patronymic only is recorded, as is the customary case with the former but not with the latter, it is likely that we have another reference to Onnophris s. Onnophris.

14 In P.Cair.Mich. I 359, 52 and 950 the papyrus is broken after his papponymic.

15 The papyrological documentation about Gemellus alias Horion has been discussed by Draycott (2015) as a case study for the lived experience of disability in antiquity.

16 Translation from APIS catalogue.

17 Translation adapted from the edition.

18 Wealthy and prominent villagers, subject to specific public duties: see Lewis (1993).

19 Translation from Barns (1949).

20 See Chantraine (1999, 898), *s.v.*

21 Translation adapted from Winter (1933, 106).

22 See Caldara (1924). Another physical defect that was used as a personal identifier was κεκαμμένος δάκτυλος ("bent, stiff finger"): CPR I 170, 4 κεκαμμένου δακ[τύλ]ουϲ τρεῖϲ χειρὸϲ δε[ξιᾶϲ (contract, Ars., 103–117 CE); P.Tebt. II 397, 6 κεκαμμένον δάκτυλον μικρὸν χειρὸϲ ἀριϲτερᾶϲ (contract, Ptolemais Euergetis, 198 CE). Moreover, κυλλόϲ appears to be a generic term indicating deformity, used as a general identification signal (P.Bingen 31, 10 τετ]ᾳνὸϲ κυλλώϲ: official list of people, Ars.?, second half 3rd BCE; P.Coll.Youtie II 105, 4 ὁ κυλλόϲ: mummy label, Panopolites, 2nd–4th CE; P.Yale III 137, 152 Νεμεϲᾶϲ κυλλόϲ: land register, Philadelphia, Ars., 216/7 CE; perhaps P.Herm. 7, 13 Ψόϊϲ κυλλόϲ: letter, Lykopolis, after 381 CE [*l.* Κύλλου *ed.pr.*]). In a future contribution I will be dealing with another interesting attestation of impairment in the papyri, deafness.

23 P.Hamb. I 117, 14 τῆι χωλῆι (account, Philadelphia, mid-3rd BCE); CPR XXVIII 9, ii 13 Παϲχειῦϲ χῳ(λόϲ?) (tax report, Tebtynis? 3rd/2nd BCE); BGU VII 1515, 9 ὁ χωλὸϲ Θαμμ. . . φοϲ (account, Philadelphia, 210–204 or 193–187 BCE); BGU VII 1559, 6 ὁ χωλ(όϲ?) (list of workmen, Philadelphia, 210–204 or 193–187 BCE); UPZ II 180a, xxiv 7 Ψενθώ(τηϲ) χωλόϲ (contract, Hermonthis, 113 BCE); SB I 428, 5–6 χωλ[οῦ (sale contract, Krokodilopolis, 99 BCE); BGU XVI 2614, 12 Ἡρακλῆν τὸν χωλὸν (official letter, Her., 21 BCE–5 CE); BGU IV 1196, iv 67 Πεταῦϲ Ταθ[ο]ῆτοϲ χωλόϲ (list of priests, Busiris, 11/10 BCE); P.Corn. 22, i 13 Ἐργεῦϲ χωλόϲ (census list, Philadelphia, early 1st CE); P.Mich. V 323, 9, 14, 36 Ἡρακλοῦν χωλήν (division of slaves, Tebtynis, 47 CE; duplicate: PSI VIII 903); BGU VII 1620, viii 2 C[ε]νπ̣ρώνιο[ϲ] χωλ̣ὸ̣ϲ (Philadelphia, first half 2nd CE); BGU IX 1893, xv 493 Ἑκῦϲιϲ χωλὸϲ (tax report, Theadelphia, 149 CE); P.Haw. 196, 17]αϲ ἡπητ(ὴϲ) [και] χωλὸϲ (account, Ptolemais Euergetis, 160 CE); P.Berl. Leihg. I 7, iii 54 Μιῶϲιϲ Μύϲ̣θου χολ(οῦ) (tax report, Ars., 162 CE); BGU IX 1896, xiv 320 Cύροϲ υἱὸϲ Cαμβοῦτοϲ χωλῆϲ (land report, Theadelphia, 166 CE); P.Mich. IV 223, xcvii 2933 Ἀπ]ολλωνίο(υ) χώλο(υ) (tax report, Karanis, 172 CE); P.Cair.Goodsp. 30, xxxi 21 χωλῷ Γ̣αίῳ (account, Karanis, 192 CE); P.Lond. II 189, vii 78 Ἶϲαϲ χωλόϲ (list of names, Karanis, second half 2nd CE); BGU III 712, i 8 Γα[ί]ῳ χωλῷ (account, Ars., 2nd CE); BGU XX 2873, 2–4 με|τὰ τοῦ χωλοῦ Ποῦ̣τ̣|τι Π̣τέϲ (work report, Elephantine, late 2nd to early 3rd CE); O.Narm. I 72, 18 κα̣τ̣ὰ Ὡ̣ρίωνοϲ χωλοῦ (memorandum, Narmuthis, 2nd/3rd CE); P.Oxy. XIX 2240, ii 32 Ναρώουϲ χωλὸϲ (account, Oxy., 211 CE); P.Col. VIII 230, ii 41 Πτολεμαῖοϲ Χαιρή(μονοϲ) χωλὸϲ (list of nominees, Karanis, early 3rd CE?); O.Mich. II 952 Πανῖλοϲ χωλόϲ (single name, Karanis, 3rd CE); P.Köln. XIII 540, 14 Cερήνου χωλ (account, u.p., 4th CE?); P.Bad. IV 95, v 94 Ἀνδρέαϲ χωλῶ, ix 199 Ἀνδρέ̣ο̣υ χωλῶ, xiv 304 Ἀνδρέου χωλῶ (account, Hermopolites, early 6th CE); SPP X 207, 4 Ποῦϲιϲ χωλ(ὸϲ) (list of names, u.p., 6th CE); P.Lond.Herm., folio 20v, 9 Ἰ̣ϲ̣ὰκ χωλόϲ (tax register, Hermopolis, 546/7 CE?); P.Oxy. XVI 1911, ii 29 δι(ὰ) Πέτρου

χωλοῦ (account, Ox., 557 CE); P.Oxy. LV 3804, v 99 δι(ὰ) Πέτρου χωλοῦ (account, Ox., 566 CE); SPP XX 222, 11 Γεώργιος χωλὸς (account, Memphites, 6th/7th CE); P.Oxy. XVI 1917, 4r, 71 Ἀνοῦπ χωλὸς, 4v, 99 δ(ιὰ) Ἀνοῦπ χωλοῦ (account, Ox., early 6th or early 7th CE); SB XXII 15244, I 4 ἄπα Ἰουλ(ίου) χωλ(οῦ) (list of workmen, u.p., 7th CE); P.Mon.Apollo I 27, 10 δ(ιὰ) Ἰωσὴφ χωλός (list of payments, u.p., 7th/8th CE); SB I 4168, 2–3 Ταπιὰμ(?) τὴν | χωλὴν (mummy label, u.p., unknown date).

24 P.Leipz. 11r, 7 Ἄρειος Πετειμώτου λινο(υργὸς) χωλόπ(ους) (account, Memphis, 3rd CE).

25 CPR XVIII 24, 42 χωλαίνων τὸ δεξιὸν σκέλος (contract, Theogonis, 232 or 206 BCE); P.Freib. IV 55, 29 χωλένων ἐν δ[εξιῶι. . . . .] (repayment of loan, Philadelphia, 71 CE); P.Oxy. III 634, 18 χωλαίνουσα τὸν (will, Ox., 126 CE); SB XXII 15353, 13 χωλαίνων (census declaration, Ox., 146/7 CE); P.Brook. 8, 10 χωλαίνω(ντος) (divorce agreement, Ptolemais Euergetis, 177 CE).

26 CPR XVIII 19, 13 ἐ[π]ισκάζων (contract, Theogonis, late 3rd BCE); SB XX 14471, i 5 [ἐπισκα]ζούσηι (contract, Ars., 160 BCE); BGU III 997, ii 5 ἐπισχάζων τὸν πόδα δεξιὸν (contract, Pathuris, 103 BCE); BGU III 998, i 5 ἐπισ[κάζω]ν τὸν πόδα δεξιὸν (contract, Pathuris, 101 BCE).

27 BGU IV 1196, v 97 μονοφω perhaps for μονόφ(θαλμος) (list of priests, Busiris, c. 11/10 BCE); P.Brux. i 10, 20–21 μονόφθ(αλμος) (census declaration, Prosopites, 174 CE); P.Oxy. LXI 4126, 3–4 τὸν ἀσ|τρολόγον \τὸν μονόφθαλμ(ον)/ (private letter, Ox., 3rd/4th CE).

28 A leucoma is a scar on the cornea of the eye formed after an injury, infection or inflammation. It appears as a white or grayish area on the clear tissue covering the front of the eye, which can cause blurred vision or loss of sight depending on the severity and location.

29 SB XX 144471, ii 10 λεύκω(μα) ὀφθαλ(μῷ) δεξ(ιῷ) (contract, Ars., 160 BCE); SB XX 14481, 5 λεύκω(μα) ὀφθαλ(μῷ) δε(ξιῷ) (contract, Ars., 158 BCE); P.Grenf. I 33, i 14 λεύκωμα ὀφθαλμόν (*sic*) (contract, Thebais, 103 BCE); BGU III 834, 12 [ο] (ὑλὴ) λεύκωμα ὀφθαλμὸν δεξιὸν (contract, Bubastos, 125 CE); P.Grenf. II 51, 9–10 λεύκωμα ὀ|φθαλμῷ ἀριστερῷ (contract, Soknopaiou Nesos, 143 CE); SB I 4414, 6 λεύκωμα ὀφθαλμῷ δεξιῷ (contract, Karanis, 143 CE); P.Berl.Frisk 1, xxii 17 λεύκ(ωμα) ὀφθ(αλμῷ) δεξιῷ (bank receipts, Ptolemais Euergetis, 155 CE).

30 P.Alex. 629 *descr.* (private letter, u.p., Roman age) ἐκ λευκώματος (untranscribed context); P.Oxy. XXXI 2601v, 1 ἵνα θεραπευθῇ τὸ λευκωμάτιον "so that the small leucoma can be cured" (private letter, Alexandria?, early 4th CE). For mentions of λευκώματα in medical prescriptions on papyrus see PSICongr. XXI 3, ii 1 πρὸς τὰ λευκώμα[τ]α (Tebtynis, 1st BCE); P.Strasb. inv. G 90, ii 10 πρὸς λευκ[ώματα (u.p., 2nd CE); likely also O.Bodl. II 2188, 3 [ ]ς λευκο.[.] perhaps for [πρὸ]ς λευκόμ[ατα] (Thebes, 4th CE?). See in general Isabella Andorlini, *Scritti sui papiri e la medicina antica*, ed. Nicola Reggiani (Florence: Le Monnier, 2017), 181 and 212; on the Strasbourg receptarium, Andorlini, *Scritti*, 265–85; on the Theban *ostrakon*, Claire Préaux, "Les prescriptions médicales des ostraca grecs de la Bibliothèque Bodléenne," *CE* 61 (1956): 135–48, 146–47.

31 In P.Giss. I 17, 10 οὐ βλέπομέν σε καθ' ἡμέραν (private letter, Apollonopolites Heptakomias, 113–120 CE) does not refer to a physical shortcoming but to the absence of the addressee.

32 P.Enteux. 25, 9 (petition, Ghoran, 222 BCE); UPZ II 180a, i 6 and 180b, i 6 (contracts, Hermonthis, 113 BCE).

33 P.Mich. XI 618, 11–12 (petition, Bakchias, 165–169 CE).

34 P.Stras. II 81, ii 17 (contract, Thebes, 115 BCE); P.Adl. 17, 5 (contract, Krokodilopolis, Pathurites, 99 BCE); P.Lond. III 678, 6 (id., 99/8 BCE); P.Wisc. I 3, 22–23 (petition, u.p., c. 256–259 CE).

35 CPR XVIII 15, 322 (contract, Theogonis, late 3rd BCE); P.Enteux. 26, 3 τοῖς ὀφθαλμοῖς ἀδυνατοῦντος (petition, Magdola, 221 BCE); P.Lond. II 219b, verso, 4 τοῖς ὀ]φθαλμοῖς (will, Thebais, 2nd BCE).

36 PSI X 1103, 14 (petition, Ptolemais Euergetis, Ars., 192–194 CE); P.Rein. II 113, 9–10 (petition, Kaminoi, Ars., c. 263 CE).

37 P.Mich. V 321, 3 ὑποκεχυμένος τὸν ἄλλον ἀριστερὸν ὀφθαλμὸν, left margin 5–6 ὑποκεχυμένος | το (= τῷ) ἀριϲτερῶι ὀφθαλμ(ῷ) (division of property, Tebtunis, Ars., 42 CE); P.Coll.Youtie I 19, 3 ὑποκεχυμένη τὰϲ ὄψειϲ (land cession, Ptolemais Euergetis, Ars., 44 CE).

38 P.Oxy. I 39, 9 = II 317, 7–8 (copies of a certificate of release from military service, Alexandria, 52 CE).

39 P.Oxyrhyncha 30, 21 [Ὦ]ρ̣ο̣ϲ μ̣έ̣γ̣α̣ϲ Πετοϲίριοϲ τυφλοῦ (account, Ars., 2nd BCE); P.Corn. 22, iii 73 Cωβθίτηϲ τυφλόϲ (census list, Philadelphia, early 1st CE); P.Mich. IV 223, 1360 Ὥρο(υ) τυφλο(ῦ), 1805 Χαιρήμ(ων) τυφλό(ϲ) (tax register, Karanis, 172 CE); P.Mich. IV 224, 1470 Ὥρου τυφ(λοῦ), 2789 υἱὸϲ Παπεῖϲ τυφλοῦ, 5471 Ἰϲᾶϲ τυφλόϲ, verso 6257 Ἰϲί⟨δ⟩ωροϲ τυφλόϲ (tax register, Karanis, 172/3 CE); P.Mich. IV 225, 2452 υἱοῦ Παπέιτοϲ τυφλοῦ (tax register, Karanis, 175 CE); SB XXVI 16675, i 8 Ἰϲᾶτοϲ Ὥρου τυφλοῦ (land register, Ars., c. 161–210 CE); P.Köln. IV 198, 6–7 Διόδωρον τὸν | τυφλὸν (business letter, u.p., 3rd CE); SB I 1974 ἐπράθη γερδίῳ ἐν πόρῳ τυφλῷ (account, Ox., 3rd CE); P.Ross.Georg. III 1, 19 ὁ Ἀπολλώνιοϲ ὁ τυφλὸϲ (private letter, Alexandria, c. 270 CE); O.Mich. I 104, 2 .[.] τυφλὸϲ (list of payments, Karanis, late 3rd to early 4th CE); CPR VIII 49, 3 Ἀτιώει τυφλῷ (account of payments, Hermopolites? 4th/5th CE); SPP VIII 1101, 1 Μαρ\κρίνᾳ/ τυφλ(ῇ) (receipt, Ars., 7th CE); CPR IX 50, ii 8 τ[υ]φλό(ϲ), 30 τυφλο̣ϲ̣ (tax register, Hermopolites, mid-7th CE); CPR IX 51r, 21 .τ̣υ̣φ̣λ̣(όϲ) (id.); SB XX 14246, 9 τυφλὸϲ (tax list, Hermopolites, 7/8th CE). In BGU XIV 2425, Τυφλὸϲ ἀλέτηϲ (list of names, Her., 1st BCE) and O.Elkab 147, 3 Τύφλοϲ Ἀρ̣ϲ̣(ιήϲιοϲ) (list of names, Eileithyiopolis, 1st/2nd CE) it seems used as a proper name. The marginal sentence in P.Oxy. XXXVI 2783 (private letter, Ox., 3rd CE) τὸν τυφλὸν ὁ ἀδελφόϲ ϲου ἀνήκαϲαί (=ἠνάγκαϲέ) μαι (=με) πωλῆϲαι "Your brother forced me to sell the blind one" is perhaps referred to an animal.

40 P.Petr.[2] 14, 26 ὑπ]όϲκνιφο[ϲ (will, Krokodilopils, 238/7 BCE); P.Petr.[2] 17, ii 33 ὑπόϲκνιπ[οϲ (will, Krokodilopils, 236/5 BCE); P.Petr.[2] 27, i 5 ὑπόϲκνιποϲ (will, Ars., 226/5 BCE); SB XII 10859, 6 ὑπόϲκνειφοϲ (will, Ghoran, 220 BCE); CPR XVIII 8, 15 ὑπόϲκνιφο̣ϲ̣ (contract, Theogonis, late 3rd BCE); P.Tebt. III 816, i 18 ὑπόϲχνιφοϲ (contract, Tebtynis, 192 BCE); P.Heid. VIII 413, 1 ὑπόϲκνιποϲ (contract, Herakleopolis, 179 BCE); P.Mich. III 190, 33 ὑπόϲκνιφοϲ (contract, Philadelphia, 172 BCE); P.Tebt. III 972 (4)r, 34 ὑπόϲκν]ιφοϲ (contract, Tebtynis, late 2nd BCE); P.Adl. 7, 6 ὑπο̣ϲ̣κνιφο̣ϲ̣ (contract, Pathuris, 104 BCE); P.Adl. 8, 3 ὑπόϲκνιφοϲ (id.); P.Mil. I 2, 4 ὑπόϲκνιφοϲ (id.); SB I 428, 5 ὑποϲκνίφο[υ] (contract, Krokodilopolis, Pathurites, 99 BCE); P.Grenf. II 35, 5 and 6 ὑπόϲκνιφοϲ (contract, Pathuris, 98 BCE); BGU III 911, 8 ὑ̣πόϲκνιφοϲ (contract, Soknopaiou Nesos, 18 CE); PSI IX 1057, 6 [ὑπ]όϲκνειφοϲ (receipt, Euhemeria, 32 CE); PSI VIII 907, 23 ὑπόϲκνιφοϲ (contract, Tebtynis, 42 CE).

41 P.Tebt. III 972 (1)v, 39 ϲ̣τρα(βὸϲ) (abstract of contract, Tebtynis, late 2nd BCE); O.Wilck. 93, 3 Βιήνχιοϲ ϲτραβὸϲ (receipt, Elephantine or Syene, 114 CE); P.Fuad.Univ. App. II 120, 8 ϲ]τραβ(ὸϲ) (contract, u.p., 2nd/3rd CE); SPP X 207, 2 Cαραπίων ὁ ϲτραβόϲ (list of people, u.p., 6th CE). In one instance from Ptolemaic age the verb ϲτραβίζω is used: PSI XIV 1402, 16 ϲτραβίζ[οντοϲ (contract, Herakleopolis, 125/4 BCE).

42 Chantraine (1999, 1000), *s.v.*

43 An even more generic term, ἀδύνατοϲ "unable", is excluded from discussion for space reasons.

44 O.Claud. I, 78.

45 Translation adapted from El Mosallamy (1981).

46 This appears to partially contrast Jane Draycott's statement that "in antiquity there was no such official category of person" (Draycott 2015, 191). On this topic see also Arzt-Grabner (2012), discussing certain individuals who demanded tax exemption based on their physical impairments, but none complained about discrimination. I am grateful to Mara Rescio for this bibliographical suggestion and some other helpful indications about this topic.

Bibliography

Adams, Ellen, ed. *Disability Studies and the Classical Body: The Forgotten Other*. London: Routledge, 2021.

Arzt-Grabner, Peter. "Behinderung und Behinderte in den griechischen Papyri." In *Disability and Impairment in Antiquity*, edited by Rupert Breitwieser, 47–55. Oxford: Archaeopress, 2012.

Bagnall, Roger S., and Bruce W. Frier. *The Demography of Roman Egypt*. Cambridge: Cambridge University Press, 1994.

Barns, John W. B. "Three Fayûm Papyri." *CE* 24 (1949): 295–305.

Breitwieser, Rupert, ed. *Disability and Impairment in Antiquity*. Oxford: Archaeopress, 2012.

Caldara, Alessandra. *I connotati personali nei documenti d'Egitto dell'età greca e romana*. Milan: Aegyptus, 1924.

Chantraine, Pierre. *Dictionnaire étymologique de la langue grecque*. Paris: Klincksieck, 1999.

Claytor, W. Graham, and Roger S. Bagnall. "The Beginnings of the Roman Provincial Census." *GRBS* 55 (2015): 637–53.

Dasen, Véronique. *Dwarfs in Ancient Egypt and Greece*. Oxford: Oxford University Press, 1993.

Draycott, Jane. "Reconstructing the Lived Experience of Disability in Antiquity: A Case Study from Roman Egypt." *G&R* 62 (2015): 189–205.

El Mosallamy, Abdalla H. S. "Public Notices Concerning Epiteresis of the One Zyteras." In *Proceedings of the Sixteenth International Congress of Papyrology*, edited by Roger S. Bagnall, Gerald M. Browne, Ann E. Hanson, and Ludwig Koenen, 215–29. Chico and New York: American Society of Papyrologists, (1980) 1981.

Garland, Robert. *The Eye of the Beholder: Deformity and Disability in the Graeco-Roman World*. Ithaca: Cornell University Press, 1995.

Hombert, Marcel, and Claire Préaux. "Certificat d'exemption de laographia." *CE* 12 (1937): 259–64.

Hombert, Marcel, and Claire Préaux. *Recherches sur le recensement dans l'Égypte Romaine*. Leiden: Brill, 1952.

Jördens, Andrea. *Statthalterliche Verwaltung in der römischen Kaiserzeit. Studien zum praefectus Aegypti*. Stuttgart: Steiner, 2009.

Laes, Christian, ed. *Disability in Antiquity*. London: Routledge, 2017.

Laes, Christian, ed. *A Cultural History of Disability in Antiquity*. London: Routledge, 2020a.

Laes, Christian. "How and Whether to Say 'Disability' in Ancient Greek and Latin." In *A Cultural History of Disability in Antiquity*, editedd by Christian Laes. London: Routledge, 2020b.

Laes, Christian, C. F. Goodey, and Martha L. Rose, eds. *Disabilities in Roman Antiquity. Disparate Bodies a Capite ad Calcem*. Leiden: Brill, 2013.

Lewis, Naphtali. "Εὐcχήμονεc in Roman Egypt." *BASP* 30 (1993): 105–13.

Nelson, Carroll A. *Status Declarations in Roman Egypt*. Amsterdam: Hakkert, 1979.

Ogden, Daniel. *The Crooked Kings of Ancient Greece*. London: Duckworth, 1997.

Reggiani, Nicola. "Identifying People in Official Reports: The Administrative Practice in Roman Egypt." In *Accounts and Bookkeeping in the Ancient World*, edited by Andrea Jördens and Uri Yiftach, 188–223. Wiesbaden: Harrassowitz, 2020.

Rose, Martha L. *The Staff of Oedipus: Transforming Disability in Ancient Greece*. Ann Arbor: University of Michigan Press, 2003.

Samama, Evelyne. "The Greek Vocabulary of Disabilities." In *Disability in Antiquity*, edited Christian Laes, 121–38. London: Routledge, 2017.

Sneed, Deborah. "The Life Cycle of Disability in Ancient Greece." PhD diss., University of California, 2018.

Southwell-Wright, William. "Past Perspectives: What Can Archaeology Offer Disability Studies?" In *Emerging Perspectives on Disability Studies*, edited by Matthew Wappett and Katrina Arndt, 67–95. New York: Palgrave Macmillan, 2013.

Wilcken, Ulrich. "ΑΠΟΓΡΑΦΑΙ." *Hermes* 28 (1893): 230–51.

Winter, J. G. *Life and Letters in the Papyri*. Ann Arbor: University of Michigan Press, 1933.

19 "Go Away Baldy"

Two Cross-Cultural Tales of Baldness

Rosalind Janssen

It is not often that inspiration for a contribution to a volume on disability in ancient Egypt is the result of having listened to a long Sunday morning sermon, while sitting on a hard church pew. The more so when the preacher chose to ignore the very reference to that perceived disability, namely the baldness of the biblical prophet Elisha. Yet such was the case with a sermon on 2 Kings 2 heard by chance in Oxford.[1] The aim of this chapter is to probe attitudes to natural baldness as a disability in the ancient Near East, and what might thereby be revealed about the masculine body in terms of both physical and psychological wellbeing. While the corpus of ancient Near Eastern texts form an outstandingly rich archival source, it is also one that is hegemonic.[2] The intention is to transgress narrative boundaries and engage in the type of interdisciplinary discourse advocated by Bal, in order to retrieve a feminist voice.[3] Indeed, Pilch has acknowledged that a feminist methodology "will fare best by recognising its task as basically cross-cultural."[4]

This ambitious objective will be achieved by simple storying. A recounting of the tale of the bald Elisha from the Hebrew Bible is followed by that of two balding workmen whose stories take up two vignettes on ancient Egypt's Turin Erotic-Satirical Papyrus. Each of these cross-cultural tales from the ancient past concludes with a brief contemporary scenario, before the two stories are drawn together in a final discussion section. The rationale is that civilizational "disciplinary separation is an artificial one maintained to protect the territory of the interpreter, not the fictive world of the story."[5] Crossing cultures and time periods, we therefore step into *Star Trek*'s Atavachron with the added objective of making illuminating connections between "all our yesterdays" and the twenty-first-century present.[6]

Methodology

To undertake this journey, it is necessary to adopt the interdisciplinary and feminist approach highlighted in the introduction. Rather than being grounded solely in Egyptology, my contribution simultaneously embraces biblical studies, ancient Near Eastern studies, early textile studies, and gerontology. As such it is a methodology that replicates the mission of the starship *Enterprise*: "to explore strange new worlds; to seek out new life and new civilizations; to boldly go where no one has gone before."

DOI: 10.4324/9781003440369-22

In 2020 Repko and Szoztak published the fourth edition of their comprehensive guide to the process of doing interdisciplinary research.[7] Reflecting in their preface on the number of developments in the field since the publication of the third edition four years earlier, these authors refer to interdisciplinarity as "an emerging paradigm of knowledge formation whose spreading influence can no longer be denied, discounted, or ignored."[8] So what then are its potential advantages and disadvantages?

Friedman neatly encapsulates these pros and cons by means of a spatial metaphor, which has connotations with *Star Trek*'s interstellar exploration; it envisages the researcher as journeying from his or her home base to other disciplines, and then returning home again.[9] The end result of such "epistemological travel" is that it "dislodges unquestioned assumptions and produces new insight, new questions to ask, new solutions to intellectual impasses at home."[10]

On the other hand, Friedman highlights the considerable dangers inherent in such foreign travel, because of "the tendency to misunderstand the 'other', appropriate the other, or decontextualize the other."[11] Prominent art historian Mitchell similarly warns that, in order to produce fresh insights, interdisciplinary ideas need to be synthesised rather than simply borrowed.[12] Spitz argues that such appropriation is by no means easy; every discipline has developed its own sense of territoriality in "a need to protect the ground it has tilled and cultivated lest invaders come to plunder and destroy."[13]

However, Friedman goes on to say that, instead of taking "quick trips across disciplinary borders," such travel risks can be diminished by "full immersion in the other for longer periods of time."[14] She also argues for the mitigating effect of guides, or "native informants," who are capable of making "a big difference on how much can be learned."[15] In recent years, I have painstakingly laid the ground work by immersing myself in other disciplines.[16]

Third-wave biblical feminism continues to expand on its repertoire of forgotten and absent subjects.[17] Moving away from a 'great women' narrative, it is increasingly men who, as in this chapter, are put under the feminist spotlight.[18] Moreover, third-wave biblical feminism considers women, men, and third-gender in relation to other axes of identity; those of disability, age, class, and sexuality are most relevant for this chapter. Biblical feminists have often described their strategy as a subversive reading against the grain of a text.[19] Bach neatly suggests that "turning the text on its head is what feminists do."[20] Elsewhere she advises us "to step outside the reader's appointed place" as "ideal reader" to become instead a "suspicious narratee."[21] In this connection, Bach identifies three challenging questions to ask the narrative: who speaks, who sees, and who acts?[22] It is a strategy which we will take up in our storytelling.

Key Definitions

Androgenetic alopecia, or male pattern baldness, constitutes the most common type of natural hair loss in men and is characterised by a receding frontal hairline and loss of hair from the crown.[23] It affects about 50% of men over the age of fifty.[24]

The 2010 UK Equality Act, which relates to workplace discrimination, has nine principles.[25] Relevant to this chapter are those of age and sex. The disability principle does not apply to baldness since facial conditions not amounting to disfigurements are not covered under the Act "unless they have a substantial and long-term adverse effect on an individual's ability to carry out normal day to day activities."[26]

Disability in this chapter refers to the societal stigma that immediately focuses on the unattractiveness of difference. This in turn causes emotional stress to the individual. The more positive aim of the contribution is to explore the dichotomy of a disability which, in ancient Egypt, although perceived as visually unattractive, simultaneously denoted an ageing body which, rather than being forgotten and othered, was still actively engaged in its society.[27]

Ancient Near Eastern Evidence

Androgenetic alopecia seems to have been widely accepted as a natural occurrence in the ancient Near East. This is attested by Indo-European cosmogonic myths, in which plant applications – such as grass – were put on the head to treat baldness.[28] That a similar attitude pertained in ancient Egypt is confirmed by the prescriptions in Papyrus Ebers 464–75, in which use is made of the bristles of a hedgehog and, on another occasion, an expensive concoction of fats, sourced from a variety of animals, which was smeared on the head as a greasy ointment.[29] Scurlock has confirmed that "despite their propensity for standing the hair on end," baldness was never blamed on Mesopotamian ghosts.[30] In Leviticus 13:40–41, androgenetic alopecia is twice stated to be "clean."[31] Querying why it was necessary to point this out, Niddith concludes that "the writers feel the need to note that sometimes baldness is just baldness."[32]

This in turn leads us to note that the main focus of Leviticus 13 is on *tasra'ath*, which has been habitually referenced in modern translations of both the Hebrew Bible and the New Testament as leprosy.[33] However, the presence of mycobacterial leprosy (Hansen's disease) disease in ancient Israel has now been contested, with Hulse firmly stating that "there are no indications whatsoever that the disease known as leprosy was present in the Near East in Old Testament times."[34] It is therefore strange that German scholars, engaged in a palaeopathological investigation of Old Kingdom skeletal material from Elephantine, should have made preliminary claims to have identified isolated cases of leprosy.[35] In the absence of a definitive publication this must remain tenuous.

What is certain is that Hulse reinterpreted *tasra'ath* as "a repulsive scaly skin disease," while Lloyd Davies subsequently identified it as the skin condition neurodermatitis.[36] For our purposes alopecia leprosa of the scalp, occurring secondary to mycobacterial leprosy, is confirmed by dermatologists to be rare; the bacillus prefers to inhabit the cooler areas of the body rather than the higher temperatures of the scalp.[37] Concluding this somewhat negative excursus into the vexed question of leprosy and its connection with baldness, we turn to our main topic by focusing on natural androgenetic alopecia as represented in our two tales.

The Tale of the Bald Elisha, Some Bad Boys, and the Bethel Bears

2 Kings 2 starts with the famous account of the ascent into Heaven of the prophet Elijah by means of a spectacular horse-drawn chariot of fire and an effective whirlwind. The event is witnessed by his disciple Elisha who immediately picks up the miracle-working mantle belonging to his mentor. Our short story concerning the bald Elisha is confined to verses 23 and 24, and concerns his encounter with a large gang of unruly boys in Bethel.[38] In verse 23, the boys twice jeered at Elisha: "Go away baldhead; go away baldhead."[39] The denouement to the story occurs in verse 24 when the prophet turns round, sees the jeering youths, and curses them in the name of Yahweh. The divine response is that two she-bears emerge from the woods, and proceed to maul forty-two of the boys.[40]

Ziolowski notes, "The horrific effect of 2 Kings 2:23-24 is intensified by the mode of its telling, which is cool and detached."[41] The purpose of this tale of mockery and punishment is to gain the reader's respect for Elisha as Elijah's legitimate successor.[42] This is confirmed by putting Bach's three questions to the text: it is the jeering boys who speak, or in this case mock, but it is Elisha who turns around and sees them and then acts in a decisive manner.[43]

Bearing in mind the treatment of the bald Elisha at the hands of these bad boys, it is not surprising that baldness dissatisfaction is a contemporary cause of psychosocial distress for men, to the extent that it is frequently being described as a 'disease.'[44] This neatly ties in with the May 2022 ruling of a Yorkshire employment tribunal, which upheld the claim of a sixty-four-year-old man who had been called "bald" by his factory supervisor on the grounds that the claimant had experienced sexual harassment.[45] The judge noted that baldness was "much more" prevalent in men than women and was "inherently related to sex."[46] However, the tribunal dismissed the former employee's claim for age discrimination, since his baldness did not prevent him from carrying out his daily job as an electrician (see pp. 4–5). As a result, the claimant in this litigation tale will be entitled to future monetary compensation at some future date. By contrast, Elisha's recompense in the form of the Bethel bears was much swifter and was moreover divinely given.

A Tale of Two Bald Workmen

The customary interpretation of the twelve explicit vignettes of sexual intercourse on the recto of the Turin Erotic-Satirical Papyrus (P. Turin 55001) from western Thebes is one of ridicule.[47] Balding older men, with accompanying 'middle-aged spread,' are being mocked for the marked flagging of their sexual energies. Thus, it is here that the intersection of baldness with age becomes of prime significance for this volume, in showing that it is vital to unpack the impact of disability on other axes of social disadvantage in ancient Egypt.[48]

Manniche has argued for a more precise Deir el-Medina provenance for this 19th Dynasty papyrus, based on comparative satirical ostraca deriving from this artisans' village.[49] Brawanski and Fischer-Elfert agree that this attribution is relatively certain on the basis that the supportive hieratic texts – added later in the Ramesside period by an unknown, but high-ranking, scribe – contain names corresponding to real personalities from the village.[50] If these authors are correct, the unknown master draughtsman who produced this valuable document was poking fun at his hard-working subordinate colleagues.

Female desire and orgasmic pleasure are certainly at the forefront of these scenes. It was Wenig who first suggested that the location was a brothel with the women as prostitutes.[51] It goes without saying that this is now a very outdated and highly sexist view. By contrast, O'Connor opted for the female singers, dancers, and musicians who entertained the elite, whereas Brawanski and Fischer-Elfert have subsequently argued for just one educated woman who was socially acceptable.[52] Omlin, author of the first definitive publication, envisaged the Turin Erotic Papyrus[53] as an adult sexual manual on a par with those produced in China and Japan. In their recent re-evaluation of the texts, Brawanski and Fischer-Elfert have instead argued that the purpose of the papyrus[54] was moral instruction rather than erotic stimulation. They envisage it as an entertaining yet didactic play, its real-life adventures narrated aloud at an official religious festival to emphasise the importance of potency.[55]

In support of the accepted reading that women are the dominant partner at the humorous expense of an underperforming balding male, we hone into the scene which has been centrally placed in what is a highly organised layout.[56]

Balding, unshaven, and displaying a prominent hooked nose, an unkempt older man has fallen out of the bed (Figure 19.1).[57] Exhausted and looking decidedly

Figure 19.1 An exhausted balding man taunted by his female lover in the Turin Erotic-Satirical Papyrus. The Museo Egizio in Turin.

dejected, he prepares to crawl away. The young woman leans over, holding her lover's balding head in both her hands.[58] The ancient draughtsman has associated his colleague's hair loss with a resulting loss of libido. However, the man may be intoxicated, rather than exhausted, as evidenced by the two vessels suspended above his body.[59] This and his huge erect phallus put a slightly more positive light on the scene in terms of male masculinity. On the other hand, since the woman looks down on her worn-out companion from a higher level, the viewer is left in no doubt as to who holds the power. Moreover, she speaks first in the accompanying caption, and begs the man not to leave their bed.[60] Both bemoan his impotence.[61] In reference to Bach's three questions, it is the woman who first speaks, sees, and then acts.[62]

If we turn to the second vignette, the accepted satirical reading of the papyrus is even less clear cut. It is one of the seven scenes in the papyrus which show actual sexual intercourse taking place (Figure 19.2). In contrast to Figure 19.1, the balding man is now very much in control of the sexual act, and far from plotting his escape.

Standing on tiptoe, a bald man penetrates a bending woman from the rear. He uses his right hand to grasp her long hair; with his left he clutches a bag that hangs over his back. O'Connor views this hair grasping as possible coercive sex.[63] Exceptionally in this vignette, the draughtsman has applied bright red pigment to the cheeks of the woman, with Omlin noting that "the woman's face is very strongly red-tinted (not as a line, but as a tint)."[64] Meanwhile, the text to the right refers

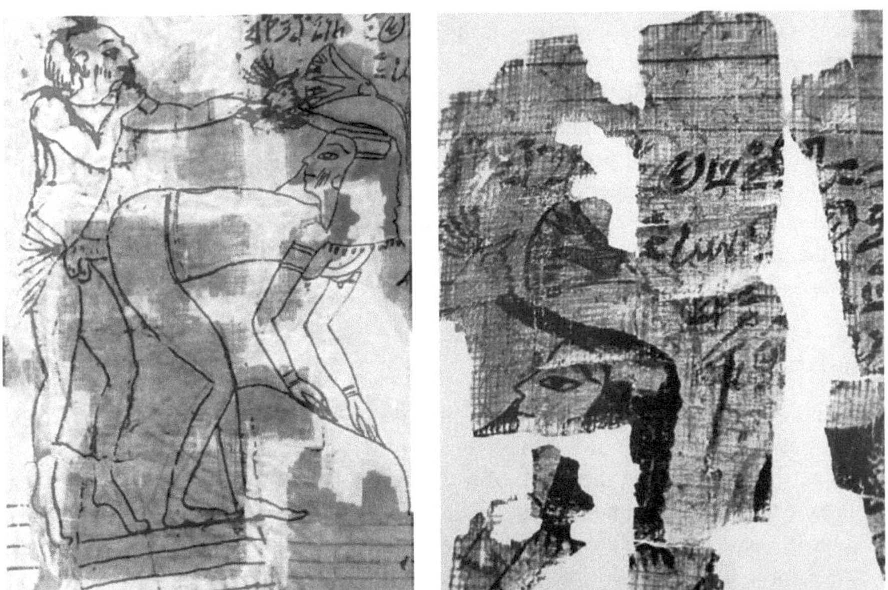

Figure 19.2 A balding man enables a woman to achieve orgasm in the Turn Erotic-Satirical Papyrus, and a close-up of the woman's rosy coloured cheeks.

to the scribe Amenhotep reading a memorandum from the woman declaring that she is successful and reliable, albeit at the expense of her partner's weakness or perhaps impotence.[65] The logical conclusion is that the man has enabled her to achieve orgasm, as evidenced by her orgasmic flush. This argument is strengthened by Stol's reading of Ugaritic texts; here it was the heat aroused in orgasm which was essential to procreation, coming either from the female or possibly from both partners.[66] That the ancient Egyptians themselves were aware of female orgasm is evidenced by a poem in Papyrus Chester Beatty I; this appropriately states: "You will enflame her passions and complete her in one night."[67]

Since the external signs of such heating are dramatically represented in our second vignette, and we have confirmatory accompanying text, there can be little doubt that the balding man is far from impotent. Further confirmation comes from Brawanski and Fischer-Elfert who note that this scene seems to represent an iconographic turning point, in that the man has recovered and is active again.[68] In terms of Bach's three questions, the woman speaks, both parties see, but it is left to the man to perform the (possibly coercive) sexual act.[69]

It is therefore possible that rather than simply mocking older men, the papyrus is simultaneously dealing with another aspect altogether.[70] Could the ancient draughtsman have been unknowingly painting a picture of Havinghurst's activity theory of ageing?[71] This claims that in order to achieve 'productive' or 'successful' ageing, older people need to continue to be active in the same way as they were at middle age. With this theory in mind, the papyrus can be interpreted in a far more positive manner: its balding older workmen are achieving 'productive' ageing, in that they are still perfectly capable of getting drunk, hiring much younger prostitutes or entertainers, and engaging in the sexual activities of their youth, albeit not always completely successfully.

An Australian medical study has sought to test the old wives' tale that bald men are more virile than their "well thatched" contemporaries.[72] Using data from an impressive statistical population, the authors concluded that bald men were no more virile than their peers. On the contrary, they were less likely to have had more than four female sexual partners. We can only speculate whether that was also the case for the balding Deir el-Medina workmen ridiculed on the Turin Erotic-Satirical Papyrus.

The Tales Juxtaposed

The aim of this final section is to align our two tales to tease out what they have to say about the dichotomy of baldness as disability. It argues that, on the one hand, androgenetic alopecia is the mark of a weak and unattractive body but, the same time, one that can be immensely powerful.

One of the symbols of masculine power and beauty in the Hebrew Bible is thick, heavy hair on the head.[73] Moreover, its ideal colour was raven black.[74] While Esau's body was defined by its hairiness, Samson and Absalom were charismatic heroes both lauded for the attractiveness of their long hair.[75] Of more direct relevance to Elisha is the fact that in 1 Kings 1:8, his predecessor Elijah is described as what can be translated as "lord of hair" or simply "a hairy man."[76] In contrast to this praise for thick hair, baldness may well have been conceived of as unattractive and even ugly.[77] Whether this had psychological implications is impossible to establish, but Elisha's swift reaction and our contemporary anecdote makes this possible. What is certain is that the prophet's lack of hair has negative connotations, because "to be bald is to be other."[78] Graybill engages in a queer reading of the passage, since the prophet's body "does not meet the norms of embodiment."[79] The same negativity is evidenced in the Turin Erotic-Satirical Papyrus in which the deficiency of the balding men is further emphasised by their negative facial expressions, unattractive hooked noses, and the flabby pot-bellied bodies which are synonymous with older age. It is therefore not surprising that didactic literature, such as the Ramesside *Instruction of Amenemope*, condones the ridiculing of those with physical and mental disabilities and the reviling of older people.[80]

In relation to the few biblical references, baldness was always a masculine trait. That this was also the case in ancient Egypt is confirmed by Kamal's recent survey of baldness as represented in Egyptian private tombs dating from the Old Kingdom to the end of the Late period.[81] From an extensive inventory of 122 such depictions, she identifies 94 as depictions of older men who are invariably agricultural labourers.[82] That there are many more references when compared with the Hebrew Bible perhaps relates to the explicit societal link between baldness, ageing, and class in ancient Egypt. Indeed, Rose is the only biblical scholar who links Elisha's baldness to age with a throwaway sentence at the very end of her article: "The passage from the Book of Kings describes an old man's despair at the loss of his master."[83]

Consistent with a lack of hair on the head as being rooted in gender and equating to a loss of masculinity, Elisha has to rely on the arrival of female animals – nicely referred to by Niditch as "two presumably very hairy she-bears" – who enact violent punishment on his behalf.[84] This can be aligned with the fact that he hardly ever touches a woman.[85] Similarly, in the Turin-Erotic Papyrus it is women, pictured with long, luxurious dark hair, who have the upper hand. On the basis that it supposedly mercilessly taunts men, Janák and Navrátilová have imaginatively proposed that the papyrus represents a commercially produced woman's magazine, its audience of literate women seeking erotic entertainment and, above all, amusement at the expense of older men.[86] Writing in relation to the Hebrew Bible, Niditch would agree: "Stories, portraying a loss of power, to those who really hold the power in actual everyday life would certainly amuse women."[87] Given the precise nature of the drawings, I would additionally argue that the literacy necessary for reading the accompanying hieratic captions was not essential, thereby considerably broadening its potential female audience.

We have already seen how, following Elijah's ascent into Heaven, Elisha picks up his mentor's miraculous mantle, conceivably a hairy cloak, made from an animal skin or hide.[88] Niditch questions whether Elijah thereby passes on his holiness to his bald successor.[89] On a purely practical level Elisha's wearing of this inherited garment directs attention to his own differences in that "his smooth head stood in sharp contrast to his rough hairskin mantle."[90] This becomes the source of mockery

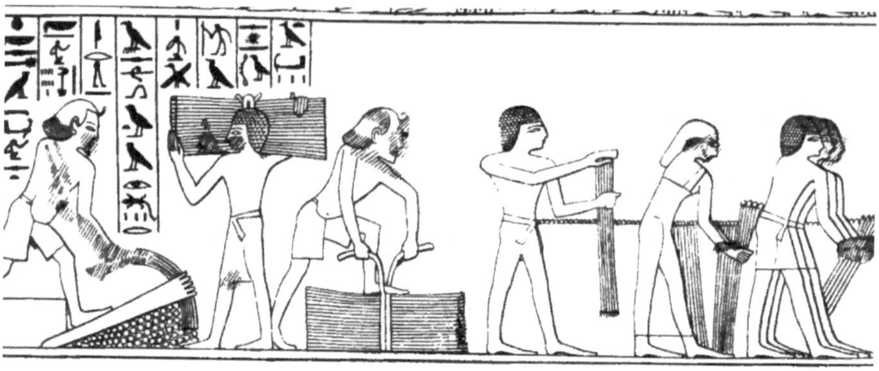

Figure 19.3 Flax harvesting scene from the 18th-Dynasty tomb of Paheri at el-Kab.

for the boys of Bethel who twice refer to him as "baldhead"; this insult means that Elisha had no choice but to defend his honour and establish his credentials.[91]

A remarkably similar insult occurs in a flax harvesting scene in the 18th-Dynasty Tomb of Paheri at el-Kab, in which an older balding man is operating a foot-operated, long-toothed, wooden comb to strip the seed heads from the stalks (Figure 19.3).[92] In the accompanying hieroglyphic caption, his younger colleague tells him in no uncertain terms, "Buck up, don't gabble, you bald old man of a fieldworker!"[93] Perhaps we can link this incident to the Turin Erotic-Satirical Papyrus, in which it is the perceived loss of libido associated with balding older men that becomes the butt of female mockery. These negative attitudes can be aligned to Oliver's social model of disability, which argues that it is the way society is structured in terms of barriers and attitudes which constitutes the disability.[94]

However, alternative histories are simultaneously evidenced in our tales, in that baldness is also a sign of a powerful body. The potency of Elisha's curse demonstrates his power over life, while the sexual performance of the men from the Turin Erotic-Satirical Papyrus shows that, as far as the second man is concerned, he has power over the procreation of new life.[95] In Egypt, the young were similarly mocking their elders who had the power to respond by cursing. This is evidenced from an instruction from Deir el-Medina which reads, "Do not ridicule an old man or an old woman when they are bent double with age; beware lest they place a curse on your old age."[96]

On a more mundane level, both our tales are about bald men in a hurry. Elisha is walking along the road from Jericho to Bethel when, dressed in his hairy mantle, he encounters the boys who have come out of the town. The Egyptian workman is still carrying his sack of tools, as do several of his colleagues. Moreover, the men on the Turin Erotic-Satirical Papyrus are not wearing "kilts twisted backwards" as stated by O'Connor, but rather their working loincloths which are tied around the waist and left open at the front.[97] In other words, both they and Elisha have entered their respective scenes straight after a solid day's work. This can be linked to the inspiring work ethic of the balding labourer on Paheri's estates (p. 302). Significantly, James draws attention to the fact that, "alone among the labourers shown in this register, the old man throws himself into his work with apparent enthusiasm, shouting to the man who brings the bundle: 'If you bring me 11,009 (bundles), I shall comb them.'"[98]

Spitz tells us that "the peripatetic scholar wanders perilously but in anticipation of unique rewards."[99] The benefits of engaging in an interdisciplinary and feminist approach in the preceding pages has far outweighed the possible pitfalls. Following Fewell and Gunn, "we have learned to seek out the different and the discordant . . . and to build a reading around it."[100]

Conclusion

While ancient Egyptian didactic literature stresses that the disabled should not be laughed at, the foolish boys of Bethel did exactly that on encountering the bald prophet Elisha. As far as the Hebrew Bible was concerned, daring to deride the unattractive nature of baldness necessitated a swift and sharp dose of divine intervention. Despite having a disability which may well have affected his psychological wellbeing, Elisha managed to confirm his legitimacy as Elijah's successor by means of a powerful curse. As a result, the Bethel boys became premature victims of what Macbeth saw as life's inevitable fate: "All our yesterdays have lighted fools/The way to dusty death."[101] Millennia before the 2010 Equality Act, it was not politically correct to mock bald men in ancient Israel.

As far as disability in ancient Egypt is concerned, if our reading of the two balding Deir el-Medina workmen on the Turin Erotic-Satirical Papyrus as sexually and professionally active is correct, its twelve vignettes can be reinterpreted. They display a nuanced attitude to ageing, and by extension age-associated disability. It is one of mockery, but at the same time of grudging respect. As such this seamlessly aligns with the interpretation of Brawanski and Fischer-Elfert, who see the entire meaning of the Egyptian papyrus as, "Don't rely on outward appearances."[102] The conclusion is that the ancient Egyptians had what might seem to us to be a surprisingly enlightened attitude to baldness as disability. Despite any stigma surrounding their appearance, older men were far from "The Forgotten Other" of the Classical World. Instead, they were fully valued and actively engaged participants in Egyptian society.[103]

Notes

1 Sermon, June 19, 2022. I have deliberately refrained from giving the name of the preacher, the church, or the denomination. While focused on 2 Kings 2:1–25 in its entirety, the Oxford cleric in question devoted considerable attention to the story concerning the bald Elisha in verses 23 and 24.

2 As demonstrated by the classic volume edited by James B. Pritchard, *Ancient Near Eastern Texts Relating to the Old Testament*, 3rd ed. with Supplement (Princeton: Princeton University Press, 1969).

3 Bal (1988, viii). Bal here talks about how "we will discover the importance, the urgency of that [interdisciplinary] approach by way of the limits of the disciplinary discourse, whose inadequacy will become progressively manifest as we proceed."
4 Pilch (1997, 308).
5 Bach (1997, 27).
6 The Atavachron was a time portal in "All Our Yesterdays," directed by Marvin Chomsky, written by Jean Lisette Aroeste, in *Star Trek: The Original Series*, Season 3, Episode 23 (March 14, 1969; Los Angeles: Paramount Television, 1966–1969), television episode. By strange coincidence, I would have watched this episode around the same time that I was having to memorise Macbeth's soliloquy, from which the title of the episode was derived (see fn. 101).
7 Repko and Szostak (2020).
8 Ibid., xvii.
9 Friedman (2001, 507).
10 Ibid., 508.
11 Ibid.
12 Mitchell (1995, 543).
13 Spitz (1995, 552).
14 Friedman (2001, 508).
15 Ibid.
16 By means of an MSc in life course development, an MTh in theology, and an MSt in literature and arts.
17 Sherwood (2017, 1–11).
18 Koosed (2017, 223–39).
19 Exum (1995, 68).
20 Bach (1999, xxvi).
21 Bach (1997, 14–15).
22 Bach (1999, xxv).
23 British Association of Dermatologists, "Hair Loss Male Pattern (Androgenetic Alopecia)," last updated March 2019, accessed June 13, 2023, https://www.bad.org.uk/pils/hair-loss-male-pattern-androgenetic-alopecia/.
24 Ibid.
25 Equality and Human Rights Commission, "Protected Characteristics," last modified July 6, 2021, accessed June 13, 2023, https://www.equalityhumanrights.com/en/equality-act/protected-characteristics.
26 UK Parliament, "Facial Disfigurement: Discrimination," last modified April 3, 2018, accessed June 13, 2023, https://questions-statements.parliament.uk/written-questions/detail/2018-03-26/134180#.
27 Adams (2021).
28 Lincoln (1991, 87–118).
29 Nunn, *Ancient Egyptian Medicine* (1997, 95, 149–50). Interestingly, a minoxidil liquid treatment, said to be expensive and not available on the NHS, is highlighted by the British Association of Dermatologists (see fn. 24).
30 Scurlock (2005, 19).
31 "If anyone loses the hair from his head, he is bald but he is clean. If he loses the hair from his forehead and temples, he has baldness of the forehead, but he is clean."
32 Niditch (2008, 112).
33 Hulse (1975, 101–2).
34 Ibid., 91. Followed by Margaret Lloyd Davies and Trevor Arthur Lloyd Davies, "Biblical Leprosy: A Comedy of Errors," *Journal of the Royal Society of Medicine* 82 (1989).
35 Alexandra D. Kozak, et al., Paper presented at the 17th European Meeting of the Paleopathology Association, Copenhagen, Denmark, August 25–27, 2008, accessed June 12, 2023, https://www.academia.edu/30386041/Leprosy_in_the_Old_Kingdom_Elephantine_Egyptian_Nubia_by_Kozak_A_D_Gresky_J_Roumelis_N_Schultz_M.

36 Ibid., 103; Davies (1985). Iterated in Margaret Lloyd Davies and Trevor Arthur Lloyd Davies, "Biblical Leprosy," 623.
37 Macedo et al. (2016, 71).
38 Most scholars have taken the noun *qērēah* to indicate physical baldness. For a discussion see Rhiannon Graybill, "Elisha's Body and the Queer Touch of Prophecy," *Biblical Theology Bulletin* 49, no. 1 (2019): 35, https://doi.org/10.1177/0146107918818042.
39 While my title takes "baldy" from the NIV, my text – as is the custom – uses the original 1989 edition of the NRSV. In the latter version, 2 Kings 2:23 reads, "He went up from there to Bethel; and while he was going up on the way, some small boys came out of the city and jeered at him, saying, 'Go away, baldhead! Go away, baldhead!'"
40 2 Kings 2:24. "When he turned around and saw them, he cursed them in the name of the Lord. Then two she-bears came out of the woods and mauled forty-two of the boys."
41 Ziolowski (1991, 334).
42 Neufeld (2015, 116).
43 Bach (1999, xxv).
44 Jankowski and Frith (2022, 2161–80).
45 Julie Temple, "Finn v The British Bung Manufacturing Company Ltd," last modified May 13, 2022, accessed June 9, 2023, https://www.birkettlong.co.uk/site/library/commercialclient/employment/tribunal-finds-calling-a-man-bald-is-sexual-harassment.
46 Ibid.
47 Notably Patrick F. Houlihan, *Wit and Humour in Ancient Egypt* (London: Rubicon Press, 2001), 130–36. A satirical remit remains the most likely, especially in view of the animal scenes portrayed on the verso.
48 Janssen and Janssen (1996, 13), Janssen and Janssen (2007, 149–50).
49 Manniche (1987, 107).
50 Brawanski and Fischer-Elfert (2012, 86). "Deir el Medinah als Herkunftsort damit relativ sicher bestimmen."
51 Wenig (1967, 21, 43). For a rejection of organised prostitution in the village, see Jana Toivari-Viitala, *Women at Deir el-Medina: A Study of the Status and Roles of the Female Inhabitants in the Workmen's Community During the Ramesside Period, Egyptologische Uitgaven 15* (Leiden: Nederlands Instituut voor het Nabije Oosten, 2001), 148–53.
52 O'Connor (2011, 361–80), Brawanski and Fischer-Elfert (2012, 86). "Anspielungen in den Mund gelegt werden, sie also Bildung genossen hat. Also ist sie nicht die billige Dirne aus niedrigstem Stand oder gar eine rechtlose Ausländerin."
53 Omlin (1973, 24). Although the papyrus was initially discovered in the 1820s, it was considered so graphically shocking that 150 years were to elapse before this its first (illustrated) publication. Omlin's plates were republished in colour by Pascal Vernus, "Le Papyrus de Turin et la Pornographie dans l'Égypte Ancienne," in *L'Art du Contour: Le Dessin dans l'Égypte Ancienne*, ed. Guillemette Andreu-Lanoë, Sophie Labbé-Toutée, and Patricia Rigault (Paris: Musée du Louvre Éditions, 2013), 108–17.
54 Brawanski and Fischer-Elfert (2012, 89).
55 Ibid.
56 O'Connor (2011, 367, 370).
57 Jos A. Omlin, *Der Papyrus 55001 (Bild 6)* (Turin: Edizioni d'Arte Fratelli Pozzo, 1973), 34–35, pls. XI and XIII.
58 Myśliwiec (2004, 123). "Most likely she wishes to help her partner up to join her on the bed."
59 Houlihan (2001, 133).
60 Brawanski and Fischer-Elfert (2012, 81).
61 A comparative rebuke – "Why is your triumph-cry as bad as (that) of a little child?" – can be found in Akkadian love literature. Nathan Wasserman, *Akkadian Love Literature of the Third and Second Millennium BCE, Leipziger Altorientalistische Studien 4*, ed. Michael P. Streck (Wiesbaden: Harrassowitz, 2016), 264–65.

62 Bach (1999, xxv).
63 O'Connor (2011, 380).
64 Omlin (1973, 35). "Das Gesicht der Frau ist sehr stark rot getönt (nicht mehr als Strich, sondern als Tönung)."
65 Brawanski and Fischer-Elfert (2012, 75). "Ich bin erfolgreich und zuverlässig(?) . . . deine [Schwäche/Impotenz(?)]."
66 Stol (2000, 6).
67 Landgráfová and Navratilova (2009, 78, 165). The authors offer a relatively recent English translation of this papyrus which is now in the Chester Beatty Library in Dublin. The verses in question are from Collection III, recto 16,9–17,13. The first poem is recto 16,10–16,11. The original hieratic edition is Alan H. Gardiner, *The Library of A. Chester Beatty: Description of a Hieratic Papyrus with a Mythological Story, Love-songs, and Other Miscellaneous Texts* (Oxford: Oxford University Press, 1931), pl. XVI.
68 Brawanski and Fischer-Elfert (2012, 82). "Turning point" is here in English.
69 Bach (1999, xxv).
70 Janssen and Janssen (1996, 150), Janssen (2006, 6).
71 Havinghurst (1961, 8–13). Developed in response to disengagement theory, which asserts that it is natural for older people to disengage from society as they come nearer to death.
72 Sinclair, English, and Giles (2013, 811–12).
73 Olyan (2008, 16).
74 Song of Songs 5:11 reads: "His head is the finest gold; his locks are wavy, black as a raven."
75 Respectively Genesis 25:25; Judges 16:17; 2 Samuel 14:26.
76 2 Kings 1:8. "They answered him, 'A hairy man with a leather belt around his waist.' He said, 'It is Elijah the Tishbite.'"
77 Olyan (2008, 20). The association of baldness with mourning is an aspect beyond the remit of this chapter, since a deliberate shaving of the head does not fall into the category of natural hair loss.
78 Graybill (2019, 33).
79 Ibid., 35.
80 Lichtheim (1976, 160–61).
81 Kamal (2019, 127–79).
82 Ibid., 130. Of the remainder, sixteen were identified as young, with twelve uncertain cases.
83 Rose (1981, 41).
84 Niditch (2008, 113).
85 Graybill (2019, 38).
86 Janák and Navrátilová (2008, 69). These authors also put forward the balanced suggestion that the papyrus was "primarily aiming at the amusement of its readers, without any special religious or political satire."
87 Niditch (2008, 117).
88 Ibid., 112.
89 Ibid., 113.
90 Ziolowski (1991, 334).
91 Neufeld (2015, 129–30).
92 James (1985, fig. 9 on 123).
93 Ibid., 122–23.
94 Oliver (1983).
95 In this connection, 2 Kings 2:19–21 sees Elisha's miracle purification of a spring in Jericho that had been causing miscarriages.
96 McDowell (1999, 142).
97 O'Connor (2011, 13–14).
98 James (1985, 122–23).

99 Spitz (1995, 552).
100 Fewell and Gunn (1993, 16).
101 I finally reference the subtitle of the present volume in its original Shakespearean sense. Shakespeare (1967, 5.5.22–23).
102 Brawanski and Fischer-Elfert (2012, 87). "Verlasse dich nicht auf den äußeren Anschein."
103 Adams (2021).

Bibliography

Adams, Ellen. "Disability Studies and the Classical Body: The Forgotten Other." In *Routledge Studies in Ancient Disability,* edited by Ellen Adams. London: Routledge, 2021.

Bach, Alice. *Women, Seduction, and Betrayal in Biblical Narrative.* Cambridge: Cambridge University Press, 1997.

Bach, Alice. "Introduction. Man's World, Women's Place: Sexual Politics in the Hebrew Bible." In *Women in the Hebrew Bible: A Reader*, edited by Alice Bach, xiii–xxvi. New York: Routledge, 1999.

Bal, Mieke. "Murder and Difference: Gender, Genre, and Scholarship on Sisera's Death." In *Indiana Studies in Biblical Literature*, translated by Matthew Gumpert. Bloomington, IN: Indiana University Press, 1988.

Brawanski, Alexander, and Hans Fischer-Elfert. "Der 'Erotische' Abschnitt des Turiner Papyrus 55001: Ein Lehrstück für das Männliche Ego?" *Studien Altägyptischen Kultur* 41 (2012): 67–97.

Equality and Human Rights Commission. "Protected Characteristics." Last modified July 6, 2021. Accessed June 13, 2023. https://www.equalityhumanrights.com/en/equality-act/protected-characteristics.

Exum, J. Cheryl. "Feminist Criticism: Whose Interests are Being Served?" In *Judges and Method: New Approaches in Biblical Studies*, edited by Gale A. Yee, 65–90. Minneapolis: Fortress Press, 1995.

Fewell, Danna Nolan, and David M. Gunn. *Gender, Power, and Promise: The Subject of the Bible's First Story.* Nashville, TN: Abingdon Press, 1993.

Friedman, Susan Stanford. "Academic Feminism and Interdisciplinarity." *Feminist Studies* 27, no. 2 (2001): 504–9.

Gardiner, Alan H. *The Library of A. Chester Beatty: Description of a Hieratic Papyrus with a Mythological Story, Love-songs, and Other Miscellaneous Texts.* Oxford: Oxford University Press, 1931.

Graybill, Rhiannon. "Elisha's Body and the Queer Touch of Prophecy." *Biblical Theology Bulletin* 49, no. 1 (2019): 32–40. https://doi.org/10.1177/0146107918818042.

Havinghurst, Robert J. "Successful Aging." *The Gerontologist* 1, no. 1 (1961): 8–13.

Houlihan, Patrick F. *Wit and Humour in Ancient Egypt.* London: Rubicon Press, 2001.

Hulse, E. V. "The Nature of Biblical 'Leprosy' and the Use of Alternative Medical Terms in Modern Translations of the Bible." *Palestine Exploration Quarterly* 107, no. 2 (1975): 87–105.

James, T. G. H. *Pharaoh's People: Scenes from Life in Imperial Egypt.* Oxford: Oxford University Press, 1985.

Janák, Jiří, and Hana Navrátilová. "People vs. P. Turin 55001." In *Sex and Gender in Ancient Egypt. 'Don Your Wig for a Joyful Hour'*, edited by Carolyn Graves-Brown, 63–70. Swansea: The Classical Press of Wales, 2008.

Jankowski, Glen S., and Hannah Frith. "Psychology's Medicalization of Male Baldness." *Journal of Health Psychology* 27, no. 9 (2022): 2161–80.

Janssen, Rosalind M. "The Old Women of Deir el-Medina." *Buried History* 42 (2006): 3–10.

Janssen, Rosalind M., and Jac J. Janssen. *Getting Old in Ancient Egypt.* London: Rubicon Press, 1996.

Janssen, Rosalind M., and Jac J. Janssen. *Growing Up and Getting Old in Ancient Egypt.* London: Golden House Press, 2007.

Kamal, Samar Mostafa. "Baldness Scenes in Ancient Egyptian Private Tombs; as an Indicator of Social Class, Activity and Physical Ability." *International Journal of Tourism and Hospitality Management* 2, no. 2 (2019): 127–79.

Koosed, Jennifer L. "Moses, Feminism, and the Male Subject." In *The Bible and Feminism: Remapping the Field*, edited by Yvonne Sherwood, 223–39. Oxford: Oxford University Press, 2017.

Kozak, Alexandra D., Julia Gresky, Nikolaos Roumelis, and Michael Schultz. "Leprosy in the Old Kingdom Elephantine (Egyptian Nubia)." Paper presented at the 17th European Meeting of the Paleopathology Association, Copenhagen, Denmark, August 25–27, 2008. Accessed June 12, 2023. https://www.academia.edu/30386041/Leprosy_in_the_Old_Kingdom_Elephantine_Egyptian_Nubia_by_Kozak_A_D_Gresky_J_Roumelis_N_Schultz_M.

Landgráfová, Renate, and Hana Navratilova. *Sex and the Golden Goddess I: Ancient Egyptian Love Songs in Context.* Prague: Czech Institute of Egyptology, 2009.

Lichtheim, Miriam. *Ancient Egyptian Literature: A Book of Readings. Vol. II: The New Kingdom.* Berkeley: University of California Press, 1976.

Lincoln, Bruce. *Death, War, and Sacrifice: Studies in Ideology and Practice.* Chicago: University of Chicago Press, 1991.

Lloyd Davies, Margaret. *Leprosy and Leviticus: Uncleanness and the Psyche.* Oxford: Pusey House Library, 1985.

Lloyd Davies, Margaret, and Trevor Arthur Lloyd Davies. "Biblical Leprosy: A Comedy of Errors." *Journal of the Royal Society of Medicine* 82 (1989): 622–23.

Macedo, Raila de Brito, Paulyare Bezerra Sampaio Ramos Santos, Daniela Mayumi Takano, and Virginia Sampaio Madeiro Leal. "Leprosy on the Scalp." *Anais Brasileiros Dermatologia* 91, no. 5 (2016): 69–71.

Manniche, Lise. *Sexual Life in Ancient Egypt.* London: Kegan Paul International, 1987.

McDowell, Andrea G. *Village Life in Ancient Egypt: Laundry Lists and Love Songs.* Oxford: Oxford University Press, 1999.

Mitchell, W. J. T. "Interdisciplinarity and Visual Culture." *Art Bulletin* 77, no. 4 (1995): 540–44.

Myśliwiec, Karol. *Eros on the Nile.* Translated by Geoffrey L. Packer. London: Duckworth, 2004.

Neufeld, Dietmar. "Mocking Boys, Baldness, and Bears: Elisha's Deadly Honour (2 Kings 2.23-24)." In *Not Sparing the Child: Human Sacrifice in the Ancient World and Beyond*, edited by V. Daphna Arbel, Paul C. Burns, J. R. C. Cousland, Richard Menkis, Dietmar Neufeld, and Studies in Honor of Professor Paul G. Mosca, 114–30. London: Bloomsbury T&T Clark, 2015.

Niditch, Susan. *"My Brother Esau is a Hairy Man": Hair and Identity in Ancient Israel.* Oxford: Oxford University Press, 2008.

Nunn, John F. *Ancient Egyptian Medicine.* London: British Museum Press, 1997.

O'Connor, David. "Satire or Parody? The Interaction of the Pictorial and the Literary in Turin Papyrus 55001." In *Ramesside Studies in Honour of K.A. Kitchen*, edited by Mark Collier and Stephen Snape, 361–80. Bolton: Rutherford Press, 2011.

Oliver, Michael. *Social Work with Disabled People.* Basingstoke: Macmillan, 1983.

Olyan, Saul M. *Disability in the Hebrew Bible: Interpreting Mental and Physical Differences.* Cambridge: Cambridge University Press, 2008.

Omlin, Jos A. *Der Papyrus 55001 und seine Satirisch-erotischen Zeichnungen und Inschriften.* Turin: Edizioni d'Arte Fratelli Pozzo, 1973.

Pilch, John J. "Family Violence in Cross-Cultural Perspective: An Approach for Feminist Interpreters of the Bible." In *A Feminist Companion to Reading the Bible: Approaches, Methods and Strategies*, edited by Athalya Brenner and Carole Fontaine, 306–23. Sheffield: Sheffield Academic Press, 1997.

Pritchard, James B. Ancient Near Eastern Texts Relating to the Old Testament. 3rd ed. with Supplement. Princeton: Princeton University Press, 1969.

Repko, Allen F., and Rick Szostak. *Interdisciplinary Research: Process and Theory.* 4th ed. Thousand Oaks, CA: Sage, 2020.

Rose, Patricia. "Bears, Baldness, and the Double Spirit: The Identity of Donatello's *Zuccone.*" *The Art Bulletin* 63, no. 1 (1981): 31–41.

Scurlock, JoAnn. *Magico-Medical Means of Treating Ghost-Induced Illnesses in Ancient Mesopotamia, Ancient Magic and Divination 3.* Leiden: Brill, 2005.

Shakespeare, William. *Macbeth*. Edited by G. K. Hunter. London: Penguin Books, 1967.

Sherwood, Yvonne. "Introduction." In *The Bible and Feminism: Remapping the Field*, edited by Yvonne Sherwood, 1–11. Oxford: Oxford University Press, 2017.

Sinclair, Rodney D., Dallas R. English, and Graham D. Giles. "Are Bald Men More Virile than their Well Thatched Contemporaries?" *Medical Journal of Australia* 199 (2013): 811–12. https://doi.org/10.5694/mja13.11360.

Spitz, Ellen Handler. "Warrant for Trespass/Permission to Peer." *Art Bulletin* 77, no. 4 (1995): 550–52.

Stol, Marten. *Birth in Babylonia and the Bible: Its Mediterranean Setting, Cuneiform Monographs 14.* Groningen: Styx, 2000.

Temple, Julie. "Finn v The British Bung Manufacturing Company Ltd." Last modified May 13, 2022. Accessed June 9, 2023. https://www.birkettlong.co.uk/site/library/commercialclient/employment/tribunal-finds-calling-a-man-bald-is-sexual-harassment.

Toivari-Viitala, Jana. *Women at Deir el-Medina: A Study of the Status and Roles of the Female Inhabitants in the Workmen's Community During the Ramesside Period, Egyptologische Uitgaven 15.* Leiden: Nederlands Instituut voor het Nabije Oosten, 2001.

UK Parliament. "Facial Disfigurement: Discrimination." Last modified April 3, 2018. Accessed June 13, 2023. https://questions-statements.parliament.uk/written-questions/detail/2018-03-26/134180#.

Vernus, Pascal. "Le Papyrus de Turin et la Pornographie dans l'Égypte Ancienne." In *L'Art du Contour: Le Dessin dans L'Égypte Ancienne*, edited by Guillemette Andreu-Lanoë, Sophie Labbé-Toutée, and Patricia Rigault, 108–17. Paris: Musée du Louvre Éditions, 2013.

Vogelsang-Eastwood, Gillian. *Pharaonic Egyptian Clothing.* Leiden: Brill, 1993.

Wasserman, Nathan. *Akkadian Love Literature of the Third and Second Millennium BCE, Leipziger Altorientalistische Studien 4.* Edited by Michael P. Streck. Wiesbaden: Harrassowitz, 2016.

Wenig, Stefan. *Die Frau im Alten Ägypten.* Leipzig: Edition Leipzig, 1967.

Ziolowski, Eric J. "The Bad Boys of Bethel: Origin and Development of a Sacrilegious Type." *History of Religions* 30, no. 4 (1991): 331–58.

Television Episode

"All Our Yesterdays." directed by Marvin Chomsky, written by Jean Lisette Aroeste, in *Star Trek: The Original Series,* Season 3, Episode 23. March 14, 1969; Los Angeles: Paramount Television, 1966–1969, television episode.

20 Archaeology of Genital Mutilation

Disabled Masculinity of Libyan Enemies in the Egyptian New Kingdom*

Uroš Matić

Introduction: On War and Disability

Studies of war and violence in ancient Egypt and Nubia have been traditionally androcentric; that is, androcentrism is understood as a projection of modern white middle-aged ableist heterosexual experiences or adaption of these experiences as a proxy.[1] Egyptologists and Sudanologists have focused on bodies of Egyptian and Nubian soldiers, per default, considered able in the modern sense of this word. Disability Studies in Egyptology are not yet fully considered in studies of war and violence in ancient Egypt and Sudan, studies which can be described as "spectacles of able-bodied heteronormativity."[2] Recently, Disability Studies has been utilized in Egyptology, primarily as a foil to the medical model, which focuses on pathologies interpreted through a modern medical lens while neglecting culturally relative attitudes to bodily differences and the individual experiences of the people having different bodies.[3]

Similarly, although Gender Studies is not new to Egyptologists,[4] they have rarely examined gender in relation to violence.[5] This intersection has been explored only recently, in archaeology and Egyptology.[6] Additionally, studies of ancient Egyptian notions of masculinity are rare;[7] so too are the more nuanced studies of masculinities as diverse, dependent upon age, class, and occupation.

Whereas Egyptologists are reticent to consider battlefields as arenas in which masculine identity can be both confirmed and contested, this has been argued historically by anthropologists and sociologists.[8] Consequently, war can lead to both masculinization and emasculation. Furthermore, deliberate disabling and mutilation of enemies in war and the taking of human body parts as trophies are cross-culturally attested practices.[9] Sexual violence against men, including rape and genital mutilation, occurs more often than is usually thought or reported.[10] This form of violence against men is often considered unorthodox and impossible by our modern society, whereas boasting of sexual violence conducted to women by combatants is more frequent.[11] Therefore, we can say that gender is one of the most common frames of war that serve to selectively carve up experience and

* Trigger warning. This article discusses extreme forms of violence and includes graphics (line drawings and photos) of violence, combat, and mutilation. Please engage in self-care as you read this article.

DOI: 10.4324/9781003440369-23

conduct of war through media.[12] These frames tend to contain, convey, and determine what is seen in the media that report on war.[13] Frames of war have a normative function, structuring and differentiating lives and diverse forms of living for those who observe reports on war.[14] Through gender as a frame of war normative ways of being a man or a woman are structured and certain bodies are framed as less male, less able or even less human, than others.[15] That gender was a frame of war in ancient Egypt and Sudan, and that it ultimately relates to deliberate mutilation of enemies, has also been argued recently.[16] Bearing all of this in mind, this chapter will explore whether the well-known custom of the cutting off the phalli of Libyan enemies in the New Kingdom can be considered as one of these physical interventions leading to gendered disability through emasculation. This will be done by examining this military practice within gender as a frame of war, and viewing disability through the lenses of Crip theory, which insists on intersection of disability with gender and sexuality. Crip theory appeared within the intersection of interdisciplinary fields of Disability Studies and queer theory in the early decades of the twenty-first century and tackles the intersections in which gender, race, sexuality, and disability converge.[17] Although emerging from lived experiences of the twenty-first century, its applications are not limited to this historical period. Crip theory finds its place in different historically contingent intersections of gender, sexuality, and disability, such as the male-centred and able-bodied ideology of New Kingdom Egyptian military.

The sources analyzed in this chapter consist of texts found on royal stelae and temple walls and images found on temple walls. The context of these texts and images in ancient Egypt indicates that they are not to be understood as representing the reality of the battlefield as such, but rather as framed in the sense of Judith Butler's use of this concept. This does not mean that none of the described or depicted events ever happened, but that the way these events are described and depicted influences the way the audience gains knowledge of them. Those who were not on the battlefield could either gain accounts from battle participants, or from the texts and images in question, provided that they had access to them and enough knowledge to read them, properly or not.[18] One can therefore even go so far as to argue that whether or not something actually happened does not change the fact that it was recorded and depicted and therefore read or seen. The audience of the presumed actual event was different from the audience of its record, textual or visual. In ancient Egypt the visual and the written material often co-occur.[19]

Phalli Cutting in the New Kingdom

The earliest New Kingdom evidence for cutting of the phalli of enemies is found in the text of the Athribis stela of king Merenptah now kept in the Egyptian Museum in Cairo. According to the Athribis stela, Merenptah fought against the Libu (*Rbw*), Libyans, and "their phalli were brought" (*jnj=tw nꜣy=sn ḥnn.w*).[20] The Great War inscription from the Temple of Ramesses III at Medinet Habu describes the campaign in his fifth regnal year and mentions "hands and phalli with foreskin beyond numbering" (*kp.w ḳrn.t nn r-ᶜ=sn*) next to the prisoners.[21] Decorating the walls of

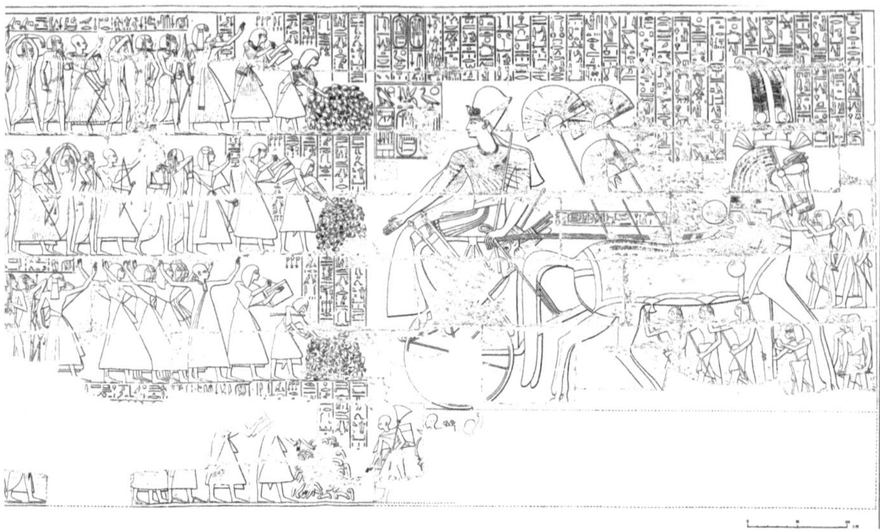

Figure 20.1 Aftermath of the First Libyan War of Ramesses III, Medinet Habu temple, scene of counting of the cut-off hands and phalli, south wall of the second court, lowest register of first scene from the east (Nelson 1930, pl. 23).

Medinet Habu are representations of soldiers presenting cut-off hands and phalli to the king in the aftermath of the First Libyan War.[22] On the right side of the scene depicting the aftermath of the First Libyan War, the king sits backwards in his chariot, looking left towards four registers of incoming soldiers bringing prisoners of war who can be identified as Libyans (Figure 20.1). To the right of the Egyptian soldiers and closer to the king are two officials counting the cut-off body parts of dead enemies in each register; the official on the left holds a papyrus roll and writes the tally while the other handles and counts the body parts. In each of his hands, he holds a cut-off hand by its thumb. None of the soldiers are depicted as actually carrying the cut-off body parts, although the piles are on the very end of the register before the seated king.

On the far right of the fourth register from above is a pile of mixed cut-off hands and cut-off phalli, with two hands visible and approximately 16 phalli. The phalli are depicted with scrotum but without foreskin showing. They look like the sign in the hieroglyphic script used to write phallus and having the designation D52 𓂸 in the sign list of Alan Gardiner. Every register is followed by the same inscription that states these are spoils brought to the king. Also listed are "1000 men, 3000 hands, 3000 phalli with foreskin" (*jr.n 1000 s jr.n 3000 kp jr.n 3000 ḳrn.t*).[23]

Another presentation of the spoils in the aftermath of the First Libyan War is depicted in the third scene from the west on the north wall outer side (Figure 20.2).[24] The king is depicted leaning on a parapet topped by a cushion, the main element of the so-called Window of Appearance, a special palace window through which the king interacts with his subjects. Behind the king is his chariot. Above the chariot is

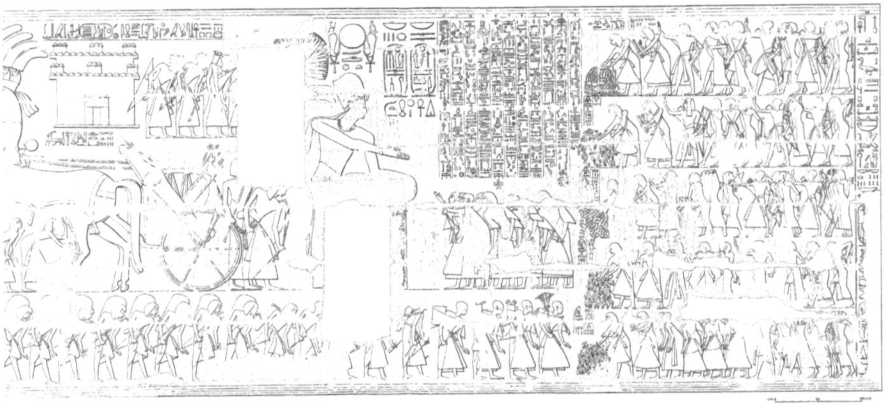

Figure 20.2 Aftermath of the First Libyan War of Ramesses III, Medinet Habu temple, scene of counting of the cut-off hands and phalli, third scene from the west on the north wall (outer side). Note the presence of the town-fortress "Usermaatre-Meriamun is the Repeller of the Temeh" (Nelson 1930, pl. 22).

the fortress. The accompanying text states that Libyan prisoners of war are in front of the town "Usermaatre-Meriamun is the Repeller of the Temeh," in which Temeh refers to another group of foreigners Egyptologists call Libyans. The king is clearly outside the town. Incoming soldiers are depicted in five registers bringing prisoners of war and before them, closer to the king, officials counting the cut-off hands and phalli with foreskin. The defeated enemies attested here are *Tmḥ Spd Mᶜšwš* "Temeh, Seped and Meshwesh," referred to as Libyans in Egyptology. The pair of officials in each of the five registers share the task as we saw earlier; the one on the right writes the tally on a papyrus roll while the one on the left counts the hands.

The number of body parts in the piles of each register can be counted. The pile on the far left of the first register contains approximately 54 cut-off phallus shafts with foreskin. The depiction is followed by inscription stating "total phalli with foreskin 12535" (*dmḏ ḳrn.t 12535*).[25] The pile in the third register has approximately 49 cut-off phallus shafts with foreskin, with an inscription stating "total phalli with foreskin 12860" (*dmḏ ḳrn.t 12860*).[26] Such high numbers of cut-off body parts stand for the entire campaign or war; however, the number might also be an exaggeration on the part of the Egyptians.

In another part of the Great War inscription, cut-off phalli are mentioned in the description of the army's triumphal return.[27] After a *lacuna,* the text mentions "donkeys before them, laden with phalli with foreskin of the land of Libu together with the hands of all the foreign lands which had accompanied them" (*[ᶜ]ꜣ.w ḫr.j-ḥꜣ.t=sn ꜣtp(.w) m-ᶜ ḥnn.w ⟨m⟩ ḳrn.t ḫꜣs.t Rbw ḥnᶜ kp.w n ḫꜣs.t [nb] wn.w ḥnᶜ=w*).[28] The fact that the text refers to *ḥnn.w ⟨m⟩ ḳrn.t* "phalli with/as *krn.t*" indicates that indeed phalli were cut off and that *ḳrn.t* is part of them. Cut-off phalli are further mentioned in the part of the text giving the list of spoils of war as *ḥnn.w m ḳrn.t* "phalli with *ḳrn.t*."[29]

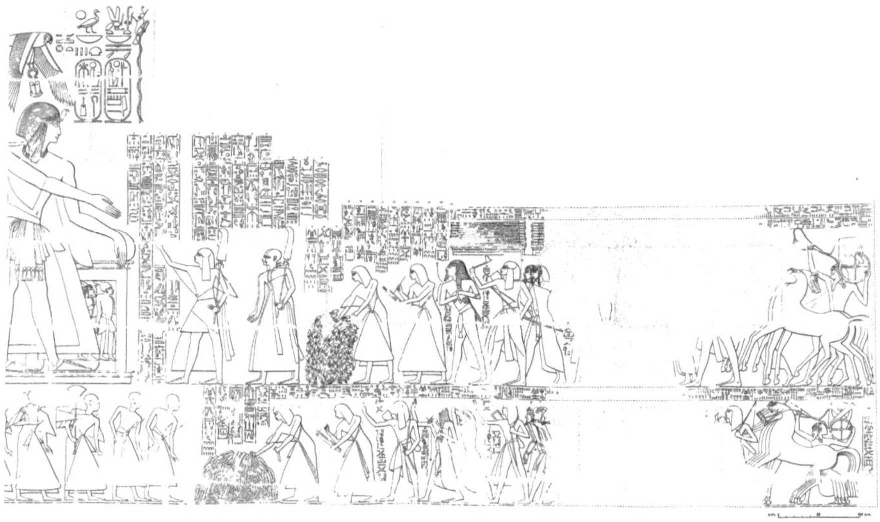

Figure 20.3 Aftermath of the Second Libyan War of Ramesses III, Medinet Habu temple, scene of counting of the cut-off hands and phalli, the east wall of the first court, to the north of the entrance (Nelson 1932, pl. 75).

The list of spoils of war in the Great War inscription of Ramesses III is similar in composition to the one of the Athribis stela of Merenptah. Both are fairly long, and they state that a total of 6,359 phalli with foreskin were brought from Libu. The text also mentions "[Sh]erden, Shekelesh, Aqaywasha, of the foreign countries of the sea, who had no f[oreskin]" (*[Š]rdn.w Škrš.w Jḳwš.w n nꜣ ḫꜣsw.t n pꜣ ym n.tj bn n=w ḳ[rn.t]*) and "Aqaywasha, who had no foreskin, slain, whose hands were brought [because they had no foreskin?]" (*[Jḳ]wš.w n.tj mn m-dj=w ḳrn.t ẖdb.w jny=t(w) nꜣj=sn kp.w*).[30]

Phalli were cut off from Libyan enemies in the Second Libyan War as well. We are informed about this from the reliefs of Ramesses III in the Temple at Medinet Habu, and specifically on the east wall of the first court, to the north of the entrance (Figure 20.3).[31]

The third register depicts six Egyptian soldiers to the left just beneath the king. They are facing right, approaching a pile of approximately 92 cut-off phallus shafts. To the right of the pile is an Egyptian official leaning forward towards the pile, holding one phallus shaft in each of his hands. Another Egyptian official to his right writes on his papyrus scroll. The scene is followed by an inscription stating "total *ḳrn.t* 2175" (*dmḏ ḳrn.t 2175*).[32]

What is *ḳrn.t*?

In the text above I refer to *ḳrn.t* as foreskin. This is the most common understanding of the word attested in the texts from the reigns of Merenptah and Ramesses III. The traditional understanding of the word is based, firstly, on the interpretation of the objects seen in the piles counted by scribes as phalli with foreskin and, secondly, the understanding of the word *ḳrn.t* as a Semitic loan word meaning "foreskin" or "phallus with foreskin."[33] We find it as *urullu* in Akkadian, *oral* in Hebrew, *urlā* in Syrian, and *gurlat* in Arabic.[34] Additionally, in the part of the text of the aforementioned Athribis stela referring to the Libyan enemies against whom Merenptah fought, it is stated that "their phalli were brought" (*jnj=tw nꜣy=sn ḥnn.w*). Although a representation of phalli-counting does not accompany the text, there is no doubt that the word *ḥnn* (singular) means phallus.[35] Judging by this text alone one could argue that however one understands the word *ḳrn.t*, the *ḥnn.w* (phalli) were cut off from the Libyan enemies during the reigns of Merenptah and Ramesses III.

Édouard Naville and Friedrich von Bissing have argued against reading the word *ḳrn.t* as foreskin or phallus with foreskin.[36] First Naville, and then von Bissing – who relied on Naville – interpreted the depicted objects in the piles not as phalli but phallus sheaths. More recently, Alexander V. Safronov questioned the understanding of *ḳrn.t* as foreskin or phallus with foreskin, providing philological, iconographic, culture-historical, and ethnographic arguments to support his interpretation of *ḳrn.t* as phallus sheath. Therefore, in the following section I will discuss the arguments presented against the interpretation of *ḳrn.t* as phallus with foreskin. I will argue that they do not stand the weight of evidence and I will present evidence which indicates the contrary.

Safronov argued that the identification of the word *ḳrn.t* with the Semitic words that have the root *grl* and mean foreskin is erroneous. According to him, the reading of the grapheme group *nꜣ*/𓈖𓄿 [hieroglyph]𓄿 (found in different written forms of the lexeme *ḳrn.t*) as Semitic phoneme /*l*/ cannot be sustained because this group is read as /*n*/ in Late Egyptian. Late Egyptian prefers the graphemes 𓂋 or 𓈖, also groups [hieroglyphs] or [hieroglyphs] for the Semitic phoneme /*l*/.[37] The word *ḳrn.t* in Egyptian texts is written in syllabic orthography which means that weak consonants such as *ꜣ*, *j*, or *w* are written too.

In all of the different writings of the word grapheme *ḳ(ꜣ)* is followed by an *r* followed by a *n(ꜣ)* followed by a *tj* (or *ṯ* in one case). In all cases except one, the word is determined with a sign for flesh, F51 in Gardiner's list. When the ending *tj* is removed one is left with *ḳ(ꜣ)-r-n(ꜣ)*. The sign or the group of signs *r*, which can be read as /*l*/,[38] are not in the final position where one would expect them in order to read the root as *grl*. This would be possible in the case of metathesis (rearranging of sounds or syllables) of radicals (one of the three consonants in a Semitic root). As argued by James E. Hoch, two thirds of the examples of metathesis in Egyptian contain *r* and in 76% of the cases, the metathesis of the second and third radical.[39] According to Hoch, there are limited cases in which the sign *n(ꜣ)* is standing for *r*.[40] Therefore, it is possible that *ḳrn.t* derives from the Semitic root *grl* meaning foreskin.

The arguments on the appropriate reading of certain grapheme groups aside, one must consider that if the word *ḳrn.t* has Semitic origins, it is used to label a Libyan body part. This can be explained by the predominance of Semitic words in the military language.[41] Nevertheless, it is instructive to consider the possibility not only that *ḳrn.t* is a Libyan word. However, we do not know much about the language of the Late Bronze Age people Egyptologists label as Libyans.

Great War inscription of Ramesses III, Karnak	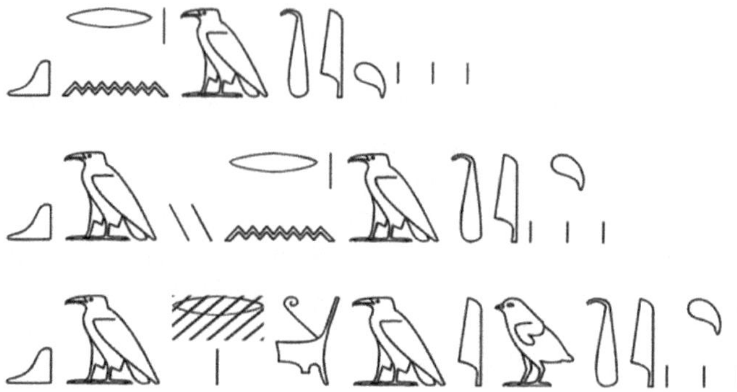
Presentation of the spoils of war, First Libyan War of Ramesses III, Medinet Habu	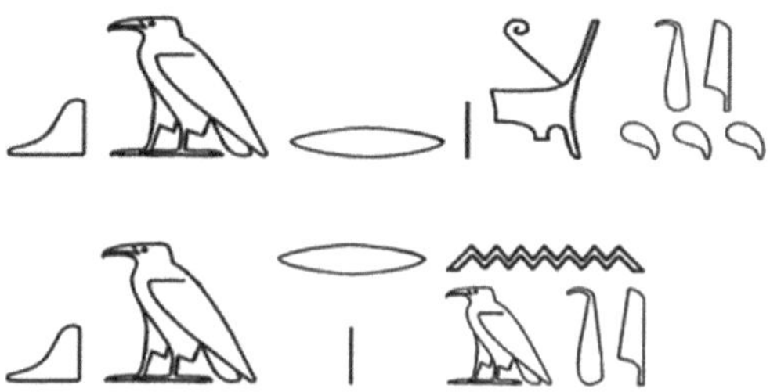
Presentation of the spoils of war, Second Libyan War of Ramesses III, Medinet Habu	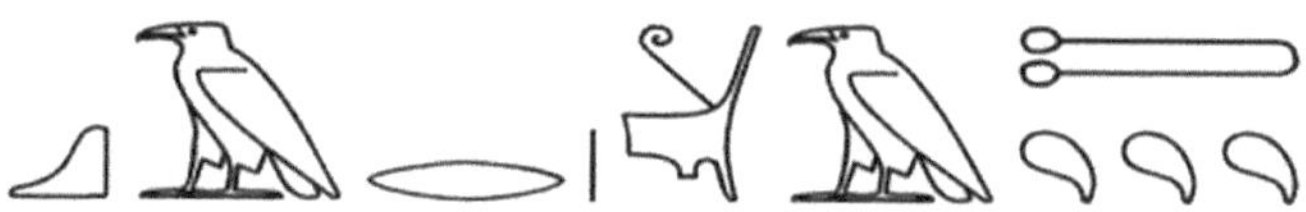

Safronov's iconographic and ethnographic evidence is based on comparing the depicted cut-off and piled phallus shafts with the sheaths worn by Bantu people in Cameroon.[42] Naville and Frans Jonckheere previously proposed similar ethnographic analogies,[43] which von Bissing accepted.[44] This is a very simple formal analogy. These scholars did not consider that the piled body parts do not resemble what Egyptologists usually identify as Libyan phallus sheaths.

Safronov argued that the fact that Aqaywasha are described in the Great War inscription from Karnak as not having *ḳrn.t* would mean that they did not have foreskin, and von Bissing saw this to be problematic. Both von Bissing and Safronov identify Aqaywasha with Ahhiyawa, attested in Hittite texts and identified with the Homeric Achaeans, ancestors of classical Greeks.[45] They supposedly did not practice circumcision. The problematic line of argumentation leading from Aqaywasha to classical Greeks and their Indo-European background is beyond the scope of this chapter.[46] Even if the identification of Aqaywasha with Ahhiyawa is correct, this still does not mean that the identification of Ahhiyawa with Homeric Achaeans is correct. Additionally, this identification argues for a coherent unchangeable identity over a thousand years. If, for the sake of argument, we accept that Aqaywasha can be related to mainland Greece and Mycenaeans, the problem remains that there is a lack of enough representations of nude mature males in Aegean art through which we could check whether or not they practiced circumcision.[47]

Another possibility is that *ḳrn.t* comes from the Semitic word for horn (Proto-Semitic *qarn*, Akkadian *qarnu*, Old Babylonian *qar.num*, Ugaritic *grn*, Biblical Hebrew *qeren*, Arabic *qarn*). This possibility is especially interesting from the iconographic point of view, to which I turn next.

I have shown that the arguments against the identification of *ḳrn.t* as phallus with foreskin, and as phallus sheath instead, are unconvincing. Instead, I offer an additional iconographic argument that *ḳrn.t* was understood as phallus with foreskin, more precisely a shaft of an uncircumcised phallus.

The cut-off phallus shafts depicted in the piles are of the same form as the shafts still attached to the living Libyan enemies' scrota on the Medinet Habu battle reliefs. There are numerous attestations of Libyan enemies in their long robes, which are slightly open to reveal their flaccid phalli (Figure 20.4). Examples of Libyan enemies depicted like this appear in the second scene from the west end of the north exterior wall at the temple at Medinet Habu.[48] Comparing the *de facto* phalli of the Libyans, when these are depicted as still attached to their bodies, with the cut-off body parts (phallus shafts) in piles, we have a striking match. Furthermore, in connection to the possibility that the word *ḳrn.t* used to label the cut-off body parts derives from the Semitic word for horn, it is important to mention that hieroglyph signs for horn and phallus are graphically similar. In fact, phallus was

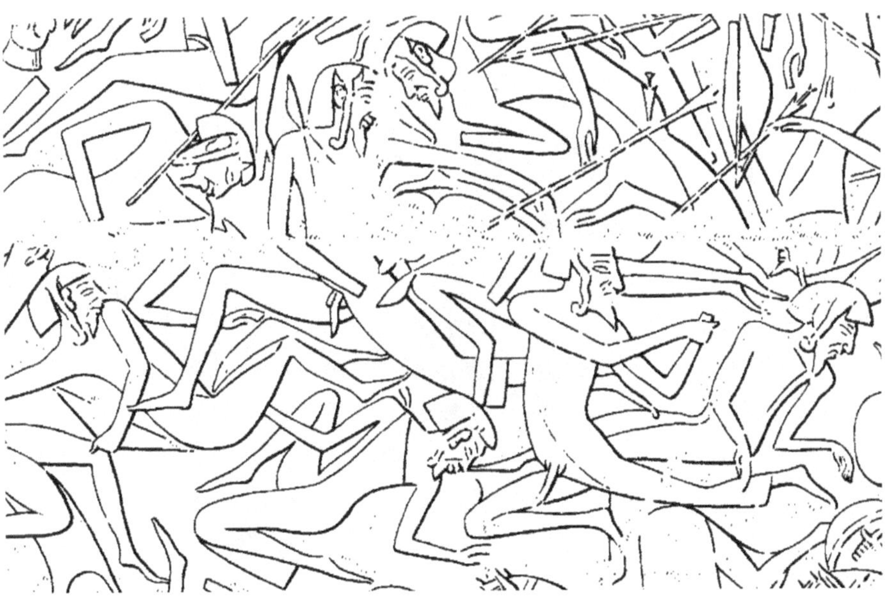

Figure 20.4 Libyan enemies depicted with long robes and flaccid phalli shafts still attached to the scrota, Medinet Habu temple, second scene from the west end of the north exterior wall (Nelson 1930, pl. 18).

considered to be a kind of a horn, as indicated by writing of the name Ab-kau on Stela Louvre C15 from Abydos dating to the end of 11th Dynasty (early second millennium BCE). Here the shaft of the phallus sign in the writing of the word *kꜣ* (bull) has been depicted as a horn[49] attached to the scrotum, just as in Medinet Habu depictions of the Libyan enemies.

The shafts of the Libyan phalli look the same as the cut-off shafts piled in the registers of the scene discussed earlier. However, the reliefs at Medinet Habu were painted, and unfortunately the colour has been lost in most representations of Libyan enemies with visible phalli. As such, we do not know if there was once paint over the phalli, which could indicate that they were covered by a form of dress, such as a phallus sheath. The solution to this problem is found on an earlier representation of Libyan enemies dated to the reign of Akhenaten (Figure 20.5).

The papyrus from Amarna kept in the British Museum in London (EA74100) depicts two Libyan soldiers beating an Egyptian who is kneeling on the ground.[50] Traces of a third Libyan figure on the right are also present. The two better-preserved Libyan figures are dressed as the Libyan enemies at Medinet Habu, mentioned previously. On the Amarna papyrus, they are depicted with their phalli clearly visible. The way the phallus shaft is shown attached to the scrotum is similar to that on the Medinet Habu battle reliefs, but contrary to the reliefs, the colours on the Amarna papyrus are excellently preserved. Here, a darker red colour is used to outline the

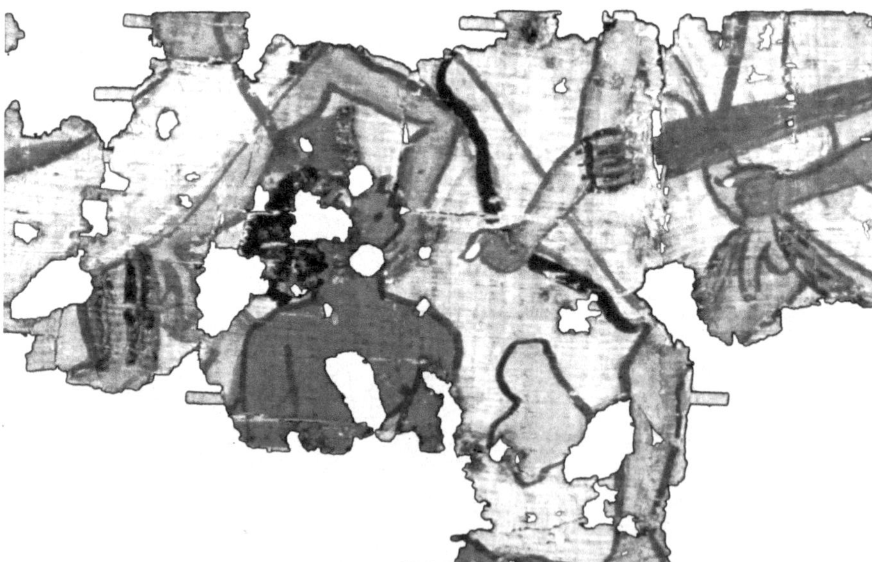

Figure 20.5 Libyan men in long robes and flaccid phalli shafts attached to their scrota, papyrus EA74100, originally from Amarna, currently in British Museum in London, line drawing of the author based on a photo detail (Image by Uroš Matić).

phalli, while a yellowish colour fills in the gaps. The rest of their flesh is filled with the same colour, while the same red is used to outline body parts and clothes. The Libyan robes are coloured white. A continuous field of colour denoting skin runs from the abdomen of the Libyans to their scrota and phalli, indicating that they do not wear anything to cover their phalli. If the phalli were dressed in some phallus sheath, one would expect a line of division for whichever colour was used for this fabric, as was done with the white robes they wore. We can, therefore, argue that the phalli of the Libyans are not covered by a phallus sheath. On the contrary, they are nude and exposed. Whether the Libyans dressed like this and fought with their phalli exposed is another issue; for us, what is important is how the Egyptians depicted them, and how they understood or constructed their Libyan enemy.

Judging from the Amarna papyrus depictions of the Libyans in long robes and exposed phalli, the Libyan enemies on the battle reliefs of Medinet Habu, wearing the same type of robe, can be said to have their phalli exposed too. Indeed, this is the same iconographic type of the Libyan enemy. Consequently, their phalli were not covered by phallus sheaths. Therefore, the cut-off and piled phallus shafts in the registers depicting the presentation of spoils of war once belonged to them, as indicated by accompanying texts. Namely, these phallus shafts are, as we have seen, followed by inscriptions listing their total number and referring to an individual cut-off phallus shaft as *ḳrn.t*. Thus, *ḳrn.t* is undoubtedly a cut-off shaft of a phallus. Bearing in mind that these cut-off phalli are depicted without the penile glans and that the *ḳrn.t* is most probably a Semitic loan word meaning foreskin, phallus with foreskin, or horn, one can argue that the traditional understanding of the word *ḳrn.t* as foreskin or phallus with foreskin (uncircumcised) is correct. These uncircumcised phallus shafts were only removed from Libyan enemies.

Disabled Masculinities

The written and visual attestations for phalli cutting are not explicit in its purpose and meaning. There are no administrative texts in which the practice of phalli cutting or other forms of mutilations of enemies are attested. Evidence from human remains is also absent. One explanation may be that the iconographic and textual evidence indicates that phalli cutting was conducted during the war and not in Egypt. Conditions under which human tissue is preserved to the point of accurate recognition are taphonomically extraordinary and it is unlikely that actual remains of cut-off phalli will ever be found. Nevertheless, some authors argue that the New Kingdom practice of hand cutting is archaeologically confirmed upon finding disarticulated human hands in the 15th Dynasty palace at Tell el-Dab'a (area F/II).[51] However, one should be careful in interpreting amputated hands in archaeological contexts as evidence of military hand cutting, since sources indicate hand amputation was also punishment for criminals (Papyrus Salt 124).[52]

Only Libyan enemies had their uncircumcised phallus shafts cut off, piled, and counted. These cut-off shafts are the same as those still attached to the Libyan enemies depicted on the battle reliefs at Medinet Habu. There are no known representations of Egyptian soldiers cutting off the phalli of Libyan enemies, but there are representations of soldiers cutting off the hands of enemies.[53] Neither are there representations of Egyptian soldiers carrying the cut-off phalli as they do with the hands. The only people in war reliefs who are depicted handling the cut-off phallus shafts are scribes. These elements allow us to think of the custom of phalli cutting in relation to representations of gender and understanding of masculinity of soldiers and scribes.

The Egyptian elite paid attention to the way it was represented in visual arts. From the Early Dynastic period, a decorum ordered compositional dominance and gender hierarchy in Egyptian art, placing men in privileged positions vis-à-vis women.[54] Male nudity was more often than not avoided since it would have to show a flaccid phallus (understood as lack of virility, power, and sexual potency and usually depicted with children, field workers, and enemies) or an erect phallus (powerful and sexually potent and usually depicted with deities).[55] Exceptions are found in informal art and texts produced by the general populace, such as ostraca or papyri with erotic scenes or official state-sponsored representations of ithyphallic deities such as Min or Amun.[56] Because only ithyphallic deities are depicted with erect phalli with exceptions solely from informal erotic art, one could argue that depicting an elite male with a flaccid or erect phallus in official contexts, such as his tomb, was against the rules of decorum. As Richard B. Parkinson argued, in most Egyptian contexts, an erect phallus is not only a manifestation of sexual arousal but stands for male power, resurrection, creation, and fertility.[57] The lack of a phallus was the lack of power. This is why powerful goddesses are also depicted with erect phalli.[58] The phallus was essential for New Kingdom elite masculine identity. Losing a phallus meant losing masculinity. We have evidence for this notion of loss and its disabling consequences in the *Tale of Two Brothers* preserved on the 19th Dynasty Papyrus D'Orbeney. In the story, Bata, one of the two brothers, cuts off his phallus to prove he did not sleep with his older brother's wife.[59] Later in the story, Bata tells his wife that she should not go outside to avoid being taken by the Sea. He says he could not defend her in that case "because I am a woman like you" (*pꜣ-wn tw=j* ⟨*m*⟩ *s.t-ḥm.t mj-ḳd=t*).[60] Thus, losing a phallus in this way would emasculate a man, and he would lack the power to defend his wife, being genderly disabled. This episode from the 19th Dynasty Papyrus D'Orbeney is chronologically close to the evidence for the cutting the phalli off from Libyan enemies and urges us to think about disabilities intersectionally, from a gender perspective.

Emasculation of enemies is well attested in the New Kingdom.[61] Cutting off phallus shafts could have had the connotation of depriving enemies of the privilege of masculinity and power. Gender was one of the frames of war as evidenced by written and visual accounts.[62] For example, Nubian boys on the war reliefs at the Derr and Beit el-Wali temples of Ramesses II in Nubia are depicted welcoming fleeing and injured soldiers with local women. The boys use gestures of mourning, indicating their vulnerability.[63] Indeed, in the battle with the Nubians depicted on the Medinet Habu temple it is said about Ramesses III that "he is looking at Bowmen like women" (*mꜣꜣ=f pḏ.tj.w mj ḥm.wt*).[64] Furthermore, and more importantly for this discussion, Libyans are described in the eleventh year of Ramesses III during the Second Libyan War as being made limp, *jry.w ḥdy.*;[65] the word *ḥdy* "to become limp"[66] is here determined with a woman in childbirth sign B3.[67] Similarly, the Libyan leader Meshesher is described as spread out on the ground, *pḵ{pgꜣ} ḥr tꜣ*,[68] with the word *pgꜣ* "to open up"[69] here written with a woman in childbirth sign B3 as its determinative like in the case of *ḥdy*. This indicates that the scribes intended to refer to the Libyan enemies as vulnerable. In relation to such gender transformations, David O'Connor even suggests a sexual background behind the decorative programme of the Eastern High Gate at Medinet Habu.[70]

When contextualized in the gender frame of war, the cutting of phalli of Libyan enemies is seen as a direct intervention on the already discursively feminized body of the enemy. Removing the phallus of a Libyan enemy physically removes his masculinity, and his body is materialized as both less male and less able than the body of an Egyptian soldier. Unlike hands, which are depicted being cut off by victorious soldiers, paraded on spears or hanging on ropes, and then piled and counted by scribes,[71] the cut-off phalli are only depicted as being counted by scribes. Evidence suggests that, at least in the visual representations, hands were cut off from enemies that were alive, but how the actual practice of this dismemberment was conducted is uncertain.[72] If Libyans fought with their phalli exposed, as indicated by ancient Egyptian representations of their dress, then it is possible that they were cut off while alive. If they fought without their phalli exposed, it is difficult to imagine how the Egyptian soldiers would have cut the phalli off during battle. Hence, these mutilations had to happen in the aftermath of the battle when the enemies were dead. This could explain why we do not have depictions of such acts. Indeed, soldiers' actions directly after battle are not depicted in Egyptian representations of war. Instead, they concentrate on the spoils of war. It is possible that the act of phalli cutting was also not depicted for reasons of sensitivity. Only scribes are shown handling cut-off phalli; depicting Egyptian soldiers handling the enemy's phalli was probably against the rules of decorum. While the audience on the battlefield differed from the audience privy to battle representations in Egypt, we should not assume their ignorance. If the soldiers cut off the phalli, people would have known that. The omission could have been a way to not affect their masculinity in the eyes of the audience. One could even consider the possibility that the scribes themselves performed the mutilation of the enemies after battle. The animosity between the soldier and scribal class is moreover well attested in the Ramesside period.[73] In this way, practices such as phalli cutting and its representations could have also affected masculinity of different social groups.

Since only Libyan enemies are targeted for such an act of mutilation it is possible that this is because of the particular danger they posed for Egypt during the reigns of Merenptah and Ramesses III.[74] Indeed, there are no attestations for such mutilations of enemies after the reign of Ramesses III, and simultaneously there are no more big campaigns against them after his reign. One should also bear in mind that phalli were taken as spoils of war, a practice that does not replace the older custom of hand cutting attested in both written and visual sources since the 18th Dynasty.

It seems that during the reigns of Merenptah and Ramesses III hands were cut off and taken from those groups of enemies who did not have phalli with foreskin, which would serve to differentiate them from those having it, such as Libyans. In practical terms, it could be that this made it easier to count different enemy groups, if one presumes that Egyptians encountered them at the same time on the battlefield. However, the idea that the Egyptians under Merenptah and Ramesses III simultaneously fought against different enemy groups, such as Libyans and Sea Peoples, was recently questioned. The king's account of such encounters may be explained as an ideological statement rather than reality.[75] If this is true, the reason behind the practice of mutilation cannot be to facilitate the counting of different enemy groups who were slain or incapacitated in war.

However, other enemy groups are also feminized.[76] This begs the question, why are only the phalli of Libyans cut off? Maybe the answer is hidden in the phalli themselves, namely, they may have been perceived by Egyptians as different and less able penises. We have seen that in the text of the Athribis stela Libyan phalli are labelled with the Egyptian word for phallus (*ḥnn*). During the reign of Ramesses III, we find the first attestations of the word *ḳrn.t* both in association with the word *ḥnn* (Great War Inscription from Karnak) and standing alone. Therefore, it is possible to think of the word *ḳrn.t* as a lexicalized form of *ḥnn.w m ḳrn.t* (phallus with/as foreskin). This does not mean that the phalli of the Libyans were cut off because Egyptians considered foreskin alien. Circumcision was a widespread practice in ancient Egypt, but not the rule.[77] Maybe the reason was the cultural attitude to an enemy group who had foreskin. This is a unique intersection of a particular understanding of masculinity and ethnicity.

Conclusion

Mutilation of enemies by cutting off their phalli is attested during the New Kingdom only in the reigns of Merenptah and Ramesses III. This occurs in the context of their campaigns against the Libyans. In this period, the Egyptians cut off the shafts of uncircumcised Libyan phalli, collected, and counted them, after which their number was registered. The cut-off phallus shaft is labelled *ḳrn.t* and this meaning of this word is secure, based on reliefs at Medinet Habu depicting phallus shafts still attached to the scrota of living Libyan enemies.

The cutting act itself is never depicted, nor are any soldiers shown holding a cut-off phallus shaft. The only figures depicted handling the cut-off phallus shafts are the scribes on the reliefs at Medinet Habu. This indicates that there was a gendered frame of the decorum of war. It structured what actions by the Egyptian soldiers, or possibly scribes if they were cutting the phalli off, are depicted and left out.

The Libyans are always depicted with flaccid phalli, contrary to New Kingdom elite notions of masculinity. Furthermore, losing a phallus, according to the *Tale of Two Brothers*, meant emasculation and being identified as a woman. Since gender was one of the frames of war in Egypt, emasculation of enemies is a frequent motif in written and visual representations of war. Gender dictates that foreign men cannot have the same gender status as Egyptian men. Therefore, they were referred to as women. This simultaneously framed the normative masculinity of the Egyptian soldiers. Cutting off the phalli of Libyan enemies is a direct intervention on the already discursively emasculated bodies of the enemies. By cutting off his phallus, the Libyan is physically turned into an effeminate, less able man, unlike the Egyptian soldier. Because the practice targets only Libyans in written and visual attestations from the reigns of Merenptah of Ramesses III, it cannot be a general discursive feminization of enemies. If that were the case, other enemies would probably be mutilated too, in other periods. This strongly indicates the practice or at least its representation was historically contingent and related to certain culturally specific intersections of masculinity and ethnicity of the Libyans in the eyes of at least some Egyptians. Considering the Libyans were the primary foe of Merenptah and Ramesses III, it is possible that this produced additional animosity which resulted in actual physical interventions on dead Libyan bodies.[78] Consequently, Libyan bodies were sexually disabled by the Egyptians on the battlefield and then further in visual representations of their bodies on temple walls. These representations of flaccid penises and the penis shafts cut off solidified the Libyans' failed or less able masculinity from the male-centred and able-bodied ideology of New Kingdom Egyptian military society.

Notes

1 Skogstrand (2011).
2 McRuer (2006).
3 For a recent critique of ableism in Egyptology see Vogel and Power (2023): for intersectionality as a theoretical concept see Crenshaw (1989); for some applications in Egyptology see Matić (2020, 2021b).
4 Matić (2012), Matić (2016), Meskell (1999), Meskell and Joyce (2003), Sweeney (2011).
5 O'Connor (2005, 439–54).
6 Hue-Arcé (2017), Jensen and Matić (2017), Karlsson (2020), Matić (2017), Matić (2023).
7 Diamond (2021), Matić (2019), Matić (2021a), 153–74. Morris (2020), Parkinson (2008, 115–42).
8 Strathern (2016, 21), Malešević (2010).
9 Harrison (2012).
10 Sivakumaran (2007, 253), Taylor (1999).
11 Misra (2015, 18).
12 Butler (2009, 26).
13 Butler (2009, 10).
14 Butler (2009, 3).
15 Butler (2009, 90).
16 Matić (2021b), Matić (2021a, 113–34), Matić (2023).
17 McRuer (2006). I am aware that disabled people do not universally accept the word "crip" and its reclaiming. Nevertheless, I stress the importance of an intersectional perspective which the so-called crip theory brings to Disability Studies, without neglecting the problem some communities have with this term.
18 Baines (1994, 81, 85), Vernus (1995, 164).
19 Baines (2007).

20 KRI IV, 8, 22.
21 KRI V, 12–23.
22 The scene appears on the south wall of the second court, lowest register of the first scene (from the east), Nelson (1930, pl. 23).
23 KRI V, 18.8–18.15.
24 Nelson (1930, pl. 22).
25 Kitchen gives the number as 22535, KRITA V, 14; Other authors give the number as 12535 as I do here, BARE IV, 52; Edgerton and Wilson (1936, 14).
26 Kitchen gives the number as 22860, KRITA V, 14; Safronov gives the same number 12535, as for the previously described register, Safronov (2010, 109); Other authors give the number as 12860 as I do here, BARE IV, 52; Edgerton and Wilson (1936, 14).
27 Inside (west) of the eastern wall connecting the main Karnak temple with Pylon VII, the northernmost of the southern pylons, BARE III, 572.
28 KRI IV, 7.10–7.14.
29 KRI IV, 8.4–16.
30 KRI IV, 8.4–8.16.
31 Nelson (1932, 75).
32 KRI V, 53.14.
33 Hoch (1994, 302), Lesko (1989, 20), Schneider (2008, 197), Wb 5, 60.15–61.4.
34 Tezel (2014, 201).
35 Wb 3, 115.1–2.
36 von Bissing (1936, 75–76).
37 Safronov (2010, 108); cf. Loprieno (1995, 13), Schneider (1992, 378–79) found /l/ only in the final position of a personal name.
38 Its function as a final syllable in personal names is clear, see Schneider (1992, 381–82).
39 Hoch (1994, 420).
40 Hoch (1994, 432).
41 Schneider (2008, 181–205).
42 Safronov (2010, 113).
43 Naville (1910) and Jonckheere (1944).
44 von Bissing (1936, 75).
45 von Bissing (1936, 107–8).
46 For the problems with this identification, see most recently Redford (2018, 115–16).
47 Franković and Matić (2023, 44–68).
48 Nelson (1930, pl. 18).
49 Morenz (2021, 163).
50 Parkinson and Schofield (1993, 35).
51 Bietak (2012, 42–43), Gresky et al. (2023, 5239); for numerous problems with this interpretation, especially those concerning the context and dating of the disarticulated hands see Matić (2019); for additional perspectives see Candelora (2021, 192–99).
52 Černý (1929, 245).
53 Matić (2019), Stefanović (2010, 149–67).
54 Baines (1990, 20).
55 Robins (2008, 208–15).
56 Manniche (1987).
57 Parkinson (2008, 121).
58 Matić (2021b).
59 Papyrus D'Orbiney (Papyrus British Museum 10183, Recto), line 7, 9. Gardiner (1932, 17.2).
60 Papyrus D'Orbiney (Papyrus British Museum 10183, Recto), line 10, 2, Gardiner (1932, 19.15).
61 Matić (2021b).
62 Foreign women and children are depicted in some New Kingdom battle scenes, but appear unharmed and not violently active. They are in scenes of battles in Syria and

Nubia and in conflict with the Sea Peoples. The only men depicted hurting foreign women and children are Sea People soldiers in the Egyptian army. Matić (2021b).
63 Matić (2021b).
64 KRI V, 8.7.
65 KRI V, 63.5–6.
66 Wb 3, 205.7.
67 To the best of my knowledge this was first discussed in the context of symbolical gender reversal by O'Connor (2005, 451).
68 KRI V, 61.11–12.
69 Wb 1, 562, 1–7.
70 O'Connor (2005).
71 Stefanović (2010).
72 Abdalla (2005, 25–34).
73 Spalinger (2006, 5–49).
74 Spalinger (2011).
75 Iskander (2010, 187–93).
76 Matić (2021b).
77 Quack (2012, 561–651).
78 Echoes of failed masculinity of Lower Egyptian rulers, some of whom had Libyan origins, are found in later sources, such as the Triumphal Stela of Nubian king Piye, founder of the Egyptian 25th Dynasty, Karlsson (2020), Matić (2023).

Bibliography

Abdalla, Magda A. “The Amputated Hands in Ancient Egypt.” In *Studies in Honor of Ali Radwan*. Vol. I, edited by Khaled Daoud, Shafia Bedier, and Sawsa Abd El-Fatah. Le Caire: Conseil suprême des antiquités de l’Égypte, 2005.

Baines, John. “Restricted Knowledge, Hierarchy, and Decorum: Modern Perceptions and Ancient Institutions.” *Journal of the American Research Center in Egypt* 27 (1990): 1–23.

Baines, John. “On the Status and Purposes of Ancient Egyptian Art.” *Cambridge Archaeological Journal* 4, no. 1 (1994): 81, 85.

Baines, John. *Visual and Written Culture in Ancient Egypt*. Oxford: Oxford University Press, 2007.

Bietak, Manfred. “The Archaeology of the Gold of Valour.” *Egyptian Archaeology* 40 (2012): 42–43.

Breasted, James Henry. *Ancient Records of Egypt. Historical Documents from the Earliest Times to the Persian Conquest*. Vol. II. The Eighteenth Dynasty. Chicago: The University of Chicago Press, 1906.

Butler, Judith. *Frames of War: When is Life Grievable?* London: Verso, 2009.

Candelora, Danielle. “Grisly Trophies: Severed Hands and the Egyptian Military Reward System.” *Near Eastern Archaeology* 84, no. 3 (2021): 192–99.

Černý, Jaroslav. “Papyrus Salt 124 (Brit. Mus. 10055).” *Journal of Egyptian Archaeology* 15, no. 3–4 (1929): 245.

Crenshaw, Kimberlé. “Demarginalizing the Intersection of Race and Sex: A Black Feminist Critique of Antidiscrimination Doctrine, Feminist Theory and Antiracist Politics.” *University of Chicago Legal Forum* 1 (1989): 139–67.

Diamond, Kelly-Anne. “Masculinities and the Mechanism of Hegemony in the Instruction of Ptahhotep.” In *His Good Name. Essays on Identity and Self-Representation in Ancient Egypt in Honor of Ronald J. Leprohon,* edited by Christina Geisen, Jean Li, Steven Shubert, and Kei Yamamoto. Atlanta: Lockwood Press, 2021.

Edgerton, William F., and John A. Wilson. *Historical Records of Ramses III, the T*exts in Medinet Habu. Vols. I and II. Chicago: The University of Chicago Press, 1936.

Erman, Adolf and Hermann Grapow, eds. *Das Wörterbuch der Aegyptischen Sprache*. Berlin: Akademie Verlag, 1926–1961.

Franković, Filip, and Uroš Matić. "Boy, You Fight Like a Woman . . . Representations of Defeated Enemies, Boys and Male Nudity in the Late Bronze Age Aegean Iconography and their Role in the Expression of Masculinity." *Men and Masculinities* 26, no. 1 (2023): 44–68.

Gardiner, Alan H. *Late-Egyptian Stories. Bibliotheca Aegyptiaca I*. Bruxelles: Fondation Égyptologique Reine Élisabeth, 1932.

Gresky, Julia, Manfred Bietak, Emmanuele Petiti, Christiane Scheffler, and Michael Schultz. "First Osteological Evidence of Severed Hands in Ancient Egypt." *Nature Scientific Reports* 13, no. 1 (March 31, 2023): 5239.

Harrison, Simon. *Dark Trophies. Hunting and the Enemy Body in Modern War*. New York and Oxford: Berghahn Books, 2012.

Hoch, James E. *Semitic Words in Egyptian Texts of the New Kingdom and Third Intermediate Period*. Princeton: Princeton University Press, 1994.

Hue-Arcé, Christine. "Violence against Women in Graeco-Roman Egypt: The Contribution of Demotic Documents." In *Archaeologies of Gender and Violence*, edited by Uroš Matić and Bo Jensen. Oxford: Oxbow Books, 2017.

Iskander, Sameh. "Merenptah's Confrontations in the Western Desert and the Delta." In *Offerings to the Discerning Eye. An Egyptological Medley in Honour of Jack A. Josephon. Culture and History of the Ancient Near East 38*, edited by Sue H. D'Auria. Leiden and Boston: Brill, 2010.

Jensen, Bo, and Uroš Matić. "Introduction: Why Do We Need Archaeologies of Gender and Violence and Why Now?" In *Archaeologies of Gender and Violence*, edited by Uroš Matić and Bo Jensen. Oxford: Oxbow Books, 2017.

Jonckheere, Frans. *La Médecine Égyptienne No 1. Une Maladie Égyptienne. L'Hématurie Parasitaire*. Bruxelles: Fondation Égyptologique Reine Élisabeth, 1944.

Karlsson, Mattias. "Gender and Kushite State Ideology: The Failed Masculinity of Nimlot, Ruler of Hermopolis." *Der Antike Sudan. Mitteilungen der Sudanarchäologischen Gesellschaft zu Berlin* 31 (2020): 99–108.

Kitchen, Kenneth A. *Ramesside Inscriptions: Historical and Biographical*. Vol. I–VIII. Oxford: Blackwell, 1969–1983.

Kitchen, Kenneth A. *Ramesside Inscriptions: Translated and Annotated*. Vol. I–V. Oxford: Blackwell, 1993–2008.

Lesko, Leonard H. *A Dictionary of Late Egyptian*. Vol. IV. Berkeley: B.C. Scribe Publications, 1989.

Loprieno, Antonio. *Ancient Egyptian. A Linguistic Introduction*. Cambridge: Cambridge University Press, 1995.

Malešević, Siniša. *The Sociology of War and Violence*. Cambridge: Cambridge University Press, 2010.

Manniche, Lise. *Sexual Life in Ancient Egypt*. London: KPI Ltd., 1987.

Matić, Uroš. "Egiptologija, rod i seksualnost: kritička perspektiva." *Genero: časopis za feminističku teoriju i studije kulture* 16 (2012): 59–82.

Matić, Uroš. "Gender in Ancient Egypt: Norms, Ambiguities, and Sensualities." *Near Eastern Archaeology* 79, no. 3 (2016): 174–83.

Matić, Uroš. "Her Striking but Cold Beauty: Gender and Violence in Depictions of Queen Nefertiti Smiting the Enemies." In *Archaeologies of Gender and Violence*, edited by Uroš Matić and Bo Jensen. Oxford: Oxbow Books, 2017.

Matić, Uroš. *Body and Frames of War in New Kingdom Egypt. Violent Treatment of Enemies and Prisoners. Philippika 134*. Wiesbaden: Harrassowitz Verlag, 2019.

Matić, Uroš. *Ethnic Identities in the Land of the Pharaohs. Past and Present Approaches in Egyptology*. Cambridge: Cambridge University Press, 2020.

Matić, Uroš. "He is Looking at Bowmen Like Women. Gender as a Frame of War in New Kingdom Egypt (*c. 1539*–1077 BC)." In *Geschlecht macht Herrschaft-Interdisziplinäre*

Studien zu vormoderner Macht und Herrschaft. Macht und Herrschaft-Vormoderne Konfigurationen in transkultureller Perspektive 15, edited by Andrea Stieldorf, Linda Dohmen, Irina Dumitrescu, and Ludwig D. Morez. Bonn: Bonn University Press, 2021a.

Matić, Uroš. *Violence and Gender in Ancient Egypt.* London and New York: Routledge, 2021b.

Matić, Uroš. "Gender as a Frame of War in Ancient Nubia." *Dotawo. Journal of Nubian Studies* 8 (2023): 100–38.

McRuer. Robert. *Crip Theory: Cultural Signs of Queerness and Disability.* New York and London: New York University Press, 2006.

Meskell, Lynn. *Archaeologies of Social Life: Age, Sex, Class et cetera in Ancient Egypt.* Oxford: Blackwell, 1999.

Meskell, Lynn, and Rosemary A. Joyce. *Embodied Lives: Figuring Ancient Maya and Egyptian Experience.* London and New York: Routledge, 2003.

Misra, Amalendu. *The Landscape of Silence. Sexual Violence against Men in War.* London: Hurst & Company, 2015.

Morenz, Ludwig. "Von pointierter Maskulinität im Ägypten des späten dritten Jahrtausends v. Chr. Zur funerären Inszenierung des Potentiaten Anchtifi als übermenschlichen, Manns-Kerl." In *Geschlecht macht Herrschaft-Interdisziplinäre Studien zu vormoderner Macht und Herrschaft. Macht und Herrschaft-Vormoderne Konfigurationen in transkultureller Perspektive 15*, edited by Andrea Stieldorf, Linda Dohmen, Irina Dumitrescu, and Ludwig D. Morez. Bonn: Bonn University Press, 2021.

Morris, Ellen. "Machiavellian Masculinities: Historicizing and Contextualizing the 'Civilizing Process' in Ancient Egypt." *Journal of Egyptian History* 13, no. 1–2 (2020): 127–68.

Naville, Édouard. "Le Mot (hiero)." *Sphinx: Revue Critique* XIII (1910): 227–37.

Nelson, Harold. H. *Medinet Habu. Vol. I: Earlier Historical Records of Ramses III.* Chicago: The University of Chicago Press, 1930.

Nelson, Harold H. *Medinet Habu. Vol. II: Later Historical Records of Ramses III.* Chicago: The University of Chicago Press, 1932.

O'Connor, David. "The Eastern High Gate. Sexualized Architecture at Medinet Habu?" In *Structure and Significance. Thoughts on Ancient Egyptian Architecture*, edited by Peter Jánosi. Wien: Verlag der Österreichischen Akademie der Wissenschaften, 2005.

Parkinson, Richard B. "Boasting about Hardness: Constructions of Middle Kingdom Masculinity." In *Sex and Gender in Ancient Egypt: Don Your Wig for a Joyful Hour*, edited by Carolyn Graves-Brown and Kara M. Cooney. Swansea: Classical Press of Wales, 2008.

Parkinson, Richard B., and Louise Schofield. "Akhenaten's Army." *Egyptian Archaeology* 3 (1993): 35.

Quack, Joachim F. "Zur Beschneidung im Alten Ägypten." In *Menschenbilder und Körperkonzepte im Alten Israel, in Ägypten und im Alten Orient. Orientalische Religionen in der Antike 9*, edited by Angelika Berlejung, Jan Dietrich, and Joachim F. Quack. Tübingen: Mohr Siebeck, 2012.

Redford, Donald B. *The Medinet Habu Records of the Foreign Wars of Ramesses III.* Leiden and Boston: Brill, 2018.

Robins, Gay. "Male Bodies and Construction of Masculinity in New Kingdom Egyptian Art." In *Servant of Mut. Studies in Honor of Richard A. Fazzini*, edited by Sue H. D'Auria. Leiden and Boston: Brill, 2008.

Safronov, Alexander V. "Несуществующий Обычай Обрезания у Греков-Ахеяйцев (Значение Египетской Лексемы Ḳrnt)." *Vestnik Moskovskogo Gosudarstvennogo Oblastnogo Universiteta* 1 (2010): 109.

Schneider, Thomas. *Asiatische Personennamen in Ägyptischen Quellen des Neuen Reiches.* Freiburg and Göttingen: Universitätsverlag Freiburg und Vandenhoeck & Ruprecht, 1992.

Schneider, Thomas. "Fremdwörter in der ägyptischen Militärsprache des Neuen Reiches und ein Bravourstück des Elitesoldaten (Papyrus Anastasi I 23, 2–7)." *Journal of the Society for the Study of Egyptian Antiquities* 35 (2008): 197. Wb 5, 60.15–61.4.

Sivakumaran, Sandesh. "Sexual Violence Against Men in Armed Conflict." *The European Journal of International Law* 18, no. 2 (2007): 253.

Skogstrand, Lisbeth. "Is Androcentric Archaeology Really About Men?" *Archaeologies. Journal of the World Archaeological Congress* 7 (2011): 56–74.

Spalinger, Anthony J. "The Paradise of Scribes and the Tartarus of Soldiers." In *Five Views on Egypt. LAe. Studia Monographica 6*, edited by Anthony J. Spalinger. Göttingen: Seminar für Ägyptologie und Koptologie, 2006.

Spalinger, Anthony J. *Icons of Power. A Strategy of Reinterpretation.* Prague: Faculty of Arts, Charles University in Prague, 2011.

Stefanović, Danijela. "The Counting of the Dead Enemy's Hands." *Гласник српског археолошког друштва* 19 (2010): 149–67.

Strathern, Marylin. *Before and After Gender: Sexual Mythologies of Everyday Life.* Chicago: HAU Books, 2016.

Sweeney, Deborah. "Sex and Gender". In *UCLA Encyclopedia of Egyptology*, edited by Willeke Wendrich and Elizabeth Frood. Los Angeles: UCLA Press, 2011. *s.v.* https://escholarship.org/uc/item/3rv0t4np.

Taylor, Christopher C. *Sacrifice as Terror. The Rwandan Genocide of 1994.* Oxford and New York: Berg, 1999.

Tezel, Sina. "The Comparative Method as Applied to the Semitic Cognate Sets with Phonological Correspondences." In *From Tur Abdin to Hadramawt Semitic Studies. Festschrift in Honour of Bo Isaksson on the occasion of his retirement*, edited by Tal Davidovich, Ablahad Lahdo, and Torkel Lindquist. Wiesbaden: Harrassowitz Verlag, 2014.

Vernus, Pascal. *Essai sur la conscience de l'histoire dans l'Egypte pharaonique.* Paris: H. Champion, 1995.

Vogel, Hannah, and Ronika K. Power. "Recognising Inequality: Ableism in Egyptological Approaches to Disability and Bodily Differences." *World Archaeology* (2023). https://doi.org/10.1080/00438243.2023.2170911.

von Bissing, Friedrich. "Die Angeblich Beschnittenen Aqaiuascha." *Zeitschrift für ägyptische Sprache und Altertumskunde* 72 (1936): 75–76.

21 DisAbility, Eunuchs and the Lived Experience in Ptolemaic-Roman Egypt

Sonia R. Zakrzewski, Stephanie Evelyn-Wright and Scott D. Haddow

Introduction: Identity and Disability in Palaeopathology

Human remains, whether skeletonised, naturally desiccated or mummified, provide a tangible link between the past and the present. Palaeopathology, the study of disease processes in the past, comprises a subset of the wider study of these past people (bioarchaeology), and commonly includes the study of health, disease and trauma as found in such human remains. Bioarchaeology has been well theorised, with the intersecting nature of different aspects of identity well recognised.[1] Identity is thus recognised as fluid and dynamic. By contrast, although disability has been recognised as one strand of identity, with a few notable exceptions,[2] disability has rarely been theorised as clearly. Within much of the medical community, disability is commonly viewed in terms of medical reductionism, with emphasis placed upon impairment and limitation. Social scientists who use the social model instead view disability as a social phenomenon, with the disability not being the bodily impairment but rather the social restrictions placed upon the individual affected by the surrounding community.[3] Bioarchaeology and palaeopathology, with their intrinsic biosocial frameworks, should thus view being disabled as simply a point upon a continuum of ability, rather than an individual viewed in binary opposition to someone who is non-disabled.[4] Following such an approach, disability in this chapter is rephrased as disAbility, with the focus moved towards being able to undertake activities and thus gives the affected individual some dynamic control over the ability to participate and choose their social role.[5] DisAbility can and will change throughout the life course of the affected person in terms of its impact, expression and severity, with some bodily changes having a lifelong effect and others having only short-term or temporary effects. Viewed through this lens, disAbility is an intersectional strand within identity, with its importance varying at different stages of the life course and contingent on the local environment.

The intersectional nature of disAbility is well demonstrated in the example of the eunuch. The castrated male has historically served specific social functions for which their physicality was deemed uniquely qualified, but was also stigmatised and othered by their society. The castrated man embodies an identity conflict, between gender and disAbility, that results in a liminal status of sometimes elevated access and influence but also isolation and stigmatisation. This idea is

DOI: 10.4324/9781003440369-24

explored further using the case study of two possible eunuchs excavated from the Quesna archaeological site in Egypt, dating to the Ptolemaic-Roman period. These individuals and their archaeological context are summarised next, followed by a description of the biological implications of castration. Then, the themes of the penis and the eunuch in the Egyptian and Ptolemaic-Roman world offer a historical context. The resulting perspectives are incorporated together to conclude with a fictive narrative that briefly explores the intersectionality of gender and disAbility within the lived experience of a eunuch.

Greco-Roman Quesna and an Introduction to the Skeletal Remains

Quesna is a gezira site in the Delta area of Egypt (Figure 21.1). The gezira, or turtle back, lies 4 km to the east of the agricultural road to Alexandria on which the modern town of Quesna lies, 65 km northwest of Cairo.[6] The site was sacred, with evidence of offerings made to the falcon god Horus.[7] Recent excavations began at Quesna in 2007, under the directorship of Joanne Rowland as part of the Minufiyeh Archaeological Survey (under the wider aegis of the Egypt Exploration Society Delta Survey). Excavations in 2007 revealed burials from the Ptolemaic and Roman periods, with individuals buried in simple pits, in mudbrick constructions and in ceramic coffins. Inscriptions on a black stone sarcophagus from the

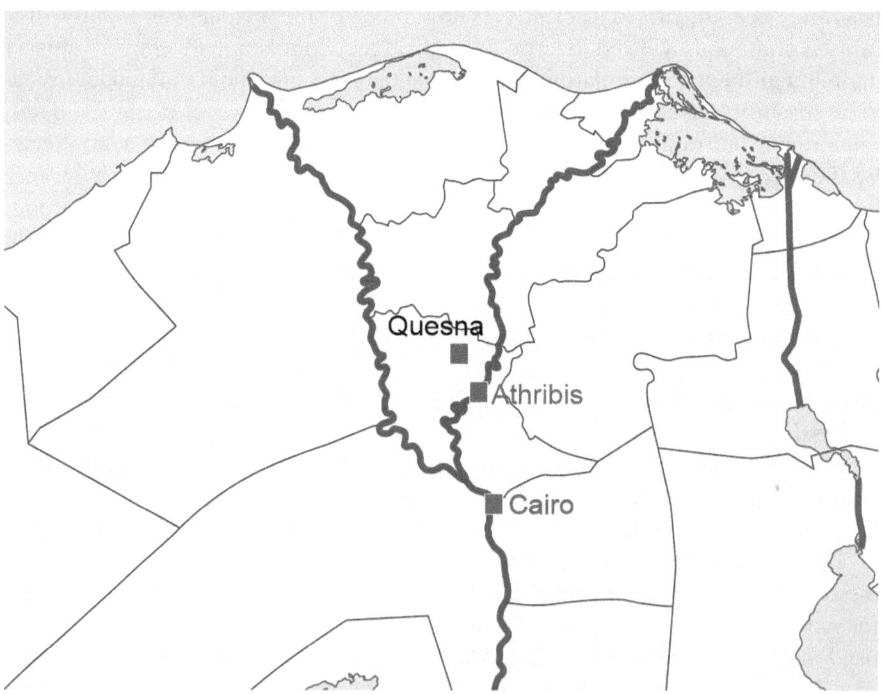

Figure 21.1 Map of the Delta highlighting the location of Quesna. Image by authors.

brick-built mausoleum in the south of the site indicated that some of the elite inhabitants and those in religious roles at nearby ancient Athribis were buried up on the Quesna gezira.[8] Ancient Athribis lies approximately 7 km from Quesna and so the Quesna gezira may have been visible from Athribis itself.[9] Overall 158 burials have been identified and/or excavated from the site.[10]

For full information about the varied pathology and unusual morphology from Quesna, please read Joanne Rowland's *Quesna*.[11] The two individuals forming the focus of this paper were found in close proximity to each other in Graves 1014 and 1019.

Grave 1014 was a large rectangular mudbrick grave that was robbed in antiquity but contained six individuals placed over each other in three layers. The uppermost individual, thus presumably one of the last to be interred, B.26, is of concern here. This body, like most of the others in this communal grave, was placed in the grave, oriented with head to the west, but unfortunately this burial was lacking the skull. The individual was laid out supine, with the right arm crossed over the left arm on the chest. Based on the pubic symphysis, B.26 was assigned to Suchey-Brooks Phase I (95% range is 15–24 years). However, the bodies of the sacrum, the heads of the ribs, spinous processes and endplates of vertebral bodies were all unfused. The epiphyses of the long bones, of the bones of the hands and feet including phalanges, metacarpals and metatarsals all remained unfused. The only bones that were united were the three bones composing the innominate and the neural arches of the vertebrae.[12] An incised Wedjat eye was found within the grave-fill although it is not known with which individual this should be associated. Reed matting may have been used to wrap at least two of individuals placed at the bottom of the grave. Additionally, blackish brown remnants of textile and dark resinous materials were found, implying some form of mummification of the individuals.[13]

In complete contrast, Grave 1019 was a simple pit dug directly into the sand, containing the extended supine skeleton of a single individual (B.21). This grave had also been robbed in antiquity. The body was oriented with the head to the south, in contrast to the dominant head-to-north orientation of this earlier phase of the cemetery, and with the arms lying along the body, with the hands on what would have been the thighs in life. The skull of B.21 was very badly damaged, with most missing. Based on the pubic symphysis, B.21 was assigned to Suchey-Brooks Phase I (95% range is 15–24 years). Dental development, and the lack of much dental attrition, also suggested an age of 16–22 for this individual.[14] However, like B.26, this individual had all the same epiphyses totally unfused, including the long bones, phalanges, metacarpal heads, sacral bodies, vertebral body endplates and innominates. This burial was also associated with many small finds of amulets etc., made of plaster (most probably gypsum) including cartonnage from around the head, several scarabs, Djed pillars, a fragmentary baboon and a Sphinx amulet.[15]

These two individuals were tall but still had completely unfused epiphyses and hence were still growing at their time of death. Using the stature estimation prediction equations established by Michelle Raxter and colleagues,[16] B.21 was 162.4 cm tall and B.26 was 168.3 cm tall compared to the cemetery average of 161.1 cm. If one assumes that their body sizes were larger than one might expect for their state of fusion of their epiphyses, assigning them to either a sex category or an age becomes problematic. Both individuals had pubic symphyses with Phase I morphology but only one of the skeletons, B.26, had teeth preserved. We therefore consider them most likely to be adolescents of indeterminate sex. Differential diagnosis for these individuals has been presented previously,[17] with possibilities including sex chromosome abnormalities, autosomal disorders such as oestrogen deficiency or hypogonadism or, as postulated by the authors, castration.

For castration to be identifiable in skeletal remains, it must be performed before epiphyseal fusion takes place, in other words before puberty. The lack of testosterone caused by the removal of the testes makes the bones develop in a similar way to females; as a result, castrates do not attain as much bone mass as an intact male because testosterone promotes an increase in bone mass.[18] Furthermore, some testosterone in the body becomes oestrogen and the latter ends bone growth. As a result, a castrate may lack sufficient testosterone to build robust bones, leading to relatively weakened muscular structure, and, additionally, may lack sufficient oestrogen to stop the bone growth.[19] This means that they develop elongated gracile long bones, which may result in extreme height and unusual body proportions.[20] Furthermore, the pelvis and skull, which develop their sexually dimorphic features during puberty, are also affected. The pelvis develops the typical male narrow form in the sciatic notch and narrow subpubic angle, but the wings of the ilia flare outwards in a more female-like shape.[21] This is associated with a more female-like body fat distribution.[22] The bones of the face also grow more slowly in castrates and so may have a childlike appearance, with an apparently heavy mandible and protruding maxilla.[23] If castrated young, the individual also retains the larynx of a boy, but develops the lungs and chest of a man, hence giving the unique quality of voice noted in castratos.[24] Castration may cause early onset osteopenia and hence make the skeleton more fragile than in other individuals.[25] Other key external traits include beardlessness.[26] The destruction of the testes is associated long term with premature aging, heart and circulation diseases and diabetes.[27] Similar bodily features are associated with congenital endocrine and/or chromosomal disorders of sexual development and complicate palaeopathological differential diagnosis. It is therefore extremely difficult to distinguish between castration and such congenital conditions because all result in similar skeletal effects and morphologies. Such congenital conditions would likely affect the individual socially in much the same way as transformation into a castrate, and thus the same issues are relevant. For simplicity and clarity of argument, we have focussed on castration as a possibility here.

The Penis in the Ancient Egyptian and Ptolemaic-Roman World

The ancient Egyptians had a series of words to refer to the male genito-urinary tract; the penis was *ḥnn*, the testicles were called *ẖrwy* (which literally means "those which are underneath") and the vas deferens was literally called the "two vessels to his testicles."[28] Furthermore, the Gardiner hieroglyph sign list contains 63 parts of the human body, including symbol D52 which is described as the "human phallus." Whilst the external nature of these hieroglyph signs might support the suggestion that there was no human dissection during the Old Kingdom, when most hieroglyphs were formalised,[29] animal dissections were undertaken, and thus their anatomy was well understood.[30] The ancient Egyptians' understanding of baboons and cattle led to the view that the penis was an object of dominion and power. Indeed, "in late times at least, the Egyptians connected the penis with the backbone,"[31] with the was staff held by gods such as Ptah suggested to derive from a bull's penis.[32] Furthermore, the ankh sign has been argued as being linked with either the penis or penis sheath.[33] Thus we see the phallus symbolism in much ancient Egyptian iconography, such as the cult of the priapic god Min who was repeatedly linked with bulls, and in actual items such as the sceptre, spear, mace and bull's horns being used as penis analogues. Of note for the Ptolemaic and Roman period are the uraeus snake, with its expanded cobra head, and oxyrhynchus fish sometimes being described as additional penis analogues.[34] The snake was also widely used as a Roman symbol of healing, with Asclepius the popular Ptolemaic-Roman healing god frequently using snakes as intermediaries for his miraculous cures.[35]

Having a complete ('perfect') body, including the penis, was required for revivification in the afterlife. Male and female genitals were always left intact in the mummification process so that sexual life would remain in the afterlife.[36] This did not preclude penile surgical procedures such as lithotomies and circumcisions. Relief evidence, like from 6th Dynasty of Ankh-ma-hor at Saqqara, has led scholars like Nunn to suggest that circumcision was undertaken as a rite of passage for ritual initiation into manhood. Indeed, a stela from Naga ed-Deir records a man called WHA who was circumcised along with 120 men.[35] It is certainly thought that circumcision in the ancient Egyptian world normally happened in late puberty, about age 16 or 17,[36] but was undertaken earlier for some by the Roman period.[37] Circumcision was not practised universally.[37] For example, the mummified remains of Ahmose I were circumcised, but those of his father and brothers were not.[38]

Lithotomy, the operation to remove bladder stones, appears to have been an area of Roman medical specialisation. Because of nutritional deficiencies, urethral calculus, or bladder stone, was relatively common in young boys and, despite the operation to excise bladder stones being complex and dangerous, "cutting for stone" is described by several ancient writers, including Celsus, Galen, Rufus of Ephesus and Paul of Aegina.[39] Certainly the removal of the stone by perineal incision is one of the longest and most detailed passages in *De Medicina* (7.26) by Celsus. "Ammonius, a hellenistic surgeon in Alexandria, developed a technique of splitting the stone. According to Celsus he was so renowned for this operation that he was surnamed 'lithotomus'–the stonecutter."[40] Although the ancient Egyptians named the bladder *sheptyt*, it is unclear how thoroughly they understood its connection with the kidneys and the penis. Despite the penis having clear importance in Egyptian thought, there is very little mention of the urinary system in the Egyptian medical papyri,[41] despite dislocation of neck vertebrae being noted as leading to penile erection in Edwin Smith Papyrus Case 31.[42]

Eunuchism and Castrates in the Ancient Egyptian and Ptolemaic-Roman World

The loss or damage of male genitalia was damaging to masculine identity in both ancient Roman and ancient Egyptian constructions of gender. The ancient Egyptian psychosocial importance of the male genitals is evident in the reception of the god Seth. In the mythical battle between Horus and Seth, Horus "tore off Seth's testicles"[43]; as a result, Seth was viewed as "the effeminate one" in Edfu texts.[44] Griffiths "saw the story of Seth's castration as 'loss of sovereignty.'"[45] In this example we see how loss of the sexual organs is equated with effeminacy, implying a reduced masculinity. The eunuch has been argued to threaten Greco-Roman values that emphasised the importance of the patriarchal family structure and its survival to the next generation.[46] The ancient Romans defined gender on the ability to procreate.[47] Eunuchs, along with groups like the Vestal Virgins, have been postulated as members of a third gender which encompassed people who did not procreate.[48] This implies possible linkage between being of a third gender and disAbility, especially when viewed in light of potential child exposure of certain infants deemed 'different' or 'other.'[49] Additionally, Roman notions of masculinity as defined through the priapic model, in which a man, *vir*, is the impenetrable penetrating agent in a sexual act, would thus cast a total castrate into the feminine, sexually submissive role and a male of failed masculinity.[50]

Despite antipathy, eunuchs likely wielded significant status and power in the Ptolemaic Kingdom and later Roman Empire. Prior to the Ptolemaic Kingdom, Alexander the Great was reputed to have taken the Persian eunuch, Bagoas, as his lover. Furthermore, the eunuch Ganymedes was the tutor of Cleopatra VII and her half-sister Arsinoe, and the eunuch Eulaeus served as a leading minister to Ptolemy VI in the second century BCE.[51] Castrates' connection to power extended to the Roman emperors, the earliest known example of which is Favorinus of Arles being a court favourite of Emperor Hadrian.[52] From the fourth century CE onward, eunuchs were known to have served in the Roman Imperial royal court, with positions like Grand Chamberlain.[53] While eunuchs may well have played a role in the upper levels of the Hellenised population, it is highly likely the Quesna individuals were not elites. There is no certainty of the likelihood of eunuchs in earlier Pharaonic Egypt, which may be a better fit for the Quesna cemetery.

The earliest reliable literary evidence of medical castration comes from Celsus, but most of our knowledge of classical medicine comes from Hippocrates of Cos.[54] Castration implies the removal, or rendering dysfunctional, of at least one of the two testicles, but this procedure may be undertaken in a variety of different ways and for a multitude of different reasons. In general, the method used and the extent of the procedure depend on the motive for the castration, with the main consequences of full castration being sterility, often accompanied by impotence and traits considered to be feminine.[55]

Francis summarises three principal methods for castration. In the first method, the testicles are removed through incisions made in the scrotum.[56] The second method has the entirety of the external genital organs removed. "This method was adopted in the case of the 'Castrati' in Roman times, and is that favoured in the Orient and Africa."[57] The final method has the testicles and septum scroti removed but leaves the upper and back part of the scrotum and the penis intact, and was the method used for the Roman 'Spadones.'[58] Francis was obviously working at a very different time and so certain aspects of his phrasing and writing might be considered somewhat problematic, such as his assertion at "the operation of castration was of Oriental origin."[59] König suggests that the methods used to remove the testicles varied from "cutting them away from the scrotum, rubbing or squeezing them to pieces, dehydration by way of unguents or plastering, to cutting off the gonads,"[60] and that sometimes the penis was also included in the procedure. Complete castration comprises total removal of the testes, scrotum and penis, whereas partial castration comprises 'only' the removal of the testicles and scrotum. Removal of the testicles alone was much less life-threatening than total castration.[61] The physiological effects could depend on the method of castration used, since if castration were undertaken by crushing (rather than removal) of the testicles, they might still be capable of some testosterone production.[62]

The rationale for castration affects the age at which the procedure might be carried out. Castration might be undertaken for medical reasons, for punishment and control, for sexual purposes, for religious reasons and/or for provision of staff for other roles, such as singing. The term eunuch is commonly associated with guardians of women and/or harems whereas castrato is associated with church and opera singers. Following Reusch, the term "castrates" is therefore preferred here since it does not imply either purpose.[63] Apart from the self-castrating Galli, castration is an emasculating process that is usually enacted by men upon other men. Whatever the rationale for the castration and whatever age the procedure was carried out, castrates occupied an ambiguous sexual position and often had the ability to pass between gendered identities.[64] Similarly, individuals with many congenital conditions, such as disorders of sexual development, would also be located outside the male-female dichotomy and could also have had the ability to pass between gendered identities.

The Galli were self-castrates who were devotees of the mother goddess Cybele and existed outside Roman normative masculinity.[65] Although the cult of Cybele was accepted as a state cult in 204 BCE, the senate refused Roman citizens the right to participate in the rites of the goddess, the Cybeline priests therefore being considered non-Roman and foreign,[66] i.e. othered by society. These individuals tended to be castrated as adults once they had reached physical maturity.[67] Unlike the other forms of castration, this was more likely undertaken by the (reasonably) clear choice of the individual concerned. In contrast, the other forms of castration were performed on others. As noted earlier, castration could take place for control and punishment. The 19th Dynasty Pharaoh Merenptah, after defeating the invading Libyan army, apparently collected 6,359 uncircumcised penises from them, their priests and their children.[68]

Ancient texts provide information regarding the medical reasons for castration. Celsus talks of afflictions that might induce cutting away of a male gonad, such as "the result of a blow, the testicle lacked nutrition; in this situation pus develops, and then all one could do, he says, is cut into the scrotum, let the pus out, and excise the testicle itself."[69] Castration was also the recommended treatment for conditions that might not immediately spring to a modern mind. Possibly because of it being a measure employed to inhibit sexual activity, castration was considered to potentially cure epilepsy; this might be because the disease was sometimes accompanied by symptoms such as unexpected sexual arousal.[70] Certainly, ancient medical authors, such as Soranus, seem to have noted some physical similarities between sexual activity and epilepsy. Furthermore, castration was also the recommended treatment for what Aëtius of Amida, in the sixth century, called elephantiasis, which is now thought to be lepromatous leprosy. Aëtius states that he met patients who had "cut away their own testicles with an iron blade. In castrated persons, you should know, the evil will not get any worse."[71] Castration was undertaken in such cases to stop the disease spreading rather than due to disease of the genitals. König also suggests that Ptolemaic-Roman doctors may have undertaken castration more frequently in the later centuries BCE than in earlier periods,[72] so suggesting an increase in the frequency of the practice at the relevant time for Quesna.

Castration and DisAbility

It is clear that from the first century CE onwards, Roman households certainly used slaves that had been deliberately subjected to castration as youths, with the operation regularly performed both by laymen and by physicians.[73] In the seventh century CE Paul of Aegina, himself a doctor, describes two methods of castration. The first is by compression and the other by excision. From his description it is clear that compression is performed on children.[74] Castration occurring before puberty affects the skeleton as it develops, although, as noted earlier, congenital conditions can lead to very similar skeletal conditions.[75] Castrates provide a compelling case study within the wider discourse of the spectrum of disAbility because, in many cases, castration was an intentional act; a person was deliberately impaired. Punitive limb amputation is another example of a deliberately created impairment, and the long-term impairment and disability associated with limb loss was a part of the punishment process. Castration can cause long-term conditions, as noted earlier; however, these impairments are secondary by-products of the main goal. Apart from singers, whose castration is intended to preserve the high-pitched voice, the main aim of castration is to render that individual sterile.

Infertility or sterility is not necessarily considered when thinking about disability today; for example infertility is not classified as a disability under the UK equality act.[76] In a Roman context, a castrate status separated the individual from the legal and social structures of citizenship and family which underpinned Roman society.[77] Still further, the slave status of many castrates separated them from their biological families.[78] Whilst imposed sterility was used as a punishment in some cases, childhood castration was undertaken to create an individual who was different from a 'normal' man.[79] For example, it was believed that castrates did not experience desire.[80] Additionally, Suetonius wrote that Emperor Nero castrated Sporus in order to turn him into a woman, suggesting that castration was seen as a process that changed a person's gender identity.[81] Eunuchs were lauded for their feminine beauty and youth, castration being viewed as a method for preserving that boyhood beauty.[82] Similarly, Roman poetry clearly indicates that eunuchs castrated as children were viewed as beautiful, youthful and physically attractive, since, for example, Earinus, the favourite of the Emperor Domitian, was considered exceptional compared with ideals of youthful male beauty.[83] A poem by Statius about him also "alludes to the fact that it is only his head hair that Earinus can dedicate; his castration means that he will not be able to grow a beard and dedicate the clippings from his first shave, such a crucial ritual in the transition from youth to manhood."[84] This gives us an upper age range for the castration process for boys and indicates that eunuch slaves were castrated before reaching puberty so that they could be appreciated for their youthful physical beauty. Castration also created a person different from other men, who did not experience the usual milestones of masculine life, like marriage and fatherhood.[85]

Castration is a rite of passage since it is a transformative process.[86] Castration thus takes a boy or man, removes them from the main social or cultural group, and places them in a liminal position, before they are re-incorporated into their social world, but "not in the same social cultural group from which they had been removed . . . [Furthermore] in some respects, the process of castration 'freezes' individuals into a liminal position–boy cannot become man, man cannot rejoin the male fraternity–which may have led to the formation of the specific, liminal, often gendered, social group of castrates."[87] Castration was used to create a different person, who existed outside the patriarchal family structure, which ideologically underpinned Roman society. The castration process thus created a liminal person and dramatically changed their position on the disAbility spectrum. The individual's paternal future was destroyed, and their perceived gender identity was altered placing them in an often-isolated position of an 'other.' Yet, there was a place in society for castrates.

Despite or perhaps because of this position, some castrates, like Earinus and Sporus, were celebrated. Eutropius was another noted eunuch, employed as grand chamberlain in the Eastern Roman Empire, and was the lover of a man named Ptolemy.[88] The castrates' liminal status made them uniquely qualified for some job roles and gave them exclusive influence and access. Since castrate slaves were separated from their family, they were seen to be entirely reliant on and invested in the success of their masters. Eunuch slaves were therefore reputed for their incredible loyalty and given enormous trust and responsibility as a result.[89] This is most apparent in the higher echelons of power, with eunuchs often necessary for the smooth court administration in the later empire. Their liminal status allowed the castrate access into spaces that non-castrated men could not go. A well-known Roman play *The Eunuch* (by Terrence, and dated to 161 BCE) emphasises the strong association and intimacy between women and eunuchs with eunuchs trusted as attendants of women.[90] This clearly demonstrates the association between castrates and the service of women, with eunuch slaves apparently in the company of men at least as much as they were in the company of women.[91] Eunuchs acted as intermediaries between high-profile men and women and, in the later empire, between a deified, sacred emperor and his subjects. Thus, eunuch slaves controlled access to the emperor and power.[92]

The castrate liminality afforded and enabled them to perform roles and have access to spaces forbidden to other men. Their liminality also made them vulnerable. "All historical eunuchs were ambiguous figures. They were necessary to the smooth functioning of society, yet they were often despised."[93] Their influence in the higher echelons of power was the cause of much hostility towards them, and their distinct otherness was an easy way to discriminate against them. Keith Hopkins describes scapegoat as a function that an emperor's eunuch advisors performed, redirecting any criticism of the emperor onto themselves. [94] Without a network beyond their master, they were vulnerable, however, easily blamed for something going wrong and with minimal recourse for support. Alongside this, castrates were physically distinct from other men, with the play by Terrence also implying that the clothing worn by eunuchs was distinctive, but the issue of clothing also links to issues of status and shame.[95] They were admired as beautiful, but also a reminder of the fragility of male sexuality and thus spurned.[96]

Despite little evidence for their presence in Egypt itself, across the Roman Empire, eunuchs or such castrates were generally non-Roman boys who had been castrated in childhood and brought into the service of the household. This service might be sexual in nature or might be guardianship (often of women in domestic contexts). They could be celebrated and praised in poetry, but were also seen, by men, as lesser individuals, to be viewed with shame and disdain. This means that our two individuals from Quesna, if they were castrates, would likely have been castrated as teenagers, and would have had a liminal position within the household. This position, both within and outside the norm, might be reflected in their burials, with one being placed in a communal grave, possibly with an incised Wedjat eye, and the other in an individual grave, with lots of funerary amulets, but positioned in a non-normative direction.[97]

Fictive Narratives as Communication

Due to bodily plasticity, life experiences are embodied and imprinted on the skeleton. Fictive narratives have been used to explore these personal and individual life experiences, both of 'normal'[98] and more unusual individuals including enslaved families[99] and disabled persons.[100] Fictive narrative allows the lived experience of palaeopathology to be explored, but also aids in communication and thus the accessibility of the study.[101] Some have dismissed fictive narratives as simply tools for use in public engagement rather than knowledge construction,[102] but we argue that fictive narrative may engender empathy and thus a new sense of understanding. Furthermore, fictive narratives may provide a mechanism to restore identity, and thus is preferable to the dehumanisation and commodification that sometimes occurs.[103] Just as there is no one true past, the bioarchaeological evidence can be interpreted in several different ways. This provides uncertainty in interpretation with many potentially different impressions of any one scenario possible. Evelyn-Wright has argued that presenting multiple different narratives depicting the same scene enables this uncertainty to be emphasised openly, with these different narratives offering different perspectives and interpretations.[104] Such narratives should be viewed as short vignettes and provide one perspective on the lived experience. Laes and Vuolanto have suggested that such an approach can "bring . . .[people] to life by means of plausible and well-informed life stories,"[105] and suggested that they might be called "faction" to demonstrate their linking of fictive narrative with careful documentation from the archaeological or historical record.

When considering skeletal palaeopathology for interpretation through faction, modern medical literature is required to determine any likely clinical symptoms and to understand the impact of skeletal lesions. A truly successful fictive narrative, however, goes beyond such an etic medical viewpoint to include emic approaches through integration of personal experience of individuals with similar skeletal change. This emic approach might include interviews with individuals living with similar socio-medical conditions, or, when this is not viable, through ethnographic research. Such an approach is obviously problematic when considering the life experience of Ptolemaic-Roman castrates due to limited social anthropological study to consult and the obvious limitations of the more recent historical record of castrates. Though one can never place oneself in someone else's shoes and thus provide their experience, the use of ethnographic study in the absence of interviews, diary entries or other suitable primary records provides the best avenue for the development of such faction.

Authors' Notes on the Fictive Narrative

The role of guardsman is a common role found for castrates across time. Their visible differences created by their castration act almost like a uniform. As noted earlier, their castration means they do not grow beards, are taller, have a unique physique, marking them as distinctive. Guardsmen roles are often to be visible, aiming to put people off from attacking, as much as protecting. The goading incidents are inspired by the taunts seen by one of the authors (SEW) that Buckingham Palace guardsman have experienced. The narrator's thoughts on gender come from ethnographic example of the Hijra, from India and Bangladesh, who describe themselves in essence as something different from men and women.[106] Eunuchs often experience social isolation and so establish a community amongst themselves, with the more experienced often looking out for and moulding the younger.

Fictive Narrative Voiced by One of the Tall Quesna Individuals

"Woman," he shouts at me. It is not the first time it's been said, and it won't be the last, all with the same venomous disdain that can only be achieved when they're deep in their cups. He says it swaying, arm flung round an actual, long-suffering woman. The arm around her shoulders that began as a loving and proprietorial gesture now has become a burden, weighing her down as she half carries this drunk along. "Woman," he shouts again louder as if I didn't hear him. He is standing close now. I cock my head to one side, quizzical, as I tower over him. I don't need to do anything else, just stand here as he takes in my full height. He sways for a moment; his companion then impatiently pulls him away, and he seems eager to go.

I am on overnight guard duty. Moments like this happen almost every night; it is part of the monotony. Guard duty is indeed tedious; it leaves a lot of time for thinking.

I was made into a guard. That was the point of my making, of that procedure years ago. My imposing height, my incorruptibility, my difference – all manufactured to perform this duty, to guard the precious cargo. My job rarely requires that I speak much, which is just as well. My singsong, boyish voice is at odds with my physique and the imposing role I have. On other occasions, people have tried to make me speak, goad me into talking so that they can laugh at the incongruous, high-pitched tones I produce. I know this, so I try not to give in to them and their provocation. I clutch the hilt of the knife at my belt; the message is soon understood.

Years ago, soon after being first cut, after a particularly violent encounter, I asked one of the others why people were so mean to us. They said that we have endured what he could not fathom. He cannot bear to imagine what we have been through and survived; the very notion of it offends him. So, he attacks. Just as the "women" he labels us as survive the birthing bed, so we have undergone a procedure they cannot bring themselves to think about, but in this case it could happen.

"Woman." I'm clearly not a woman. I still find it jarring, even now. But neither am I one of those men. I am neither man nor woman. I have been created into something else and it does not fit into either category. But it has given me a place, a purpose, a community. I see enough beggars on these streets to know the value of that. I have this role and this life.

I catch my fellow guardsman's eye. I wonder if he is having the same thoughts I am. I hear his stomach gurgling with hunger; probably not. He rolls his eyes slightly at me in mutual understanding. It is just another night.

Notes

1 Gowland and Knüsel (2006), Knudson and Stojanowski (2009), Stojanowski and Knudson (2020).
2 Battles and Gilmour (2022, 23–40), Byrnes and Muller (2017), Schrenk and Tremblay (2022), Vogel and Power (2022, 502–15), Zakrzewski and Evelyn-Wright (forthcoming).
3 Thomas (2007), Tremain (2002, 32–47).
4 Zakrzewski (2014, 57–68), Zakrzewski (2015, 157–67), Zakrzewski and Evelyn-Wright (forthcoming).
5 Zakrzewski and Evelyn-Wright (forthcoming).
6 Rowland and Hamdan (2012, 11–24).
7 Rowland et al. (2013, 53–84), Rowland and Zakrzewski (2008, 15–17), Woodman, Ikram, and Rowland (2021).
8 Rowland (2008, 69–94), Rowland and Hamdan (2012, 11–24).
9 Rowland (2008, 69–94).
10 Rowland (forthcoming).
11 Rowland (forthcoming).
12 Rowland (2008, 69–94).
13 Rowland (2008, 69–94).
14 Rowland (2008, 69–94).

15 Rowland (2008, 69–94).
16 Raxter et al. (2008, 147–55).
17 Haddow, Zakrzewski, and Rowland (2017, 206).
18 Reusch (2013, 29–47).
19 Reusch (2013, 29–47).
20 Reusch (2013, 29–47).
21 Reusch (2013, 29–47).
22 Bullough (2002, 1–17).
23 Reusch (2013, 29–47).
24 Bullough (2002, 1–17).
25 Reusch (2013, 29–47).
26 Bullough (2002, 1–17), Tougher (2013, 48–72), Tougher (2021, 2).
27 Ringrose (2007, 498).
28 Nunn (1996, 47).
29 Nunn (1996, 52).
30 Gordon and Schwabe (2004).
31 Gordon and Schwabe (2004, 127).
32 Gordon and Schwabe (2004, 117).
33 Gordon and Schwabe (2004).
34 Gordon and Schwabe (2004, 137).
35 Jackson and Leahy (1990, 271–74).
36 Halioua and Ziskind (2005, 50).
37 Montserrat (1996, 36–39).
38 Halioua and Ziskind (2005, 50).
39 Jackson (1988), Jackson (1990, 5–27).
40 Jackson (1990, 7).
41 Nunn (1996, 47).
42 Gordon and Schwabe (2004, 108).
43 Nunn (1996, 98).
44 Gordon and Schwabe (2004, 135).
45 Griffiths (1958) reported in Gordon and Schwabe (2004, 134).
46 Ringrose (2007, 496–501), Stevenson (1995, 504).
47 Montserrat (2000, 153–81).
48 Montserrat (2000, 153–81).
49 Harris (1994, 1–22), Evans Grubbs (2013, 87–88).
50 Masterson (2014, 26).
51 Tougher (2021, 2).
52 Stevenson (1995, 504).
53 Hopkins (1963, 62–80), Stevenson (1995, 504).
54 König (2021, 221–37).
55 König (2021, 221–37).
56 Francis (1926, 95–110).
57 Francis (1926, 97).
58 Francis (1926, 95–110).
59 Francis (1926, 98).
60 König (2021, 222).
61 Bullough (2002, 1–17).
62 Bullough (2002, 1–17).
63 Reusch (2013, 29–47).
64 Tracy (2013, 1–28).
65 Latham (2012, 84–122).
66 Roller (1997), Stevenson (1995, 498).
67 Tougher (2021, 4).
68 Bullough (2002, 1–17).

69 König (2021, 225–26).
70 König (2021, 229).
71 König (2021, 231).
72 König (2021).
73 König (2021).
74 Tougher (2013).
75 Aufderheide and Rodrígues-Martin (1998, 325–44), Lewis (2019, 567–84), Ortner and Putschar (1981).
76 721, Parl. Deb., H.C. (6th ser.) (2022–2023), 336WH.
77 Roller (1997, 555).
78 Ringrose (2007, 501).
79 Ringrose (2007, 501).
80 Stevenson (1995, 503), Tougher (2021, 48).
81 Bullough (2002, 10).
82 Tougher (2021, 27).
83 Tougher (2013, 50).
84 Tougher (2013, 60).
85 Ringrose (2007, 497).
86 Reusch (2013).
87 Reusch (2013, 31).
88 Tougher (2013).
89 Ringrose (2007).
90 Tougher (2021, 21–30).
91 Tougher (2021, 21–30).
92 Hopkins (1963).
93 Ringrose (2007, 501).
94 Hopkins (1963, 63).
95 Tougher (2021, 28).
96 Ringrose (2007, 501).
97 Rowland (2008, 69–94).
98 Aasgaard (2015), Boutin (2012).
99 Brooten (2015).
100 Boutin (2016), Evelyn-Wright (2021), Laes (2021).
101 Evelyn-Wright (2021).
102 Hosek and Robb (2019).
103 Buikstra (2019).
104 Evelyn-Wright (2021, 70).
105 Laes and Vuolanto (2021, 8).
106 Tripathi (2015).

References

Aasgaard, Reidar. "Growing up in Constantinople: Fifth Century Life in a Christian City from a Child's Perspective." In *Children and Family in Late Antiquity: Life, Death and Interaction*, edited by Christian Laes, Katariina Mustakallio, and Ville Vuolanto, 135–68. Leuven and Walpole, MA: Peeters, 2015.

Aufderheide, Arthur, and Conrado Rodrígues-Martin. *The Cambridge Encyclopedia of Human Paleopathology*. Cambridge: Cambridge University Press, 1998.

Battles, Heather, and Rebecca Gilmour. "Beyond Mortality: Survivors of Epidemic Infections and the Bioarchaeology of Impairment and Disability." *Bioarchaeology International* 6 no. 1–2 (2022): 23–40.

Boutin, Alexis. "Written in Stone, Written in Bone: The Osteobiography of a Bronze Age Craftsman from Alalakh." In *The Bioarchaeology of Individuals*, edited by Ann Stodder and Ann Palkovich, 193–214. Gainsville, FL: University Press of Florida, 2012.

Boutin, Alexis. "Exploring the Social Construction of Disability: An Application of the Bioarchaeology of Personhood Model to a Pathological Skeleton from Ancient Bahrain." *International Journal of Palaeopathology* 12 (2016): 17–28.

Brooten, Bernadette. "Early Christian Enslaved Families (First to Fourth Century)." In *Children and Family in Late Antiquity: Life, Death and Interaction*, edited by Christian Laes, Kataiina Mustakallio, and Ville Vuolanto, 111–34. Leuven and Walpole, MA: Peeters, 2015.

Buikstra, Jane. "Ethical Issues in Biohistory: No Easy Answers." *Bioarchaeology International* 3 (2019): 288–314.

Bullough, Vern L. "Eunuchs in History and Society." In *Eunuchs in Antiquity and Beyond*, edited by Shaun Tougher, 1–17. London: Duckworth & Classical Press of Wales, 2002.

Byrnes, Jennifer, and Jennifer Muller. *Bioarchaeology of Impairment and Disability.* Cham: Springer, 2017.

Evans Grubbs, Judith. "Infant Exposure and Infanticide." In *The Oxford Handbook of Childhood and Education in the Classical World*, edited by Judith Evans Grubbs, Tim Parking, and Roslynne Bell, 83–97. Oxford: Oxford University Press, 2013.

Evelyn-Wright, Stephanie. "Dis/ability Stories from Roman Dorset: An Integrated Osteobiography Approach." PhD thesis, University of Southampton, 2021.

Francis, A. G. "On a Romano-British Castration Clamp Used in the Rites of Cybele." *Proceedings of the Royal Society of Medicine, Section of History of Medicine* 19 (1926): 95–110.

Gordon, Andrew, and Calvin Schwabe. *The Quick and the Dead: Biomedical Theory in Ancient Egypt.* Leiden: Brill, 2004.

Gowland, Rebecca, and Christopher Knüsel, eds. *The Social Archaeology of Funerary Remains.* Oxford: Oxbow Books, 2006.

Haddow, Scott, Sonia R. Zakrzewski, and Joanne Rowland. "Two Potential Cases of Eunuchism from a Ptolemaic-Roman Cemetery in the Western Delta of Egypt: Differential Diagnosis and Social Implications." *American Journal of Physical Anthropology* 162, no. 64 (2017): 206.

Halioua, Bruno, and Bernard Ziskind. *Medicine in the Days of the Pharaohs*. Translated by M. B. DeBevoise. Cambridge: Harvard University Press, 2005.

Harris, William V. "Child-Exposure in the Roman Empire." *The Journal of Roman Studies* 84 (1994): 1–22.

Hopkins, Keith. "Eunuchs in Politics in the Later Roman Empire." *The Cambridge Classical Journal* 9. (1963): 62–80.

Hosek, Lauren, and John Robb. "Osteobiography: A Platform for Bioarchaeological Research." *Bioarchaeology International* 3 (2019): 1–15.

Jackson, Ralph. *Doctors and Diseases in the Roman Empire.* London: British Museum Press, 1988.

Jackson, Ralph. "Roman Doctors and their Instruments: Recent Research into Ancient Practice." *Journal of Roman Archaeology* 3 (1990): 5–27.

Jackson, Ralph, and Kevin Leahy. "A Roman Surgical Forceps from Near Littleborough and a Note on the Type." *Britannia* 21 (1990): 271–74.

Knudson, Kelly, and Christopher Stojanowski, eds. *Bioarchaeology and Identity in the Americas.* Gainesville, FL: University Press of Florida, 2009.

König, Jacqueline G. "Emasculating Healers. Medical Castration Practices in Greco-Roman Antiquity." *Journal of Ancient History* 9 no. 2 (2021): 221–37.

Laes, Christian. "Dysfunctional and Pitied? Multiple Experiences of being 'Disabled' in Ostia Antica and Environs." *Medicina nei Secoli* 33, no. 1 (2021): 199–216.

Laes, Christian, and Ville Vuolanto. "A New Paradigm for the Social History of Childhood and Children in Antiquity." In *Children and Everyday Life in the Roman and Late Antique World*, edited by Christian Laes and Ville Vuolanto, 1–10. London: Routledge, 2021.

Latham, Jacob. "'Fabulous Clap-Trap': Roman Masculinity, the Cult of Magna Mater, and Literary Constructions of the Galli at Rome from the Late Republic to Late Antiquity." *The Journal of Religion* 92, no. 1 (2012): 84–122.

Lewis, Mary. "Endocrine Disturbances." In *Ortner's Identification of Pathological Conditions in Human Skeletal Remains*. 3rd ed., edited by Jane E. Buikstra, 567–84. London: Academic Press, 2019.

Masterson, Mark. "Studies of Ancient Masculinity." In *A Companion to Greek and Roman Sexualities*, edited by Thomas K. Hubbard, 19–32. London: Blackwell, 2014.

Montserrat, Dominic. *Sex and Society in Graeco-Roman Egypt*. London: Routledge, 1996.

Montserrat, Dominic. *Reading Gender in the Roman World*, 153–81. London and New York: Routledge, 2000.

Nunn, John F. *Ancient Egyptian Medicine*. London: British Museum Press, 1996.

Ortner, Donald, and Walter Putschar. *Identification of Pathological Conditions in Human Skeletal Remains*. Washington: Smithsonian Institution Press, 1981.

Raxter, Michelle H., Christopher B. Ruff, Ayman Azab, Moushira Erfan, Muhammad Soliman, and Aly El-Sawaf. "Stature Estimation in Ancient Egyptians: A New Technique Based on Anatomical Reconstruction of Stature." *American Journal of Physical Anthropology* 136, no. 2 (2008): 147–55.

Reusch, Kathryn. "Raised Voices: The Archaeology of Castration." In *Castration and Culture in the Middle Ages*, edited by Tracy Larissa, 29–47. Cambridge: Boydell & Brewer, 2013.

Ringrose, Kathryn M. "Eunuchs in Historical Perspective." *History Compass* 5, no. 2. (2007): 495–506.

Roller, Lynn E. "The Ideology of the Eunuch Priest." *Gender and History* 9, no. 3 (1997): 542–59.

Rowland, Joanne. "The Ptolemaic–Roman Cemetery at the Quesna Archaeological Area." *The Journal of Egyptian Archaeology* 94 (2008): 69–94.

Rowland, Joanne. *Quesna*. London: Egypt Exploration Society, forthcoming.

Rowland, Joanne M., and Mohamed A. Hamdan. "The Holocene Evolution of the Quesna Turtle-Back: Geological Evolution and Archaeological Relationships within the Nile Delta." In *Prehistory of Northeastern Africa: New Ideas and Discoveries. Studies in African Archaeology 11*, edited by Jacek Kabaciński, Marek Chłodnicki, and Michał Kobusiewicz, 11–24. Poznań: Poznań Archaeological Museum, 2012.

Rowland, Joanne, Salima Ikram, G. J. Tassie, and Lisa Yeomans. "The Sacred Falcon Necropolis of Djedhor(?) at Quesna: Recent Investigations from 2006–2012." *Journal of Egyptian Archaeology* 99 (2013): 53–84.

Rowland, Joanne, and Sonia R. Zakrzewski. "Quesna: The Ptolemaic and Roman Cemetery." *Egyptian Archaeology* 32 (2008): 15–17.

Schrenk, Alecia, and Lori Tremblay. *Bioarchaeology of Care through Population-Level Analyses*. Gainesville, FL: University of Florida Press, 2022.

Stevenson, Walter. "The Rise of Eunuchs in Greco-Roman Antiquity." *Journal of the History of Sexuality* 5, no. 4 (1995): 495–511.

Stojanowski, Christopher, and Kelly Knudson, eds. *Bioarchaeology and Identity Revisited*. Gainesville, FL: University Press of Florida, 2020.

Thomas, Carol. *Sociologies of Disability and Illness*. Basingstoke: Palgrave Macmillan, 2007.

Tougher, Shaun. "The Aesthetics of Castration: The Beauty of Roman Eunuchs." In *Castration and Culture in the Middle Ages*, edited by Tracy Larissa, 48–72. Cambridge: Boydell & Brewer, 2013.

Tougher, Shaun. *The Roman Castrati: Eunuchs in the Roman Empire*. London: Bloomsbury Publishing, 2021.

Tracy, Larissa. "A History of Calamities: The Culture of Castration." In *Castration and Culture in the Middle Ages*, edited by Tracy Larissa, 1–28. Cambridge: Boydell & Brewer, 2013.

Tremain, Shelley. "On the Subject of Impairment." In *Disability/Postmodernity: Embodying Disability Theory*, edited by Mairian Corker and Tom Shakespeare, 32–47. London: Continuum, 2002.

Tripathi, Laxmi. *Me Hijra, Me Laxmi*. New Delhi: Oxford University Press, 2015.
Vogel, Hannah, and Ronika Power. "Recognising Inequality: Ableism in Egyptological Approaches to Disability and Bodily Differences." *World Archaeology* 54 (2022): 502–15.
Woodman, Neal, Salima Ikram, and Joanne Rowland. "A New Addition to the Embalmed Fauna of Ancient Egypt: Güldenstaedt's White-Toothed Shrew, *Crocidura gueldenstaedtii* (Pallas, 1811) (Mammalia: Eulipotyphla: Soricidae)." *PLoS One* 16, no. 4 (2021): e0249377.
Zakrzewski, Sonia R. "Palaeopathology, Disability and Bodily Impairments." In *Palaeopathology in Egypt and Nubia: A Century in Review*, edited by Ryan Metcalfe, Jenefer Cockitt, and Rosalie David, 57–68. Oxford: Archaeopress, 2014.
Zakrzewski, Sonia R. " 'Behind Every Mask there is a Face, and Behind that a Story'. Egyptian Bioarchaeology and Ancient Identities." In *Egyptian Bioarchaeology: Humans, Animals, and the Environment*, edited by Salima Ikram, Jessica Kaiser, and Roxie Walker, 157–67. Leiden: Sidestone Press, 2015.
Zakrzewski, Sonia R., and Stephanie Evelyn-Wright. "Theorising Disability in Egyptian Bioarchaeology." *Bioarchaeology of the Near East* (forthcoming).

Index

FSC
www.fsc.org
MIX
Papier | Fördert
gute Waldnutzung
FSC® C083411

Kolibri 360 GmbH
Ferdinand-Jühlke-Straße 7
99095 Erfurt, Deutschland
produktsicherheit@kolibri360.de